AF515897

INDIAN HEALTH LANDSCAPES UNDER GLOBALIZATION

Centre de Sciences Humaines (Centre for Social Sciences and Humanities): Created in New Delhi in 1989 the CSH, is part of network of research centres of the French Ministry of Foreign Affairs. The Centre's research work is primarily oriented towards the study of issues concerning the contemporary dynamics of development in India and South Asia. The activities of the Centre are focused on four main themes, namely: Economic transition and sustainable development, political dynamics, institutional set up and social transformations regional dynamics in South Asia and international relations International and regional relations, Institutional structures and political constructions of identity and urban dynamics.

Centre de Sciences Humaines, 2 Aurangzeb Road, New Delhi 110011, India, Tel: (91) 11 2301 62 59, Fax: (91) 11 2301 84 80
E-mail: public@csh-delhi.com
Website: http://www.csh-delhi.com

Institut Français de Pondichéry (French Institute of Pondicherry): Created in 1955, the IFP is a multidisciplinary research and advanced educational institute. Major research works are focusing on Sanskrit and Tamil Languages and literatures—in close collaboration with the Ecole Française d'Extrême-Orient—ecosystems, biodiversity and sustainability, dynamics of population and socio-economic development.

Institute Français de Pondichéry, 11, Saint Louis Street, PB 33, Pondicherry 605001, Tel: (91) 413 2334 168/2334 170
Fax: (91) 413 2339 534
E-mail: ifpdir@ifpindia.org
Website: http://www.ifpindia.org

Disclaimer: The views expressed in this publication are those of the respective authors and are not necessarily endorsed by the Centre de Sciences Humaines or any other institution to which the authors may belong.

Indian Health Landscapes under Globalization

Edited by

ALAIN VAGUET

MANOHAR

CENTRE DE SCIENCES HUMAINES

2009

First published 2009

© Individual contributors, 2009

All rights reserved. No part of this publication may be reproduced or transmitted, in any form or by any means, without prior permission of the editor and the publisher

ISBN 978-81-7304-722-0

Published by
Ajay Kumar Jain *for*
Manohar Publishers & Distributors
4753/23 Ansari Road, Daryaganj
New Delhi 110 002

Typeset by
Kohli Print
Delhi 110 051

Printed at
Salasar Imaging Systems
Delhi 110 035

To my wife Yvette
my daughters: Nina, Suzy, Lili, and
my son Niels

Contents

Tables

Figures

Acknowledgements

This volume is very much indebted to Centre de Sciences Humaines (CSH) of New Delhi and to his successive directors F. Grare, V. Dupont and Basudeb Chaudhuri. All of them admitted in the Centre some young researchers from the University of Rouen (Upper Normandy) dealing in matter concerning with Health Geography, four of them wrote a chapter in this book. Véronique Dupont was kind enough to support, through funding, the translation of the chapters.

Two Scientific Secretary of the Centre, namely P. Chapelet and B. Lefebvre, devoted a lot of time to organize this book. On behalf of all the contributors they should be warmly thanked. It is also to be reminded here that the very first step of this book results from an international seminar 'Health and Social Sciences' held by Pierre Chapelet, in CSH, in March 2003.

Most of the authors gathered again in another international seminar organized by Bertrand Lefebvre (CSH and University of Rouen, France) and S. Aggarwal (University of Delhi, India), in December 2006: 'Emerging Health Challenges and the Response of Indian Healthcare'.

Finally, I would like to acknowledge the inspiration I gain from the Indian colleagues, the students and from Professor S. Curtis (Durham University, UK) who accepted the charge providing the concluding remarks.

ALAIN VAGUET

CHAPTER 1

Introduction: Indian Health Landscapes under Globalization Treatment?

ALAIN VAGUET

Reports concerning health in India (e.g. Misra et al., 2004; Planning Commission of India, 2002) show that life expectancy has regularly increased in concordance with the reduction in poverty since Independence although the extent varies considerably between places and human groups. It means that independent India and its state-controlled economy was able, in spite of a reduced budget, to rapidly improve the condition of living of a part of its enormous population. But as noted by S. Menon (2004: 133): 'the doubling of life expectancy at birth in the last five decades, for instance, does not hold up against advances made in the developing countries of East Asia and Latin America, where life expectancy is the same as in developed nations'. The undeniable success of neighbouring Sri Lanka in the fields of health and education seems partly connected to the help of World Bank. Would it become a must for independent India to rely on global institutions (Menon, 2004)?

However, what kind of future is shaping up post-liberalization? Will financial developement and rapid economic growth alleviate the country from under-development and thus, its children from under-nourishment? Would free market economy and, competitive market forces be relied on to make hospitals and clinics, more efficient whenever they become privatized?

For the more optimistic globalization appears as one of the main determinants of world economic growth, not only for the profit it earns big firms, but also for improving the quality of life of millions of poor people in emerging countries. And one of the best predictors of quality of life is the health status of the people.

At the same time, if we apply systematically the process of globalization to the field of health, many disturbing questions arise. Are national health priorities more and more driven by international capital? How far does privatization of health depend upon the global market forces? Finally, is economic liberalization a chance to level the life of all Indians, or does it risk increasing health inequalities and burden the State that has become weaker in front of global forces?

As a matter of fact, behind globalization stands the question of power. When the global level compresses time and space, it reduces the role of other scales, including territorial control originally vested in the State. All the institutions operating at the world level encroach more or less upon the competencies of the State, including the orientation of the health sector. During this process, would India become weak, unable to secure any more the right to health for suffering citizens, leaving this job to global health institutions, NGOs, or to market-oriented clinics?

This volume brings together an array of perspectives on such questions in contemporary India. After liberalization can the government safeguard the autonomy of public health, promote efficiency and escape the invariable commodification of health services, this is the main question this volume raises. In this book, French and Indian geographers, sociologists, economists and lawyers use the global perspective to introduce the outcomes of the process of globalization within the field of Indian health systems. This systematic examination of costs and benefits seems a good indicator of the level of integration of an emergent country.

In a first step, this introduction tries to draw upon some definitions and presents some theoretical bases through the exploration of some selected authors. Afterwards, some general perspectives driven by theory are discussed with analyses of specific examples. Finally the table of contents is introduced to help the reader to understand how the editor has organized the chapters of the book.

Many great authors wrote essays using the concept of globalization promoted by MacLuhan in the 1960s. These permanently stimulate debate among citizens and academics. These divide people who fear a danger and want to generate a group of health activists to organize a fight against global forces from those who believe that more private funds could help to bridge the financial gap in the health budget. Of course, the two co-exist and this kind of debate could remain sterile in the sense that it refers mostly to ideology, pro or con liberal options, which is not our primary purpose here. Naturally nobody can ignore the relationship between liberalization and globalization, but we aren't fighting to impose a view and demand immediate action but attempting to organize a social sciences book that express the views of free persons in their fields of competence. Most of the contributors offer frankly their opinion and the contrasting perspectives are to be considered as a gain, not a weakness.

Globalization could be defined as a complex set of processes involving the move of capital, information, people and goods across 'the inherited map of political boundaries' (O'Loughlin et al., 2004). Of course, these clashes between the networks (transnational corporations) organizing the flux and the territories (states) are matters of great concern for geographers as in this context, spatial phenomenon are continuously reconfigured and produce some 'hyperdifferentiation at the regional levels and within metropolitan areas (. . .) in terms of capital accumulation and levels of prosperity. Winners and losers are easily identified by geographic location' (O'Loughlin et al., 2004: 7).

In terms of epidemiology, easy mobility of capital, goods and persons, would become a matter of great concern as it would multiply the interactions and the consequent risks of transmission of communicable diseases. SRAS or bird flu is a contemporary example which required worldwide effort to prevent the epidemic from becoming a pandemic. AIDS is sometimes presented as the first global pandemic, two decades were sufficient for the HIV to spread all over the world. Of course, the unequal level of development amplifies the risks, as controls and measures of prevention are not equally present in the world. More than the lack of health professionals, today the lack of veterinary professionals in the Third World could be seen as a major threat.

The numerous critics of globalization believe that there is nothing new in it, because for them the world has been open since centuries. They point to the past when the Old and New Worlds were brought into contact by the great discoverers (1492). Europeans easily invaded the American peninsula as most of its inhabitants died of chickenpox, measles, typhus and flu that arrived with them to the continent where it was totally unknown. Nevertheless, the present level of integration of economies[1] and the subsequent stream of workers, migrants and refugees paves the ground to a dangerous period in epidemiological terms.

At the same time, if globalization is seen as a potential danger for health of humanity, it could also propose more prevention measures to tackle globally the universal health questions. Unfortunately, this process is not uniform everywhere; it follows broadly the major inequalities between the underdeveloped world and the developed one. Cholera, leprosy and, polio myelitis and the so-called vaccine-preventive diseases underline the boundary between the two worlds as these diseases remain present in the southern hemisphere. No more scientific advancement is awaited to cure this kind of diseases, only a better share of wealth.

Public health is an important element of the basic precautionary measures required to keep populations safe from preventable hazards. Most countries have laws that make the States more or less in charge of the protection of the health of their citizens. In a federation like India, this role is now entrusted to the numerous states, most of which lack resources to do so and the country is suspected to have 'no real national public health infrastructure, no surveillance system, and no reporting mechanism' (Garett, 2000). This weakness, shared by most poor countries, opens the way to the concern of other nations which fear transmission of malicious microbes to their territory. For that reason, the politics of control must be collective as viruses ignore boundaries. But if a multilateral organization takes care of it, it may be accused of interference in State policies.

Nowadays, in addition to nation states and the WHO, operating since fifty years, the World Bank and many bilateral agencies suggest a greater role of a worldwide power. However, the 1993 World Bank orientation toward health was highly controversial (Ray, 2003). When the Bank proposed to invest in the health sector, it accepted the existence of a market in this field. Many critics suspect that this would lead to the commodification of health (Pellegrino, 2001). That includes making hospital and health products more attractive, thanks to marketing and advertising. The suspected end result would be the promotion of privatization of health, with the well-documented problem of supplier-induced demand.

K.V. Narayan (2003) highlighted this fact in Andhra Pradesh, 'one of the few states where the private sector in medical care has outgrown the size of public sector through direct and indirect state patronage'. He denounced the transfer of critical cases from private to public hospitals. The author also argued that in a sample of cities, 'the incidence of the Caesarian operations in the private hospitals was about 16 per cent higher than that in the public hospitals'.

In the same way, some other critics denounced how the 'epidemic of reforms', coming from international pressure, has diluted the responsibility of States and distorted national priorities. As a result, 'for the first time in independent India, the crude death rate has remained almost unchanged over the last decade' (Qadeer, 2000).

Among all the countries concerning globalization should we differentiate internationalization from globalization? As we know, in the first case, the extension of economic activities of the States across boundaries matters. Bilateral economic exchanges belong to this kind of process, for example the initiative PEPFAR.[2] In that case, US funds help selected poor countries to reduce selected illnesses, with selected methodologies. But the scale of the State still prevails and many militants criticized the moral choices made by the President G.W. Bush of USA, they highlighted how he tries to refrain the diffusion of condoms and to promote marital fidelity.

In the second case, that is globalization, the qualitative integration of the world market triumphs over the strategies of the different states. The multilateral 'Global Fund against TB and AIDS' is of this type, surpassing the interest of a single nation for the benefit of all the affected persons.

The two processes may naturally operate at the same time, for the advantage of divergent interests. Incidentally, the difference between internationalization and globalization may remain largely theoretical when some States are accused of becoming an empire. They may try to influence the decisions of multilateral agencies to promote their own interests, or the interest of their industries.

Vaccination programmes are also good examples of the mix between globalization and internationalization. WHO, as a global actor, is sometimes accused of promoting a costly policy of vaccination against polio myelitis in poor countries like India, for the benefit of the pharmaceutical industries of the West (Phadke, 2006). The argument is that in terms of public health, the level of transmission of these diseases remains very low compared to other priorities like TB. On the other hand, if the global fight against selected diseases is sustained, there worldwide eradication may be possible. Since 1998, after 2 billion children were vaccinated, the Global Polio Eradication Initiative has reduced the number of polio cases by 99 per cent. Similarly WHO and *Lancet* announced in 2007 that the number of measles death has decreased by 60 per cent since 1999, thanks to an intense campaign of vaccination. Today the polio virus remains endemic in only four countries including India. Unfortunately, in Pakistan the number is jumping as conservative clerics declare this 'infidel vaccine' an American plot to sterilize innocent Muslim children (Walsh, 2007).

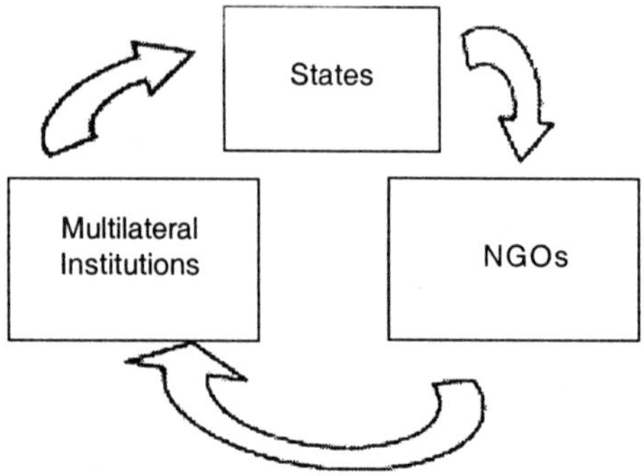

FIGURE 1.1: THE DIFFERENT ACTORS

Generally, three types of actors interfere: States, Multilateral Institutions (MIs) and NGOs (Dixneuf, 2003). Of course, these divisions are artificial; NGOs may be national organizations (TAC in South Africa) and multilateral agencies like Global Funds can be instruments of a powerful State.

WHO is not a good example of a powerful multilateral institution. So far, it has produced more recommendations than agreements and the organization has been able to change deeply since its founding. In fact, \$5 billion of multilateral aid for health (through the UN system) remains limited compared to \$55 billion of bilateral one (government to government) (Lang, 2005). Contrary to many loose statements, global public health institutions seem quite weak. More than that, they do not speak in a single voice. For instance, during the arguments about structural adjustment, UNICEF challenged the liberalization promoted by World Bank (Walt, 1998), and asks for an 'adjustment with a human face' (1987). At present, WHO as well as NGOs, question the decisions of the World Trade Organization (WTO) towards intellectual property of health products. Instead of a super power, the opinions of the world's institutions may reflect more or less the diversity of the planet.

In matters of health, as in general political matters, many actors interfere in the game, reflecting the unequal distribution of power in the world. The powerless have sometimes a chance to win when they cooperate. As health is a precious resource, an emotional affair, it becomes a matter of global citizenship where small players try to play a role.

In a scenario where the States are not equal, the most powerful would like to speak for all, or suggest a universal model to be transferred worldwide. But it can be observed that instead of concentrating power in one hand, surprisingly, globalization could sometimes be an opportunity to distribute power among small hands. That's what happened when some NGOs and some multilateral agencies organized a powerful lobby to reduce the price of some critical medicines against AIDS, in contradiction with the WTO laws. Unfortunately those successes are always challenged and the fight remains permanent. Today, as India enters the WTO, its pharmaceutical industry must give royalties to the inventors of new pills and naturally the correspondent rising cost will affect the accessibility of critical medicines to patients who need them. In the eyes of the global citizen, a country like India, perceived as friendly to poor AIDS patients[3] seems now much more global business minded. Some of its biggest industrialists are now interested in the protection of property rights as it may become an opportunity to attract big pharmaceutical laboratories in the country to impulse low cost researches.

During the formulation of the 'Patent Act' and the 'victory' of low-income countries, at the Doha round of the WTO, India was seen as the leader of the fight for affordable medicines against 'big pharma' companies (Thomas and Weber, 2004). In fact, it is a terrible paradox that some private Indian companies can produce some Antiretrovirals (ARV), but very few are accessible to Indian patients. Now, after the decision of the Indian Parliament to adopt the 'new Patent Act' and to follow the legislation of WTO, India is accused by NGOs like Doctors Without Borders of forgetting AIDs patients of Africa who depend upon Indian medicines. Some activists believe there is a market-driven agenda at the level of individual countries like India too. India attracts less direct investment than China but is able to promote more fusions abroad.

Recently, a transnational pharmaceutical company has filed a case against the Indian interpretation of intellectual property laid down by the WTO. In this context, the new version of an old pill is not protected. A coalition composed of Global funds and NGOs (Oxfam International, Doctors Without Borders) are helping India fight for flexibility of Trade-Related Aspects of Intellectual Property Rights (TRIPS) agreement which permit production of affordable medicines for the benefit of public health in low income countries. Experts estimate that more than court action, the threat to flexibility comes from bilateral agreements between northern states and southern ones. The question of governance of global public health is not fixed definitely by the WHO or by the WTO, and the states interfere in the game.

Does the interference of globalization really reduce the scope of national governments? Regardless of global tendencies such as cost containment, many authors believe that each country adapts its system in the frame of its own history (Curtis and Taket, 1996). In the case of India, Rama Baru (Baru, 2002) has concluded that contrary to some other countries in the world, India had an opportunity to develop alternative choices for his health sector, but it was not done. The decisions (of the Bhore Committee) after Independence, puting the nation on the way of a National Health System, now seems outdated. Indeed today's development of health as a tertiary sector largely through private enterprise is contrary to what the WHO has proposed for a country like India. Many official publications pay lip service to WHO advices, but the reality differs widely. The country has made choices which have facilitated the privatization of health sector and to some extent the government is responsible for it, so this tendency is not strictly 'super induced' by globalization. One interpretation could be that India would like also to take advantage of globalization, not only suffer from it. Many researchers (e.g. Gobatto, 2003) have shown that 'globalization is not a one way process' (Vaguet, 2004). It may also offer more choice to the imagination of the population (Appadurai, 1996). Citizens and industries, do not only suffer from global tendencies like liberalization of the health sector, they adapt or transform the information and use it as a new resource. It could be the responsibility of the State to orient the change toward more equity.

At present, the process of commodification of health is making medical treatment unaffordable for most Indians. Health sector is developing rapidly on market demand long before the settlement of any health insurance system. The unequal American health system model is followed by India. Who can differentiate the impact of globalization and the part of internal choice in such a situation? The Indian society known for its diversity of cast, class and so on, producing a health system which is not based on solidarity, is it so surprising.

Real improvements in the health sector since Independence cannot hide the substandard quality of services extended to most people. Indian literature depicts stories of criminal neglect (Narayan, 1945). The *Economic and Political Weekly* denounces the unhygienic conditions under which a lot of tubectomy operations are conducted in the public health system. In October 2004, the news magazine *Frontline* revealed that nearly all medical laboratories, most of them private, cannot expect to reach an international level. Contrary to its reputation, the Indian State seems reluctant to impose strict norms on private medical services and the global institutions are not powerful enough to do it.

Interestingly, in the matter of resilience of State power, R. Rosecrance's book is very helpful to interpret contemporary health mutations (Rosecrance, 1999). He demonstrated that some nation States may become virtual when, instead of territory and conflicts (weapons and military efforts) they concentrate on the global market, economy of services and mobility of capital.

The United Kingdom, Switzerland, Japan and Germany inaugurated this trend, now followed by Singapore and Hong Kong. These are 'Head Nations' who are able to invent new technologies and services and set up their productions outside their territory. The success of such virtual states depends upon their capacity to organize reliable links with the other nations that are no longer peripheral. In such a scenario, globalization is seen to push towards peaceful integration of different parts of the planet. As a matter of fact, independent sources show the present reduction of the number of conflicts in the world as the good face of globalization.

On the contrary, China and India, as 'Body Nations' are seen to become increasingly places of production[4] and their risks of conflict remain high. But the process of virtualization will satisfy the interests of the emerging middle class in these countries. Getting good education and jobs, high standard of life and consumption as well as the protection of their health capital will become the aim of this class. Of course, this minority connected with an international network will become more influential in policy matters and will push for the promotion of a mushrooming private health sector.

The main consequence of these developments will be the relative reduction of State power. The State will only be necessary to maintain some regulations, in fact to protect values, which should not be left to the market in justice and maybe health. The virtual State will have a low capacity to act on the main determinants of globalization. If in addition, economic growth is falling or not equally shared, there will be growing unrest among citizens who cannot expect a better result from any political team. For this reason U. Beck, who observed an increase of extremist non-democratic parties around the world, promotes the notion of the 'cosmopolitic'. In this concept, he tries to reject, 'old categories' as national or international. He suggests that, the present and the sometime irritating trend that gives mega power to global players may finally be a chance to create more interdependence between nations. As Beck (2002) puts it, if global problems (as global warming) did not exist, one should invent them.

Viewing this problem through a country like India was a chance to go deep into the contradictions between national sovereignty, permanently proclaimed, and an economic growth, partially dependant on the links with global trade. More than elsewhere, the rapid integration of India, in economic terms, is not only considered as a mark of shining economy, but perceived as a risk. Risk of losing a recently-won independence, suspecting the new ways of development becoming the betrayal of the values of non-alignment, self-reliance, or at least the end of the protection of the economy against old and new imperial powers.

In term of health, globalization remains incomplete. The present situation seems partially non-intentional because global governance of public health is poorly organized. In the name of collective security, each actor—international organizations, states, civil societies—is following his own way, according to the interest of the moment. Nobody conscientiously wishes the present scenario, but everyone acts according to it. Globalization displays many avatars; the role of the State remains one among others, it will not be erased easily.

The terminological choice of titles and chapters may sound strange and repetitive to those who ignore the major synthesis of our colleague S. Curtis who accepted to conclude this book. Her work was a great source of inspiration. She proposed to use the name 'landscape' in a metaphorical way. 'The concept of a landscape has often been used to convey the idea of a system of factors and processes that interact in particular settings to produce geographical variation. The elements included in a conceptual landscape depend on knowledge of the key relationships and causal pathways producing geographical variation. It is possible to imagine different conceptual landscapes of health geography, associated with different theoretical perspectives on health variation, overlaying each other in the same place'.

Five types of health landscapes where identified, namely environment, power, consumption, poverty and therapeutic, but for our purpose concerning globalization, two of these were used—the landscapes of power and of consumption derived from the work of P. Bourdieu.

As a matter of fact, the global forces have often been interpreted as market-driven. Liberal politics influenced by the US 'empire' are suspected to promote the 'industry of health', for example big pharmaceutical companies, the privatization, or 'corporatization' of clinics and so on. To some extent, each author has escaped from simple arguments and has identified a field of health where he/she has highlighted how India may be alternatively seen as victim or shareholder of global strength. That is the reason why we intensively make use of this helpful concept to advance the whole system perspective of putting health in its global and local complexity.

The book is roughly divided into two equal parts, according to the estimated speed of the globalization process going on. In the first one, 'Emerging Health Landscapes', all the contributions show recent tendencies rapidly amplified by the globalization processes. In the second one, 'Low Speed Health Landscape', it appears that some rampant tendencies still obliterate the Indian sanitary situation.

The two first papers may be interpreted as the best examples of *contrasting landscapes* because globalization always shows several faces. In his chapter, E. Eliot highlights how the spread of AIDs in India remains the best example of an almost uncontrolled pandemic, where poverty and local denial have postponed necessary prevention. Meanwhile, the 'new global yoga', starting from South Asia and considered in this chapter, as a sort of alternative medicine by A.C. Hoyez, has become a new way of curing or caring around the world. Finally, India has had to suffer a global burden but has simultaneously, been able to become a centre of diffusion of different therapies.

Entrepreneurs of emerging India competing internationally have amplified the many *landscapes of globalization.* The strategy of some important stakeholders seems now to make health care much more profit oriented. For B. Lefebvre studying the dynamics of corporatization in the field of private hospitals, the pending question remains the access of the majority of population to these networks of clinics.

The global institutions cannot be seen as culprits in this. S. Aggarwal reminds us of the WHO advice, accepted by the city of Delhi: Healthy City goals are in total opposition with the expansion of expensive tertiary establishments. The models of health promotion and empowerment (Ottawa Charter, 1984) involved in the Healthy City project are more oriented towards the provision of information and participation of citizens.

Global, international, bilateral, national, all the levels interact and no one is definitely good or bad. P. Chapelet in 'Allopathic Landscapes under Global Competition' introduces the responsibility of the Indian State in the genesis of the pharmaceutical industries, which was able, in less than 20 years, to reduce the importations of the multinationals and stimulate the volume of Indian exportations. In one sense, here the nation prepares its industries to globalize their activities, regardless of a still difficult access for a huge part of its citizens.

For J. Chaisse and S. Guennif this State industrial policy gave to Indian companies the central role in the drastic reduction of the price of ARV specialities for the benefit of millions of AIDS' patients in the world. On the contrary, the new regulations imposed by the WTO, much more respectful of intellectual property, introduced some new incertitude. Doctors Without Borders (Médecin Sans Frontieres, MSF) has denounced regularly the rising risk created by the regulated global competition resulting in unequal access to second line medicine for the world's patients. Some lobbies in India itself have slowly found some advantages in this situation: when brevets are clearly protected, direct investments of foreign origin could pave the way to develop medical or pharmaceutical researches. India would become able to go beyond the production of generics. Tomorrow, will the new and most useful pills be discovered in India? Facing these attractive arguments, the present multiplication of multilateral agreements between countries, leads the authors, to a pessimistic conclusion instead of a bright future.

One finds the same feeling in the article of R. Akhtar, who reminds us the paradox of a still poor country, which produces nevertheless more medical doctors than necessary and that fuels a 'brain drain' of professionals towards well developed countries. As a retroaction, it leads, after liberalization, to a flood of Non-Resident Indians, a 'brain tank', promoting the mushrooming of tertiary hospitals of the private sector. Unfortunately this development is of little help to the rural areas where most of the population lives. More than a classical critic of an uneven distribution of professionals between rural and urban spaces, this article depicts a chronically medical practice, which too often fails to cure and care with humanity.

The second section of the book: 'Slow Speed Health Landscape', emphasizes the fact that for citizens there is still a long way to go from emergence to development.

In the chapter 'Pending Globalization Landscapes', M. Clerc shows how the multiplication of NGOs is embedded in the global strategy of structural adjustment and is expected to help the necessary rising of civil society. At the same time the Indian State controls their role, which remains concentrated mainly on prevention work. If one remembers that many Indian private pharmaceutical companies are able to sell low-price pills to contain AIDS in Africa, in India itself, easy access for poor AIDS' patients, until recently, was denied. In this context of restriction of real treatment, the author pleads for the respect of the invaluable work done by NGOs to minimize suffering.

The same power game, global and national, interferes in leprosy care. This illness is not fatal as AIDS, but in the middle of the 1990s, WHO and the World Bank decided to launch a new programme for its eradication. The lowering of prevalence rate was also taken into consideration by the NGOs. F. Martin denounces the pressures produced by European 'bio-politics' models of bodies or disease, which orient health priorities much more towards the illness and its rehabilitation than towards the people suffering from it.

The same blind transfer of model can be found in the contribution of S. Brisset. She studied in Chennai, the interactions between water management and public health. Contrary to the expectations of a 50-year old water project and in spite of the help of the World Bank, the improvement since 1997, in terms of volume of water distributed per head, has produced a disaster in terms of environmental health. Of course, more time is needed to evaluate a process in all its actions and retroactions, but this last example shows very clearly that the process of economic take-off is taking place in cities where basic amenities are pending, at the price of poor health status of the citizens.

The 'Unequal Globalization Landscapes' has two articles. The first one exposes the poor situation of Indian women, especially at the time of motherhood. The second one treats the development of local democracy that eventually aggravates unequal access to health services.

V. Chasles points out the historical choice of Indian (male) governments to promote birth control more than an efficient reproductive health care system, proposed during the World Conference of Cairo (1994). In the same way, as a result of their status in the society, women are encouraged to undergo antenatal examination but rarely taken for postpartum visits to take care of themselves.

The risk of increasing inequality is the main threat to the global good governance rules celebrated by global institutions and governments as well. S. Tawa Lama Rewal demonstrates precisely how the key words of local democracy, decentralization and participation, percolate in Delhi. She concludes that the devolution of responsibilities does not give any more power to generate a local alternative to the prevalent privatization of health care. For that reason, in term of health services one can doubt the democratic advantages of decentralization process which far from a better service to all citizens, give much more emphasis to visible actions—multiplication of dispensaries and health camps—of the newly empowered leaders and to their will to become elected again.

To summarize, this last article exemplifies the ambiguity between global political terms and the reality in which poor health situation and poor quality of provisions are prevailing.

Finally, working within the field of health—viewed as a key component of the State and society under globalization process—allowed us to show its risks as well as its advantages through concrete case studies. A speed process, as the emergence of clinics or the pharmaceutical industry, can only take place when, during a period, global and national level interact in the same direction. Otherwise, the efforts being contrasted by societal strength lead to slow speed, as in the reproductive health sector or decentralization.

To conclude, one should remember that contrary to many places in the world, health is not a priority in Indian society. It remains invisible in the present political debates, and if the author of the 'Virtual State' is true, the growing concern of an emerging middle class will elevate the healthiness demand and stimulate privatization, commodification and finally produce more inequalities.

As a final paradox, one can highlight that health, being invisible in the domestic debates, always puts India in the centre of the global game.

NOTES

1. For the world, direct investments abroad increased to 34 per cent in 2006.
2. PEPFAR: The President's Emergency Plan for AIDS Relief, 2003.
3. According to MSF, about 50 per cent of AIDS drugs in the developing world are Indian generic.
4. Of course, as the Indian case shows clearly, those countries will also develop services, the difference between the production and services sectors is narrow; software production, for instance, is much more a service than an industrial production.

REFERENCES

Appadurai, A., *Modernity at Large: Cultural Dimensions of Globalization*, Chicago: University of Minnesota Press, 1996.

Baru, R., 'Health Sector Reform: The Indian Experience', in A. Twaddle (ed.), *Health Care Reform Around the World*, London: Greenwood Publishers, 2002.

Beck, U., *Power in the Global Age*, Bonn: Blackwell Publishing, 2005.

Curtis, S., and A. Taket, *Health and Societies: Changing Perspectives*, London: Hodder Arnold, 1996.

Dixneuf, M., 'La santé publique comme observatoire de la mondialisation', in J. Laroche (ed.), *Mondialisation et gouvernance mondiale*, Paris: Presse Universitaire de France, 2003.

Garett, L., *Betrayal of Trust, The Collapse of Global Public Health*, New York: Hyperion, 2000.

Gobatto, I. (ed.), *Les pratiques de santé dans un monde globalisé*, Paris: Khartala, 2003.

Lang, T., 'The (Re)emergence of Health as a Key Policy Driver', in F.H. Buttel and McMichael, *New Directions in the Sociology of Global Development*, vol. 11, Oxford: Elsevier, 2005.

Menon, S., *No Place to go*, New Delhi: Penguin Books, 2004.

Misra, R., R. Chatterjee and S. Rao, *India Health Report*, New Delhi: Oxford University Press, 2004.

Narayan, K.V., 'Size and Nature of Healthcare System', in C.H. Hanumantha Rao and S. Mahendra Dev, *Andhra Pradesh Development. Economic Reforms and Challenges Ahead*, New Delhi: Centre for Economics and Social Studies (CESS) and Manohar, 2003.

Narayan, R.K., *The English Teacher*, Oxford: Heinemann, 1945.

O'Loughlin, J., L. Staeheli, E. Greenberg, *Globalization and its Outcomes*, New York: The Guilford Press, 2004.

Pellegrino, E., 'The Commodification of Medical and Health Care: The Moral Consequences of a Paradigm Shift from a Professional to a Market Ethic', *Journal of Medicine and Philosophy*, 24, Oxford: 2004.

Phadke, A., 'Drops that Paralyse', *Times of India*, 2006, http://www.timesofindia.indiatimes.com/articleshow/2122225.cms

Planning Commission of India, *India Vision 2020*, New Delhi: Planning Commission of India, 2002.

Qadeer, I., 'Health Care Systems in Transition. The Indian Experience', *Journal of Public Health Medicine*, 2000, 22 (1), pp. 25–32.

Ray, C.N., *Liberalisation and Urban Social Services, Health and Education*, New Delhi: Rawat Publications, 2003.

Rosecrance, R., *The Rise of the Virtual State: Wealth and Power in the Coming Century*, New York: Basic Books, 1999.

Thomas, C. and M. Weber, 'The Politics of Global Health Governance: Whatever Happened to "Health for All by the Year 2000"', *Global Governance*, 2004, p. 10.

Vaguet, A., 'Healthcare Systems Caught in the Twists and Turns of Globalization', in Landy and B. Chaudhury (ed.), *Globalization and Local Development in India*, New Delhi: Manohar, 2004.

Walsh, D., 'Polio Cases Jump in Pakistan as Clerics Declare Vaccination an American Plot', *The Guardian*, 15 February 2007.

Walt, G., 'Globalisation of International Health', in T. Heller et al., *Working for Health: Open University Course Reader*, Milton Keynes: Open University Press, 2001.

PART I

EMERGING HEALTH LANDSCAPES

A. CONTRASTING LANDSCAPES OF GLOBALIZATION

CHAPTER 2

Spatial Dimensions and Emergence of HIV/AIDS in India: Geographic Concepts for Understanding AIDS

EMMANUEL ELIOT

Introduction

The Indian Union's gradual assimilation into what may be called the 'World System' (Brunet, Dollfus, 1990) at the beginning of the twenty-first century has had an effect on the movement of goods and products, but also on viruses that spread as people became more mobile. Rapid displacement and travel at the global level—especially since 1970–80—has had an impact upon causal organism transfers. The discovery of the first infected cases in the mid-1980s in India can be taken as the regional indicator of the trend towards the pathogenic uniformization of certain types of virus, such as the AIDS virus. T. Barnett and A. Whiteside (2002) have shown how AIDS may be deemed a macro-effect of globalization. The process underway is affecting developing countries more particularly, sometimes very strongly.

The onset of HIV in the early 1980s was a 'spatial event' (EPEES, 2000) at the global level, in the sense that it corresponded to an imbalance or transformation in a subsystem of the 'World System', with lasting effects. However, 'new properties' were generated in some areas within the 'World System'. Therefore, we may consider HIV/AIDS as one of the 'World System's' 'emerging properties', as it is caused by social and environmental interactions.

However, the notion of emergence has several connotations. Semantically, at the first level, its meaning is synonymous with onset. This means that the virus has been introduced and identified by screening certain population groups. That is, the disease has emerged, which means that it can be identified and classified. The notion of an emerging disease is therefore defined as 'the action of any newly identified or previously unknown infectious agent that has created public health problems at the local and international level'. In its second meaning, emergence defines a status change, i.e. the onset of new properties. It is usually linked to a bifurcation, i.e. an identifiable change in a given system. However, emergence is often identified after the fact. In the 'World System', the onset of HIV seems to reflect a status change in causal organisms in the global system. On this subject, M. Grmek (1983) uses the concept of pathocenosis to understand the phases of stability and swings in epidemiological situations over time. The notion is defined as 'a set of disease conditions present within a specific population at a given moment' (Grmek, 1983). 'Competition' between diseases and the notion of disease emergence can be studied through this concept when a set of diseases is being controlled, leaving a gap that others can take up. Thus, AIDS appeared and was identified in the early 1980s, at a time of increasing control over infectious, parasitic and deficiency diseases from the end of the nineteenth century to the second half of the twntieth century. In a nutshell, the term emergence defines status change, observation as well as identification of the phenomenon within a system.

AIDS was the main emerging disease in the beginning of the twenty-first century. HIV was the most 'active' infectious agent among the 36 new agents identified since 1972 (Desselberger, 2000). It has been the source of infection for nearly 35 million people and has caused 17 million deaths since it spread in human beings.

Based on data available with leading health organizations HIV/AIDS mapping reveals a north/south divide (Figure 2.1). It is in poor and developing countries that most newly identified cases of and deaths from the disease are reported. Though it was restricted to certain groups and countries when it was first identified in the 1980s, the HIV/AIDS epidemic very soon became a pandemic, severely affecting vulner-able social groups in particular. Though it remains a 'south' epidemic, even in the 'north' strong disparities can be seen between vulnerable populations and others. In spite of new generic anti-retroviral drugs in the market, treatment is still not easily accessible in developing countries. According to often incomplete data due to the States' lack of efficient information networks, the highest number of HIV positive persons is to be found in 'Sub-Saharan Africa', followed by 'South Asia' and 'Latin America', although there is a wide gap between Africa and the others. The prevalence map (Figure 2.1c) shows a rate of approximately

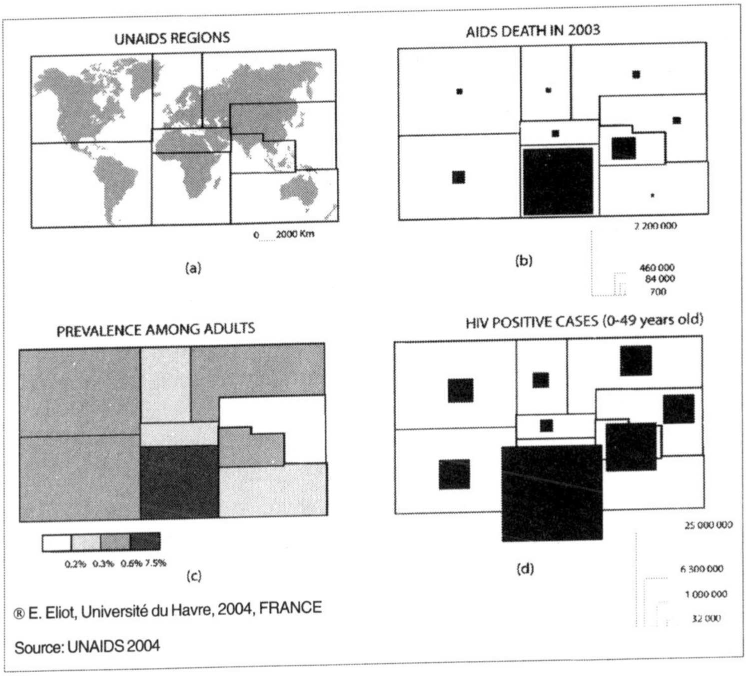

FIGURE 2.1: AIDS EPIDEMIC IN THE WORLD (2003)

0.6 per cent for most regions. However, two groups of areas tell a different story. The first consists of Western Europe, North Africa, Oceania and South-East Asia, with a rate lower than or equal to 0.3 per cent. The second is made up of Sub-Sahara Africa, with a very high rate of 7.5 per cent. This region is most affected by the epidemic.

The second most affected region is South Asia. In this region India has the highest number of cases. According to certain sources (UNAIDS, CIA) the figure stood at 5–8 million in 2004. The variance in figures is quite significant and is more than just a topic of discussion between specialists (cf. Chapter 9), for with a population of more than a billion people even a low prevalence in India translates into a very high number of infected persons.

This chapter aims at presenting key factors for a better understanding of the HIV/AIDS epidemic in India by laying special emphasis on its emergence and causes. This issue will be dealt with based on four points. The first will attempt to understand the spatial forms that facilitated the epidemic's entry into the country. Due to their specific nature, position and structure certain configurations seemed to have played a key role in introducing the epidemic into the country. The second point will deal with relations between locations at the regional level. Spatial interactions structure the epidemic's area of prevalence and spread it. The third point will deal with conditions in which the epidemic was introduced at the local level. Despite inaccurate data on AIDS cases, the rise in the mortality rate during the 1990s seems to indicate a change in the causes of death, thus leading to the hypothesis of an AIDS epidemic. Lastly, population displacement modes and the functioning of certain territorial systems have contributed to the disease's emergence. We will also be dealing with a situation of epidemic concentration in certain places and its evolution to the stage of spreading to a larger scale.

In brief, we will be returning to the start of the epidemic by 'dissecting' the places where HIV emerged and studying the epidemic's movement in the country. This analysis is based on the study of a scale mechanism, i.e. the methods by which the epidemic went from one scale to another.

The work presented here is of a geographer. He therefore gives importance to one criterion to understand health problems: space. In relation to other social sciences, geography centres on space and the specificity of places. The spatial dimension quite obviously belongs to human beings organized in societies. Time is too often the only factor taken as a reference point while studying epidemics. Indeed, epidemics too have a geography in the sense that they are linked to location and space, which in their turn are linked to time.

Various data have been taken into account to deal with the HIV/AIDS epidemic in India: serologic records,[1] the Mumbai Corporation's medical data on mortality and its causes[2] and data taken from individual private and public screening centres in Andhra Pradesh in the 1988–94 period. By collating results from different information sources we were able to gain further clarifications about the epidemic.

Crossroads and Interfaces—Two Spatial Structures in the Introduction of The Epidemic

The epidemic found the most 'permeable' or more 'porous' borders to spread into Indian territory. Certain spatial structures are thus endowed with a greater capacity to connect spaces and locations, due to their specific properties. Thus, interfaces determine both contacts as well as interpenetration between spaces at different levels. Crossroads or hubs too constitute a type of contact point—both a meeting and departure point.

NODAL AND LINEAR INTERFACES

There are several theories on the introduction of HIV into India and reveal the significant role played by population displacement as the epidemic's vectors (Figure 2.2).

The first theory has to do with the Indian mafia. It has very close links with Central and East Africa. There are ample financial flows, trafficking of human beings (prostitution) and drugs trafficking between India and these regions that harbour a large number of the Indian diaspora. Besides, the relationship between these regions goes a long way back. Arab and Indian sailors had established outposts such as

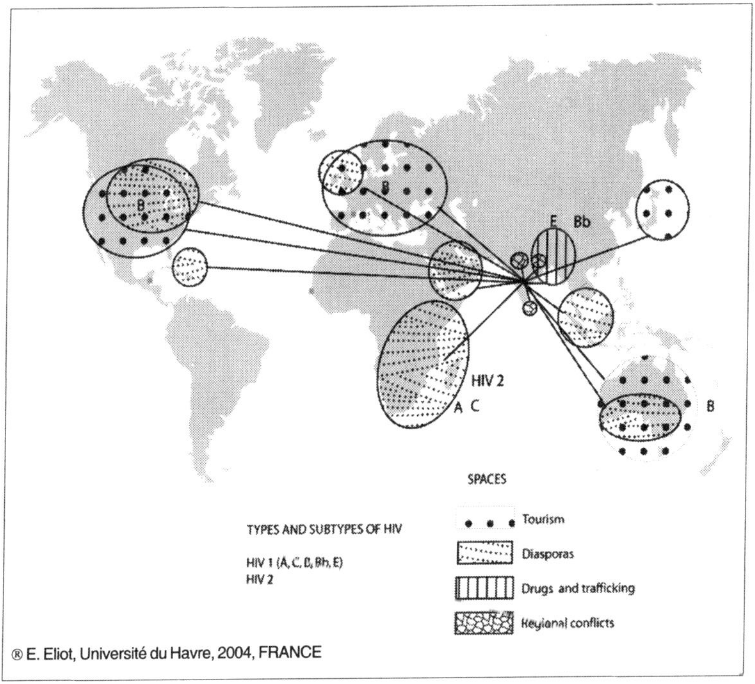

FIGURE 2.2: HYPOTHESIS OF INTRODUCTION OF HIV IN INDIA FROM SPACES TO NETWORKS

Sofala, to the south of Zambezi River as early as in the first century of our era. During the British colonization era, Indian communities were transplanted in South and East Africa. There are approximately 2,500,000 Indians (about 15 per cent having emigrated officially) living in the eastern and southern parts of Africa in the beginning of the twenty-first century (Figure 2.3).

The return of call girls after several years in East Africa where they could have contracted the virus could therefore explain the introduction of the HIV-1 C and A sub-types that are common in Africa, and also HIV-2 originating in Mozambique where this infection seems to have had a long history (Rémy, 1998).

A second theory proposes the role of cross-border migrations of people from nations like Thailand and Myanmar infected earlier by the virus. There is extensive population displacement, miscellaneous trafficking, especially drug smuggling, related to the proximity of the Golden Triangle's opium production centres, between India and its

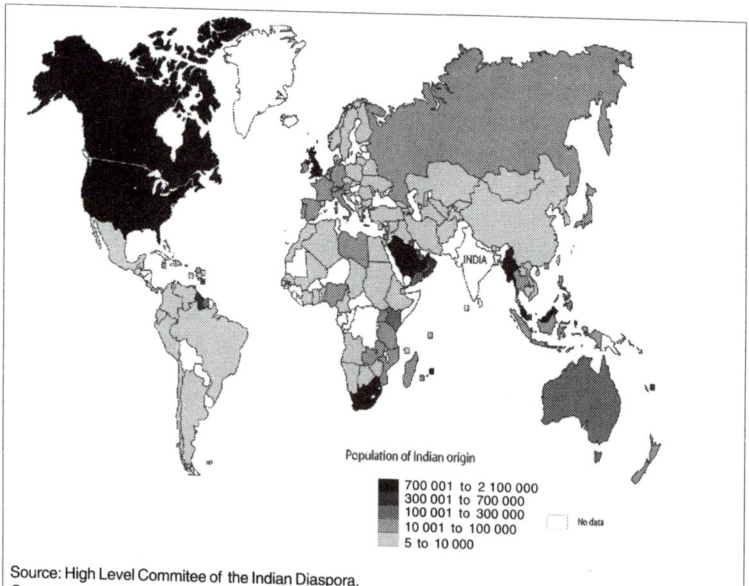

Source: High Level Commitee of the Indian Diaspora, Government of India, 2001, http://indiandiaspora.nic.in

® E. Eliot, Université du Havre, 2004, FRANCE

FIGURE 2.3: POPULATION OF INDIAN ORIGIN IN THE WORLD

eastern neighbours. The HIV-1 sub-type E as well as sub-type Bb—largely found among drug addicts—could have been introduced through such flows.

According to the third theory, conflicts have played the role of catalyst in spreading HIV. Kashmir and Assam have a large concentration of armed forces. Local conflicts can have a destabilizing effect due to the population migrations they lead to, which in turn can facilitate the spread of the virus (Smallman-Raynor and Cliff, 2004).

Finally, we come to the last theory. Migrations of tourists and workers from North America, Europe and the Gulf countries could have been responsible for the presence of a large variety of sub-types, especially sub-type B, which is often detected in these regions. Certain regional units seem to be more affected in India, such as major international tourist centres (the Delhi–Jaipur–Agra triangle, Goa, Manali, and so on) and the big metros (like Mumbai, Delhi).

INDIA—AN EPIDEMIOLOGICAL HUB

Accurate information about the first Indian AIDS patients screened is very scarce. The Indian authorities' denial of the possible propagation of the AIDS epidemic (cf. Chapter 9) and its lack of funds, particularly for serological equipment in the 1980s, partially explain this state of affairs. The first HIV-positive cases in India were identified in end 1985 in six Chennai prostitutes. The first confirmed AIDS case was identified in Mumbai a few months later. This was a businessman who had spent many years in the United States where he had undergone a coronary bypass surgery. Two more confirmed HIV-1 positive cases were identified in the beginning of 1987, at the Christian Medical College, Vellore (Tamil Nadu). But neither had received blood transfusions or travelled abroad.

However, specific information about HIV sub-types became available only in the early 1990s. Earlier serological records would have helped to better understand the ways and means of the epidemic's entry into the country. Anyhow, positive blood samples taken from patients suffering from sexually transmissible diseases in 1990 and 1991 contain a type of HIV-1 sub-type C. A sample analysed in Mumbai in 1992 contained sub-type A. In Hyderabad, a patient who had stayed in Uganda was found to be Type B positive. The first case of HIV-2 was identified in 1990 in a woman in Mumbai. Other cases were also identified the same year in Vishakhapatnam (Andhra Pradesh) and Chennai. A study done in 1996 on 16 serological samples collected before 1992 revealed proof of the presence of HIV-2 at least before 1989 (Kulshreshtha et al., 1996).

Despite the paucity of information, all known HIV types as well as all known sub-types were identified in HIV-positive persons in India (Figure 2.4). India seems to have been the epidemic's Asian hub right from the beginning of the 1990s. Its location in Asia, between Middle East and South-East Asia, gives it a very specific character. The country is the epidemic's 'host territory' and has also become a major regional dissemination centre in Asia—to the Persian Gulf countries through labour migration, to other South Asian countries (Sri Lanka, Nepal, Bangladesh) and even to the rest of Asia through the Indian diaspora's migratory networks.

Taking everything into consideration several theories can be advanced on the introduction of HIV. They overlap both in time and space and interact with each other, thus forming a set of currents that focus on certain areas. Certain spatial forms also encourage virus introduction: crossroads or hubs connecting one location to the other, as well as interfaces, in terms of discontinuities due to the strategies adopted by actors, which emphasize contacts and exchanges. Moreover these spatial forms are organized at all levels.

Urban System and Hierarchical Diffusion at a Regional Scale

The HIV epidemic seems to have emerged in locations that are densly populated and which are well connected, such as cross-border areas, international scale metros or international tourist centres. Polarities resulting from interactions also create epidemic areas at the regional level. They follow migratory channels and network clusters produced by human activities. In the 1950s, the Swedish geographer T. Hägerstrand (1952) began working on the spatial analysis of the phenomena of expansion and spread. Since then epidemiological studies have been based on a conceptual and methodological framework designed to understand its space-time dynamics. Generally two types of dissemination diffusion are recognized. The first one—called 'contagious'—structures the expansion of the phenomenon based on neighbouring localities. The second, called 'hierarchical', takes into account potential interactions between locations.

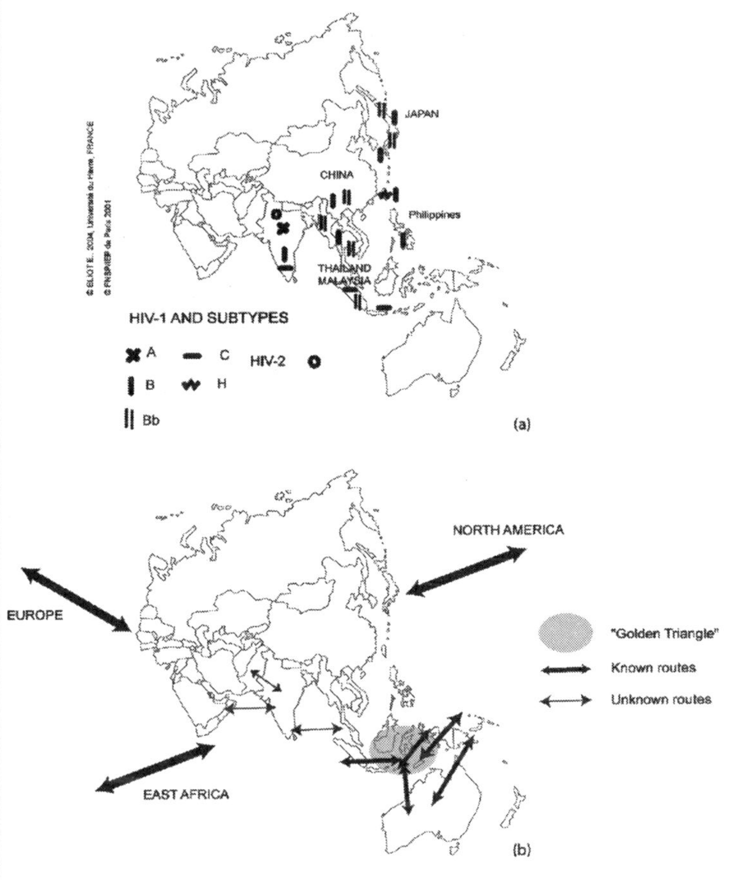

From
Bruce G *et al.*, 1992, "The molecular epidemiology of HIV In Asia", *Carc calling*, Vol.n°7, n°4, 1994
Weniger BG, Takebe Y, OuCY, Yamazaki S., 2001, "The molecular epidemiology of HIV in Asia", *AIDS*, Mar 9;15(4):545

FIGURE 2.4: TYPES AND SUB-TYPES OF HIV-1 AND HIV-2 IN SOUTH AND SOUTH-EAST ASIA

MODEL-BASED INTERPRETATION

As homogeneous serological data is not available continuously over time and space at the regional level in India, certain analytical options have to be found to understand the spread of the epidemic. Models are suitable tools in this context. In fact, comparing a model to the actual picture presented by statistical data allows us to explain and identify the differences between theoretic construction and available data.

In this perspective, a causative agent like HIV needs human beings to develop and spread. As a result, it is possible to simulate the displacement of agents by analysing the movements of human beings. The gravity model taken from the world of physics helps us to understand the intensity of interactions between particles. By analogy, in geography, two parameters are built into the model: the weight of the centre and the Euclidian distance between such centres. Gravity thus expresses the 'interactions levels' in a system of cities. The latter act through all the goods and services offered attract more people depending on their proximity and size. All said and done, this model does have its limitations, for on the one hand it supposes that individuals contracting the virus do not have a specific behaviour and that they therefore do not infect several people during their different stages of displacement and, on the other hand, it tends to exaggerate the effect of the distance between centres. However, it nonetheless has a heuristic dimension by attempting to validate hypotheses on the spread of the epidemic.

THE HIERARCHICAL COMPONENT OF THE EPIDEMIC IN ANDHRA PRADESH

The theory that some locations are characterized by their potential for a high degree of interactions—due to their size or function—can be tested through a deductive approach. In fact, they are most likely to be major epidemic epicentres and also to have been the epidemic's point of introduction because they engender large flows of goods and people to other locations in the state, the rest of India and poles in other countries. Three locations in Andhra Pradesh are a case in point for this theory. The first is the state capital—Hyderabad, with a population in excess of four million inhabitants in the beginning of the 1990s. Not unlike many other Indian state capitals, it has stronger links with other big metros than with its hinterland and therefore constitutes a centre that is very open to other Indian metros (Ramachandran, 1989). The second is the industrial port city of Vishakhapatnam, which is also the state's second largest city with more than a million inhabitants according to the 1991 Indian census figures. By its function itself it generates a high degree of movement between India's east coast and neighbouring countries in the Bay of Bengal. The third place is a Hindu pilgrimage centre (Tirupati) to which people flock from all over India.

It is possible to assess the epidemic's transmission probabilities by studying a fifteen-town urban sub-system in Andhra Pradesh and simulating the introduction of the causative agent into these cities.

Two data series were compared in this manner. The first one is serological data collected from all private and public screening centres in Andhra Pradesh between 1986–94. Despite defects in the screening systems at the time (lack of funds, small number of screening centres, doctors' failure to recognize the disease, basically passive screening of patients, etc.), the data collected helped us fill certain gaps in data, amongst other things, caused by the under-declaration of cases by health authorities. In fact, the state's AIDS cell had identified 281 confirmed cases during this period using the Western Blot test.[3] However, the sample confirms 1299 cases, i.e. four times more. The second data series is calculated following the Markovian scheme[4] based on a gravity matrix taking into account the state's fifteen most populated towns and their respective distances in kilometres. Repeating the process (iteration) helped in 'activating' the model and thereby simulating transmission.

The correlation between transmission probabilities and the data collected in the state's screening centres is very high (0.91), thereby validating the theory. Residue analysis has shown that very few towns differ from the model (Figure 2.5). The epidemic seems in fact to follow town hierarchy based on their size but also on their specific functions. Tirupati, a medium-sized town in the state, is especially attractive due its function as a pilgrimage centre. This function increases its real interaction potential much more than the number of inhabitants would have led us to believe.

As seen in studies on the United States (Gould, 1994) and Western Africa (Amat-Roze, 1993), HIV transmission in India contains a hierarchical component. It follows its own spatial logic. It has a reticular configuration, centred on the nodal locations and spreading along the major axes of movement. However, some locations have a pull disproportionate to their size due to their specific function.

The acknowledgement of these locations—as both epidemic transmission and reception centres—can be taken to a higher level. Thus we can ask how is the epidemic structured and how is it organized in these locations? What are the resulting spatial inequalities? How and where did they appear?

Attempts at finding a partial answer to these questions led us to one of the most important Indian metros—Mumbai. In fact, this city is a

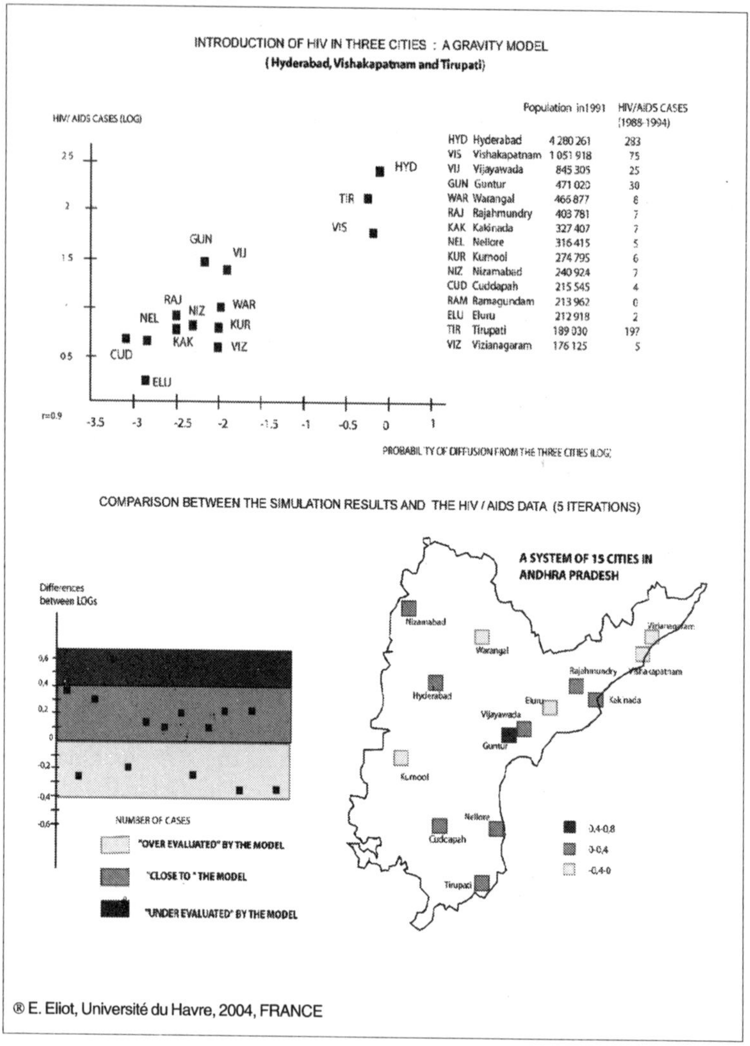

FIGURE 2.5: SIMULATIONS

laboratory for the analysis of the epidemic's spatial phenomena. It was one of the Indian cities that most worried the authorities in the beginning of 1990s and as a result the state and non-governmental organizations swung into action and conducted a number of epidemiological surveys.

The Emergence of the Epidemic: Mumbai as a Case in Point

Mumbai's Epidemiological Situation in the Middle of the 1990s

The primary question for which we have to find an answer when examining the emergence of the epidemic at the local level is: what are the identifiable changes pertaining to mortality? As only incomplete data about AIDS-related deaths is available for the mid-1990s it would be appropriate to find an answer to this question indirectly by identifying the diseases most frequently associated with AIDS: opportunistic diseases or diseases occurring in concert with AIDS.

A data series was gathered during the summers of 1995–6 by the Mumbai Corporation's health departments to find an answer to this question. The data covers the 1986–94 period and focuses on death records and the causes cited by the city's health departments. This data is incomplete in certain details as they were taken from a defective system: absence of systematic registration of causes of death, system management and organization problems and so on. However, Mumbai's death notification system is much more efficient than that of other Indian metros.[5] Thus, the collected data helps us to identify certain trends and establish certain theories.

During the 1986–94 period mortality changes by age group[6] (Figure 2.6) in Mumbai show three characteristics: a reduction of infant and child mortality, a distinct reduction in mortality in the fifty-plus age group and a marked rise in adult and youth mortality. These characteristics remain comparable for either sex (Figure 2.7). However, the male mortality rate is more clearly marked by a decrease in the age group of the elderly and an increase in the adult/youth age group. It is not suitable to discuss the variations within this period here (see Eliot, 1998 and 1999): some characteristics were amplified whereas others fluctuated highly. All said and done, we can understand the changes in Mumbai's mortality rate in the light of the epidemiological transition model.[7] This model defines changes in the nature of diseases affecting the population. As time goes by, infectious, parasitic and deficiency diseases are gradually replaced by chronic, degenerative and non-communicable diseases. The moving force behind this change in causes of death is socio-economic growth. However, the transition from one stage to another takes place at a different pace for different regions and societies. In Mumbai's case, the advancement and progress

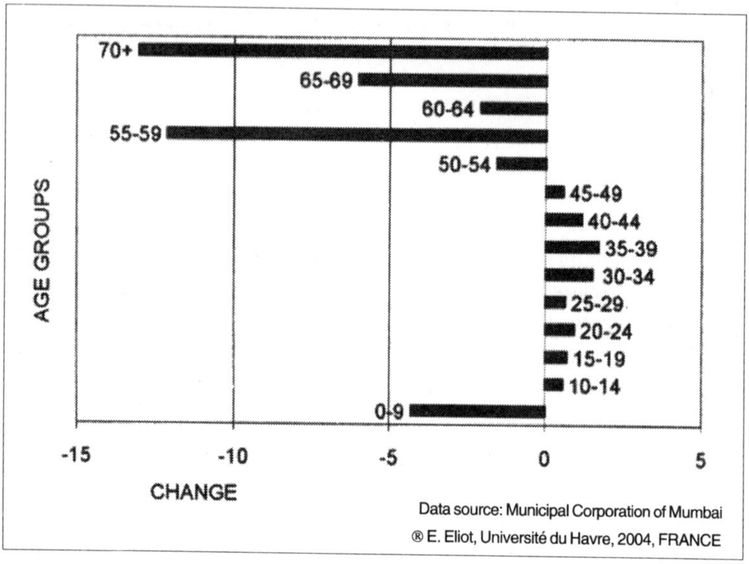

FIGURE 2.6: CHANGE IN AGE-SPECIFIC MORTALITY RATES BETWEEN 1986 AND 1994 IN MUMBAI

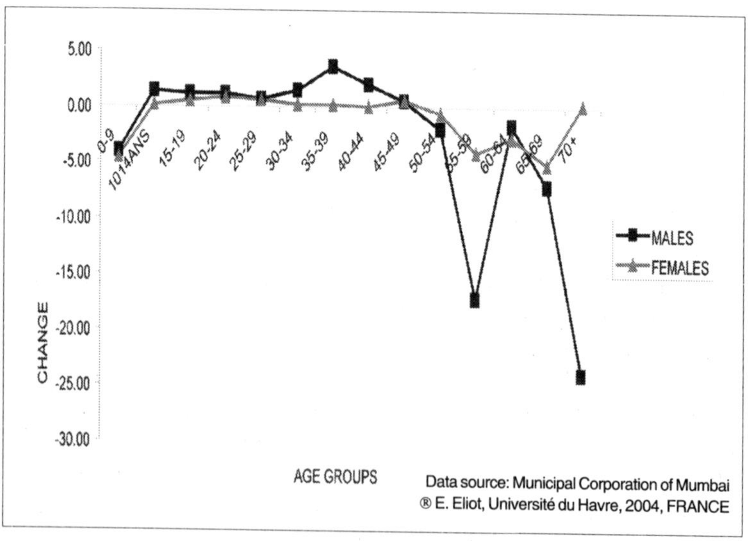

FIGURE 2.7: CHANGE IN AGE-SPECIFIC MORTALITY RATES BY SEX BETWEEN 1986 AND 1994

made in the field of hygiene, women's education, and medical care had brought about a striking improvement in the health situation after the Second World War. This resulted in the lowering of infantile and child mortality and a distinct decrease of mortality in the most aged population during the period under study. The higher mortality rate among the youth and young adults, especially males, thus appeared to be an 'anomaly' in the model. The rate should have either stabilized or increased moderately. Thus, a clear change in the mortality curve could be observed.

The epidemiological transition model designed by A.R. Omran based on mortality change studies in North American and West European societies did not seem the right filter through which we could understand the mortality situation in this Indian metro in the mid-1990s. Therefore, looking into causes of death and their changes was deemed necessary in order to take into account other indicators during this period.

Data for studying the causes of death is the most incomplete data available. The data collected is therefore classified by number of deaths per major disease group and not by mortality rate per cause of death per age group. Yet it does shed some light (Figure 2.8): an increase in degenerative diseases, sociopathies and certain infectious diseases (tuberculosis, Hepatitis B).

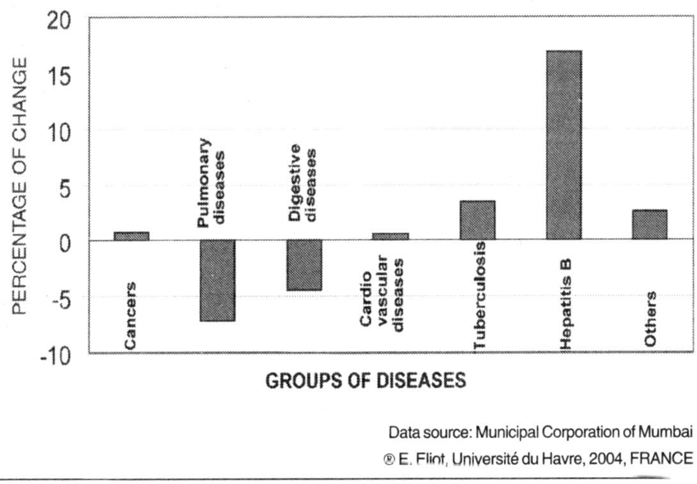

FIGURE 2.8: PERCENTAGE OF CHANGE FOR SELECTED DISEASES BETWEEN 1986 AND 1994 IN MUMBAI

An analysis of changes in mortality and causes of death in the 1986–94 period seems to show a change in the situation: an increase in the mortality rate for the adult and young adult groups as well as an increase in certain parasitic diseases. These characteristics support the finding of a new epidemiological situation that can, however, only be proved if validated for a more recent period. Nevertheless, the fact that the mortality rates became more complex is apparent in two ways: an increase in certain infectious diseases and a dual characteristic pertaining to mortality—a decrease in the age group of the elderly and an increase in the young adult age group.

CENTRAL 'PATHOGENIC SPACES'

In order to support the thesis of a combination of indices leading to a more complex epidemiological situation in the metro's population, we have to examine the location of these changes.

The gender-wise mortality rate change between 1986 and 1994 shows an increase in mortality, more so in the male population and in the central and southern[8] (Figure 2.9) wards. At the city level, mortality increased by 13.30 per cent over the period of study, i.e. 1.40 per cent per year. The southern and central wards showed the highest increase. Take the case of Ward A, for instance, where male mortality rose from 11.7 per cent in 1986 to more than 18 per cent in 1994. In other parts of the metro, the rate tended to decrease or stagnate, with the exception of Wards P/South and N.

In the case of the female population, the increase was much lower: 0.30 per cent per year. However, some wards were characterized by a high annual increase in mortality between 1986 and 1994: F/North, F/South, K/East and S (approximately 4 per cent per year).

In brief, a change did take place since 1986. Thus, excess male mortality can be observed in most of Mumbai's southern and central wards. The lack of mortality rate data classified according to age groups in each ward does hinder the identification of the classes with the highest increase, but the general curve supports the hypothesis that the increase in rate was perhaps the highest in the male adult and young adult age group in the southern and central wards.

Changes in certain causes of death were superimposed on these changes in mortality rates. Certain diseases have been selected to illustrate the rise in AIDS cases, due to the lack of confirmed AIDS patients' data and due to problems in disease identification during this

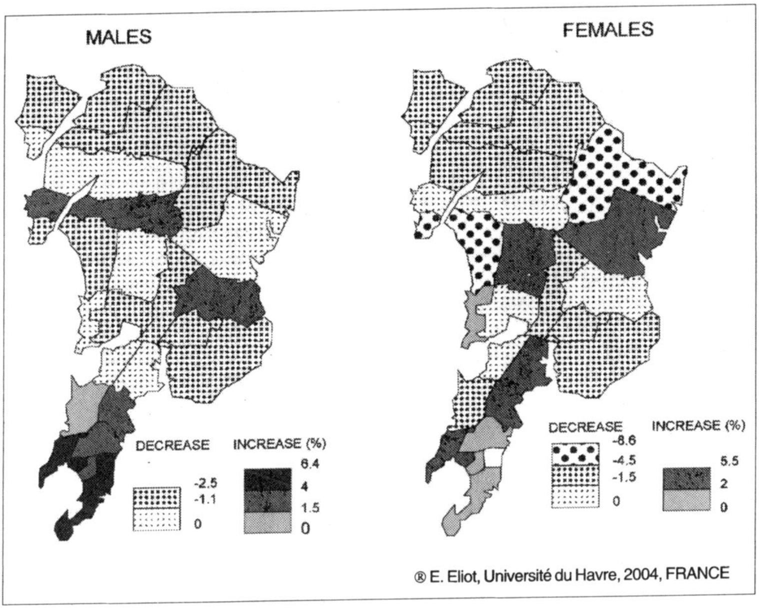

FIGURE 2.9: CHANGES IN MORTALITY BY WARD BETWEEN 1986 AND 1994

period. These diseases are known for their close links with AIDS as major opportunistic diseases. Based on the available data, the choice fell on four causes of death: tuberculosis, hepatitis B, digestive and pulmonary diseases. Some of these diseases like tuberculosis and hepatitis B show a more marked increase than others. Thus, between 1986 and 1994, the diseases likely to indicate the transformation of AIDS into an epidemic were increasingly noted as the causes of death in the southern and central wards (Figure 2.10). Ward E exemplifies this situation. These diseases accounted for 18.4 per cent of the causes of death in 1986. They rose to 42.2 per cent of total deaths in 1994.

To sum up, the emergence of AIDS in Mumbai between 1986 and 1994 seems to be supported by a range of facts. In fact, the metropolis saw a distinct increase in the young adult and adult male mortality rate during this period whereas in other age groups the rate tended to fall, though there is of course a difference between them. From the perspective of causes of death, the pathogenic causes became more complex, combining a moderate increase in degenerative diseases and a sharp rise in some parasitic diseases.

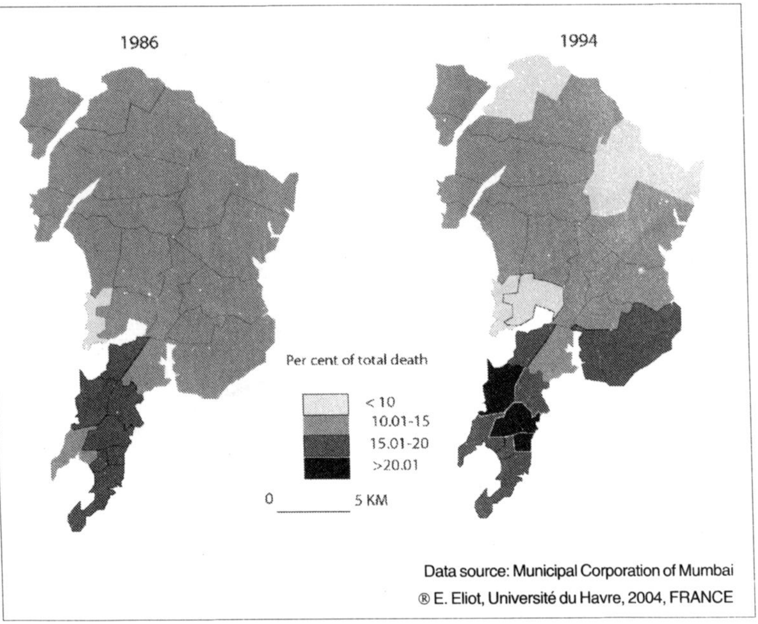

FIGURE 2.10: CHANGES IN INFECTIOUS DISEASES BY WARD BETWEEN 1986 AND 1994

At the ward level we can see that the highest increase in male mortality rate was concentrated in the southern and central wards where there was a distinct rise in parasitic diseases too. Located in the centre of the Mumbai peninsula, Ward E seems to have been the most affected by the epidemic in 1994. The health conditions in this group of neighbourhoods had always been problematic, right from their inception in the mid-nineteenth century. In fact, the British health authorities had deemed the situation 'intolerable' in the early twentieth century (Ramasuban and Cook, 1996). The mortality rate in these wards was the highest in the city and this became a permanent feature in the course of the century. Since India's Independence in 1947, the mortality rate here remained higher than in other areas and wards of the city. Thus, these areas seem to represent long-standing disease-ridden areas in which HIV seems to have infiltrated, further worsening the mediocre health conditions there. The epidemic seems to have found 'a place in the sun' in this part of Mumbai.

In this context we would like to present and define these areas in the first phase and then consider some theories about the probable origin and vectors for the spread of the disease in the metropolis. Briefly, this last section we will try and understand the set of geographical mechanisms involved in the epidemic's emergence in Mumbai's central areas.

Transitional Phases: From The Concentration to the Spread of The Epidemic

The term 'antiworld' coined by R. Brunet (Brunet, 1990) is an attempt to define the areas of secrecy, 'parallel worlds' (Brunet, 1981) and 'interlopes'[9] created by the 'World System'. This is 'the less well-known part of the world that desires to remain so, which is seen both as the world's negative and its indispensable twin' (Brunet et al., 1993). Thus, the world too has its dark side and maintains a relationship of dependency and complementarity with the 'antiworld'. All systems have their own defects that can be hidden, denied, swept under the carpet or simply tolerated. This part of the system that does not conform to norms and/or laws can be defined as the 'antiworld'. It has its own spaces, organizational logic and modes of operation. Spaces for racketeering, smuggling and 'letting off steam' (Brunet and Dollfus, 1990) which are necessary for social control, were in fact the first places where the epidemic took hold and remain its primary centres.

Central Mumbai and its Antiworld

It is in these wards, most affected by the epidemic and located at the heart of the Mumbai peninsula, that we find a cluster of areas born of the wave of urbanization at the end of the nineteenth century and in the early twentieth century. Close to the colonial era's textile mills, they were labour pools until labour strikes crippled the textile industry in 1980. Centrally located in terms of their position in the transportation network and close to the metro's major decision-making centres, these areas are the subject of massive land speculation today. However, the 1948 Bombay Rent Act that froze house rents at their prevailing level does restrict the destruction of old buildings and purchase of vast tracts of land albeit in a small way. Two areas within the central part are especially notorious: Kamathipura, which houses one of the largest concentrations of sex workers in the city, and Byculla, the Mumbai underworld's 'base camp'. Moreover, Mumbai is one of the Indian mafia's headquarters despite the fact that most leaders operate from abroad, such as from Dubai. The textile industry's crisis in the 1980s drove a section of this area's population towards greater insecurity and vulnerability, which resulted in the growth of gangs. Indeed, the mafia adopted a strategy of charity to recruit members. Thus, the gangs also have a Robin Hood effect on the have-nots (Jaffrelot, 1997). The liberalization of the gold and electronic products trade made smuggling unprofitable in the 1990s and the mafia turned to debt recovery and racketeering (Jaffrelot, 1997).

The location strategy adopted by these 'actors' is rather special. Situated at the interface between several areas, they slotted themselves into a matching area: close to the shipping warehouses in the city's east, the financial district in the south and the upmarket residential areas of the west. These sectors' are located at the metro's major communication nodes, which they also use. Nested within and confined to the metro's centre, this area represents the hidden face of power—the home of the underground economy and human and goods smuggling, with ambivalent links with the political authorities.[10]

THE EPIDEMIC'S ENTRANCE LOCKS AND COMMUTATORS[11]

Figure 2.11 attempts to offer theories on the epidemic's emergence and the swing between two epidemiological situations, and from a stage of concentration to one of dissemination. It identifies the interactions between the occurrences and locations, possible HIV delivery routes and its carriers as well as connecting points at various levels.

The non-resident mafia leaders control the flesh and illegal goods trade in Mumbai. The city's gangs 'control' people and goods at the local level. They are the local agents of the underworld's godfathers. The flesh trade could have played a role in introducing HIV. Men belonging to these gangs or clients frequenting prostitutes could also have introduced the retrovirus. Whichever be the case, the prostitute population seems especially vulnerable to the disease. Insecure living conditions, pressures by pimps and clients and the lack of protection make them a potentially high-risk epidemiological group. At the all-India level, the data given in the 2004 UNAIDS Report (Figures 2.12 and 2.13) shows that among the sentinel population, prostitutes were the most affected by AIDS in the 1987–2001 period.

Without entering into any debate on the veracity of the data (cf. Chapter 9) and even in the case of a more accurate registration of HIV

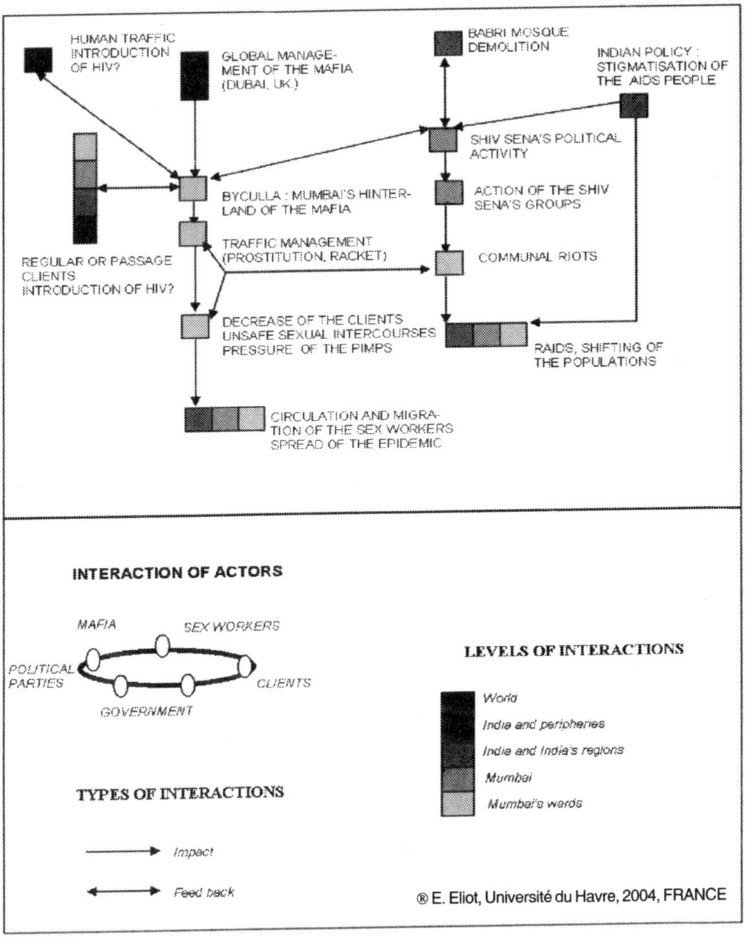

FIGURE 2.11: TRANSITION BETWEEN TWO EPIDEMIOLOGICAL SITUATIONS

carriers during the period, there was a distinct rise in the percentage of confirmed cases, reaching nearly 50 per cent in some localities in the early 1990s. And the percentage is sometimes even higher in the beginning of the twenty-first century.

In Mumbai, the red light districts are concentrated and located near major connection points with the rest of the city (Mumbai

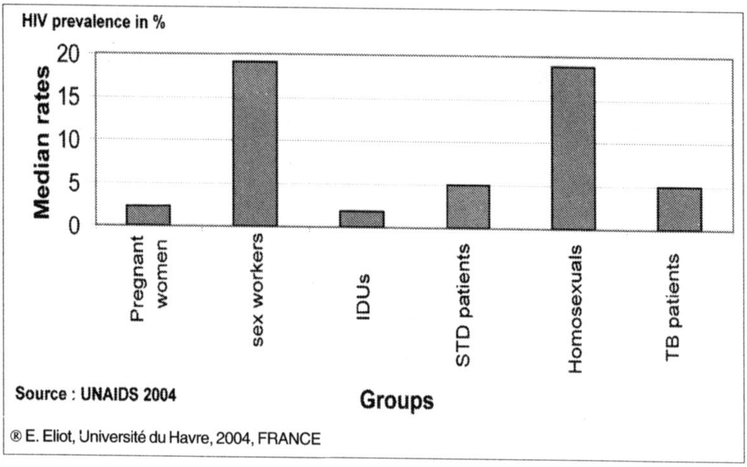

FIGURE 2.12: MEDIAN RATES AMONG SENTINEL POPULATIONS

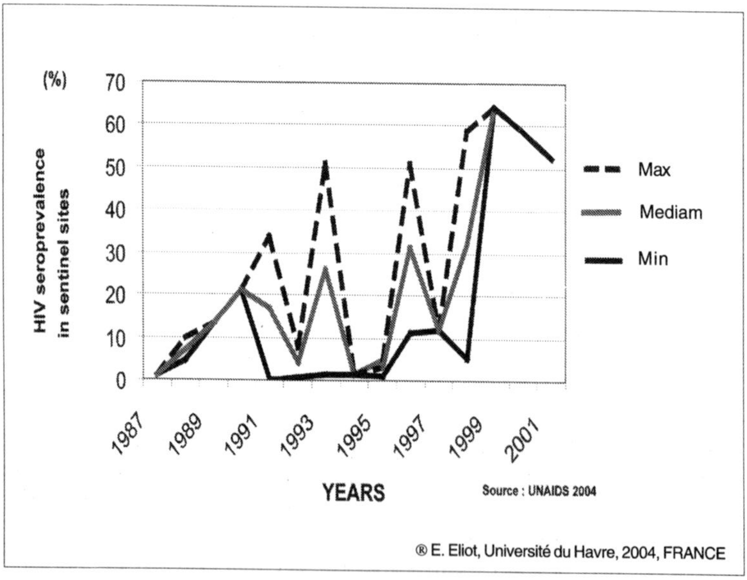

FIGURE 2.13: HIV AND SEX WORKERS TRENDS BETWEEN 1987 AND 2001

Central, Dadar, etc.). Thus, there is intense interaction between the rest of the city and this area. Clients transit through and—if they are infected here—can subsequently spread the infection to peripheral areas (contagious transmission) or more distant areas (jump transmission).

There are two other causes that promote and worsen this primary generative and accelerative effect. The first is the public health policy implemented by the authorities in the 1990s. According to some sources, the danger of AIDS was in fact denied both at the national and municipal levels. In the beginning of 1990s, the government thought it fit to hide the truth from the people since it considered AIDS as a disease that afflicted foreigners and social deviants only.

The lack of special wards in hospitals for AIDS patients, under-equipped screening centres and problems in access to health facilities are all indicators that authorities lacked seriousness in handling the epidemic. It is true that development and poverty issues made appointing quality management and supervisory staff a difficult task but the delay in establishing a good screening system and the attendant ostracism of these patients is a part of the denial process. The action taken in the first phase at the local level targeted high-risk groups. Instead of being preventive in nature they proved to be repressive, hounding and displacing the infected population to other locations. This crackdown by the Mumbai police helped to spread the disease faster to other areas. Infected women chased away from these central areas were forced to flee to other locations and in order to survive, worked in their new locations. The more they were isolated, the more they became transmission points as the epidemic grew and in proportion to the so-called 'preventive' police raids conducted at the behest of the municipal authorities.

The second factor that accelerated the spread of the epidemic was due to the communal riots that followed the demolition of the Babri Masjid by Hindu fundamentalists in Ayodhya in the winter of 1992–3. In the red light area of Kamathipura, for example, massacres, starvation, and blackmail by pimps or even police pressure had disastrous consequences on the epidemic's transmission. There was hardly any clientele even a few months after the violence. A survey conducted in 50 brothels that had closed down after the riots showed a 25 per cent fall in clientele (Gilada, 1994). The lack of clients and the fact that pimps and brothel owners started demanding more money forced 25 to 30 per cent of prostitutes to migrate to other areas. In addition, to repay the loans they had taken from their brothel owners, who had themselves sustained heavy financial losses during the riots; prostitutes may have increased the number of unprotected sexual relations. These two factors caused HIV to spread more rapidly to other city areas and other regions, increasing the number of contamination centres and spreading the disease.

Data on the number of deaths between 1986 and 1994 sheds additional light on the situation. A statistical exercise crossing the number of deaths per ward and age group was done during the following periods 1986–91 and 1991–4 (Eliot, 1999). It was aimed at identifying mortality fluctuations during the 1986–94 period. At the end of the 1980s, only a few wards showed an increase in deaths that could be attributed to AIDS (20–40 years age group). Ward E took the lead in this matter. On the other hand, between 1991 and 1994 we observe a pronounced fall in mortality in this ward, more so in the 25–39 years age group that is normally most affected by the epidemic. This could be attributed to defects in the mortality data gathering system or an ad hoc change in health conditions, but it is also possible to assume that the AIDS positive population had shifted or was shifting to other areas. This is partly borne out by the increase in AIDS-related deaths in other Mumbai wards during this period (1991–4), especially in Mumbai's eastern and north-western wards.

To sum up, the HIV epidemic seems to have first raised its head in the metro's central districts that are high-flow areas connected at different levels. Certain entry locks and transfer points later linked up these various 'nested' areas. For example, at the city level, the Mumbai Central railway station links the metro's different spaces (both individual and community spaces). There are also groups of individuals organized in different territorial groups that create contacts between different spaces through controlled strategies: human trafficking of vulnerable people, mafia gangs raids by Hindu extremist groups during the 1991–2 communal riots.[12] The city's central districts therefore acted as a 'commutator' or switch, connecting various spaces and territories and thus helping the epidemic to develop from the concentration stage to the transmission stage.

Thus, the epidemic's introduction seems to be a spatial event in so far as there was a switchover from a localized, long-standing epidemiological situation to another, through a transitory phase.

Conclusion

This analysis is an attempt to demonstrate that the emergence of HIV was due to an interactive combination of phenomena. Population displacement does indeed represent the epidemic's main carrier, but all population displacements did not have the same effect. The emergence of HIV is probably linked to uncontrolled antiworld displacements: cross-border human flows either directly or indirectly linked to the drugs trade, human trafficking, prostitution, population displacements as a result of communal riots, repressive measures by political authorities, and so on. These displacements created and organized spatial forms such as interfaces and crossroads or hubs, through which HIV was introduced and spread. Mumbai's central districts exemplify how the epidemic's introduction was facilitated by particular socio-spatial configurations. These local configurations interacted with others organized at different levels. However, these mechanics of scale that determined the epidemic's dynamics were not linear in nature, in the sense that they did not pass automatically from one scale to the other. Scale jumping could and did occur, thereby making the epidemic's spatial analysis far more complex.

NOTES

1. Data taken from individual collections by public and private screening centres in Andhra Pradesh between 1988–94.
2. Data taken from individual collections from Brihan Mumbai Municipal Health Services.
3. In the early 1990s Western Blot was the most reliable test to identify HIV positive cases.
4. Epidemic transmission probability calculations are based on methods evolved by P. Gould in P. Gould, 1993, *The Slow Plague: A Geography of the AIDS Pandemic*, Cambridge: Blackwell, p. 228.
5. For a more detailed analysis of data refer to: E. Eliot, 1997, 1998, 'Changes in Mortality in Mumbai' in *The Looming Epidemic: The Impact of HIV/AIDS in India*, New Delhi and London: Mosaic Books and Hurst and Co., 1997, 1998, p. 190.
6. The given calculation measures the difference in standardized mortality rates between 1986 and 1994.
7. A.R Omran proposed the epidemiological transition model in the early 1970s. A.R. Omran, 'The Epidemiologic Transition: A Theory of the Epidemiology

of Population Change', *Milbank Memorial Foundation Quarterly*, 49, 1971, p. 509.

8. For civic administrative purposes, Mumbai is divided into 'wards', 'sections' and 'blocks'.
9. Interloper: English word meaning 'an intruder who creeps in and settles in by your side' in R. Brunet, R. Ferras, H. Théry, *Les mots de la géographie: un dictionnaire critique*, Belin-Reclus, 1993.
10. During 1998, Bal Thackeray, the emblematic Shiv Sena chief, was involved in a corruption case along with the Indian mafia in Dubai. T. Singh, 'Plus and Minus of Shiv Sena', in *The Tribune* online edition, Saturday, 19 December 1998.
11. Commutator: 'A Configuration Connecting Two Spaces (. . .)', taken from J. Lévy, M. Lussault (dir.), *Dictionnaire de la géographie et de l'espace des sociétés*, Paris Belin, 2003. (Close to the concept of a synapse R. Brunet, R. Ferras and H. Théry, *Les mots de la géographie : un dictionnaire critique*, Belin-Reclus, 1993.)
12. To know about the Shiv Sena's role in Mumbai, refer to G. Heuzé, 'Bombay: La Shiv Shena et le territoire urbain' in *Hérodote*, no. 71 or J. Lele, 'Saffronization of the Shiv Sena: The Political Economy of City, State and Nation' in S. Patel and A. Thorner (eds.), *Bombay: Metaphor for Modern India*, OUP, 1996. On the chronology of events in Mumbai, refer to K. Sharma. 'Chronicle of a Riot Foretold' in S. Patel and A. Thorner (eds.), *Bombay: Metaphor for Modern India.*

REFERENCES

Amat-Roze, J.M., 'Les inégalités géographiques de l'infection à VIH et du SIDA en Afrique subsaharienne', in *Social Science and Medicine*, 36, 10, 1993, pp.1247–56.

Bharat, S., *Facing the Challenge: Household and Community Response to HIV/AIDS in Mumbai, India*, Geneva: World Health Organisation, 1996.

Barnett, T. and A. Whiteside, *AIDS in the Twentieth Century: Disease and Globalisation*, London: Palgrave Macmillan, 2002.

Benko, G. and U. Strohmayer, *Horizons géographiques*, Collection d'Autre part, Breal, 2004.

Bruce, G.W., Y. Takebe, O. Chin Yih and S. Yamazaki, 'The Molecular Epidemiology of HIV in Asia', *Carc Calling*, vol. 7, no. 4, 1994.

Brunet, R., 'Géographie du goulag. L'espace aliéné', *L'Espace Géographique*, 10, 3, pp. 215–32, 1981.

Brunet, R., *Le déchiffrement du monde*, Belin–Reclus, 1990.

Brunet, R. and O. Dollfus, *Mondes nouveaux*, vol. 1, Géographie Universelle, Belin-Reclus, 1990.

Brunet, R., R. Ferras and H. Thery, *Les mots de la géographie: un dictionnaire critique*, Belin-Reclus, 1993.

Desselberger, U., 'Emerging and Re-emerging Infectious Diseases', *Journal of Infection*, 2000, 40, pp. 3–15.

Durand-Dastes, F. and G. Mutin, *Afrique du Nord, Moyen-Orient, Monde indien*, Géographie universelle, Belin-Reclus, 1995.

EPEES, 'Evènement spatial', *L'Espace géographique*, 2000, 3, pp. 193–217.

Eliot, E., 'Changes in Mortality in Mumbai', in P. Godwin (ed.), *The Looming Epidemic: The Impact of HIV/AIDS in India*, London: Hurst and Co. Publishers, 1998.

Eliot, E., 'Diffusion of HIV in Mumbai', in C.Z. Guilmoto and A. Vaguet (ed.), *Essay on Space and Populations of India*, Institut français de Pondicherry, 1998.

Eliot, E., *Les lieux du SIDA dans l'espace indien*, Thèse, Université de Rouen, 1999.

Froment, A., 'Ecologie humaine et médecine tropicale', *Ecologie humaine*, 28 February 1997.

Fortin, R., *Comprendre la complexité: introduction à la Méthode d'Edgar Morin*, L'Harmattan, 2000, p. 231.

Gilada, I.S., 'The IHO Relief Story', *Aids Asia*, 2 February 1994, pp. 6–8.

Gmerk, M.D., *Les maladies à l'aube de la civilisation occidentale*, Payot, 1983.

Gould P., *The Slow Plague: A Geography of the AIDS Pandemic*, Blackwell, Cambridge, 1993.

Gould, P., 'The search for Spatiotemporal Information: Predicting the Next Map of AIDS', *Systema Terra*, 1994, 3, pp. 24–7.

Hägerstrand, T., *The Propagation of Innovation Waves*, Lunds Studies in Geography, Series B., vol. 4, 1952.

Jaffrelot, C., 'L'Inde: l'Etat de droit en procès', *Les Cahiers du CERI*, no. 36, 1997.

Kulshreshtha, R. et al., 'HIV Prevalence in Uttar Pradesh', *Indian Journal of Medical Research*, 103, March, pp. 131–3.

Lévy, J. and M. Lussault (ed.), *Dictionnaire de la géographie et de l'espace des sociétés*, Paris: Belin, 2003.

Patel, S. and A. Thorner, *Bombay: Metaphor for Modern India*, Oxford University Press, 1996.

Ramachandran, R., *Urbanization and Urban Systems in India*, Oxford University Press, 1989.

Remy, G., 'L'infection par le VIH-2 dans le monde: une mise en question géographique', *Cahiers d'études et de recherches francophones santé*, vol. 8, no. 6, November–December, 1998.

Ramasubban, R. and N. Crook, 'Spatial Patterns of Health and Mortality', in S. Patel and A. Thomas, *Bombay: Metaphor for Modern India*, New Delhi: OUP, 1996, pp. 143–69.

Smallman-Raynor, M.R. and A.D. Cliff, *War Epidemics: An Historical Geography of Infectious Diseases in Military Conflict and Civil Strife, 1850–2000*, Oxford Geographical and Environmental Studies, Oxford University Press, 2004.

Vaguet, A., 'Du système pathogène au Système-Monde?', in *Cahiers Géographiques de Rouen*, 1994, pp. 39–40.

Weniger, B.G., Y. Takebe O. Chin Yih and S. Yamakazi,'The Molecular Epidemiology of HIV in Asia', *AIDS*, 9 March 2001; 15(4), 54.

CHAPTER 3

Health, Societies and Identities in the Globalization Era: The Example of Yoga Therapy

ANNE-CÉCILE HOYEZ

It is quite easy to understand the relationship between yoga and health today. All those who practice yoga, or see it from the outside, inevitably perceive this relationship, although it may take different forms. Indeed, the link between yoga and health frequently passes through a host of filters—cultural, social, political, religious, philosophical and other interpretations—that everyone modulates according to their own desires.

There are many ways in which yoga can be interpreted: some may think that yoga is something that one can 'tinker with' on one's own.[1] Moreover, yoga also stems from a cultural and social demand and production originating in India, but not just India. We all know that yoga is Indian, even Hindu, and that the discipline developed there over two thousand years ago.

But yoga did not necessarily have an illustrious history in India. Long restricted to the ascetic practices of certain individuals, it seems to be have been given a new lease of life about a century ago, and more precisely, the last fifty years, when it was reinterpreted as a community practice, both in India and in the West.

Two major movements essentially account for the spread of this practice. On the one hand, the work done by Swami Vivekananda who, from 1893 onwards, travelled all the way to North America, Europe and even within India, played a decisive role in establishing a so-called 'universal' corpus. Indeed, Swami Vivekananda strove to spread 'India's spiritual wealth to the West', which in turn allowed him to introduce 'the West's material wealth to India'.[2] On the other hand, a host of works by Orientalists also contributed extensively to the spread of yoga, especially their translations of sacred texts, rendering them accessible to the Western public. This led to a surge of enthusiasm, that eventually culminated in the establishment of 'Yoga for Westerners' courses in the 1930s and then again in the 1950s.

In fact, yoga has often served as a pretext for the dissemination of modern forms of Hinduism, also called neo-Hinduism. Swami Vivekananda himself worked to develop a corpus of Jnana-Yoga and Bhakti-Yoga, as did other parallel movements such as the Theosophical Society,[3] which published hybrid works (mixing spirituality and science) offering the results of scientific experiments conducted within the framework of existing knowledge about the interactions between yoga and science.

Psychoanalysts from the Freudian school, as well as the Jungian school,[4] looked into the issue, as did sportspersons, intellectuals, and so on. Consequently, with its new lease of life in the West, yoga was ethnicized, becoming a component of health and culture from India. This observation was not based on a cliché, but is the result of both an internal view (by those practising yoga), as well as an external view (by those observing everything happening around yoga). Yoga, or rather 'yoga therapy', which is what we shall be examining in this paper, has long been the subject of research within a confined milieu, essentially through private initiatives. Today, it is one of the major orientations adopted by ministries of health and NGOs.

Indeed, yoga therapy is both national (when it enters various government policies) and transnational (when it overpasses national borders and policies). But above all, it has become globalized. From India to the West Coast of the US, from East Europe to South America, from the old Europe to the Asian dragons, yoga can be found among the treatments adopted by many individuals, through the transnational links that have become the via media for social and identity-building, as we shall see at the end of this article.

We shall also be taking a close look at the ins and out of this process in the health and social spheres, as it has opened up new research issues for social science researchers—for the study of a therapeutic re-interpretation of an ancient corpus in today's world.

Emergence of the Relationship between Yoga and Health

Definition of Complementary Medicine in the International Context

Complementary medicines are becoming increasingly important these days, especially in Western societies, as 'one-third of American adults have used alternative treatment and 60 per cent of the public in the Netherlands and Belgium, and 74 per cent in the United Kingdom are in favour of complementary medicine being available within the framework of the National Health Service. Moreover, a survey among Member States of the European Union in 1991 identified about 1400 herbal drugs used in the European Economic Community' (WHO, 2002).

What are these complementary medicines? Why have they been given this name? The WHO describes 'complementary medicine' as therapies that call for the use of drugs based on plants, animal parts and/or minerals, as well as therapies that do not offer any medicinal products as such, but inputs that are manual and spiritual, such as acupuncture and yoga.

Often, the term 'complementary medicine' is also used for 'traditional medicine', a comprehensive term designating 'traditional systems of medicine such as traditional Chinese medicine, India's Ayurveda and the Arab Unani medicine, with various other indigenous medicines' (WHO, 2002). These terms, which remain quite vague, could be discussed at length.[5]

The difficulty in defining these medicines stems essentially from the fact that they are part of fairly different cultural and health systems, which call for diverse interpretations and different health and healing practices. Consequently, in countries where the main health system is biomedical—i.e. everywhere—'traditional medicine' is called 'complementary', 'alternative' or 'non-conventional'. Thus, the term 'traditional medicine' is often used in the West when referring to medicines of African, Asian or Amerindian origin, and the term 'complementary medicine' is used to refer to non-biomedical therapies of European or American origin.

For the sake of convenience, the WHO uses the abbreviations 'TRM/CPM' (traditional medicine/complementary medicine). However, such a broad definition cannot be taken at face value. We are not trying to question WHO's typology, but we would like to broaden its meaning in the light of the socio-cultural realities of the world-society. In fact, if we look at it closely, it seems difficult to group all the therapies proposed together, because on the one hand, they have been modelled for the most part by transnational dynamics and, on the other, their practices are being constantly renewed, re-interpreted and re-adapted according to changing times.

RE-EMERGENCE OF COMPLEMENTARY MEDICINES IN THE WORLD

The emergence of complementary medicines can be observed both in the projects that have been launched in the health sector[6] and the analyses of social science researchers.[7] Depending on the angle of approach, these assertions may have different foundations, but they are nonetheless complementary. From the public's perspective, as R. Massé puts it, they seem to stem from a desire to prolong the biomedical approach through religio-therapeutic acts that could appear to be increasingly possible and envisaged solutions, thereby ensuring a more cultural and humane relationship between the health sector and the patient's social and family life.

From the perspective of politics and the facilities that have been provided, these assertions stem from a dual assessment, based on facts that differ from country to country. On the one hand, the re-emergence of complementary medicines would appear to be a policy line aimed at reducing health costs, as these systems of medicine require less investment by the State (fewer drugs, lower cost associated with the training of medical personnel) and for patients or, on the other hand, a policy line aimed at reinforcing a health system's cultural features as part of an inward-looking identity-related strategy, as is the case in India and China, among others.

The Western interest for complementary medicine has further reinforced its status. By using and acclaiming a given complementary medicine increasingly, the West bestows a certain intellectual authority on its country of origin, which in turn sees this as an opportunity to revitalize its traditional system.

Today, complementary medicines are no longer just fads in the West. They are digging deeper roots in the countries where they were born, following the virtuous circle offered by the globalization of their corpus.

YOGA: INSTITUTIONALIZATION AS A COMPLEMENTARY HEALTH SYSTEM IN INDIA

Everyone today is more or less aware of what yoga is, in many countries. Without defining yoga at length, let us just say that it relates to a physical and spiritual practice aimed at enabling the person practising it to attain liberation (*mukti*) in an overall state of good health. Thus, yoga is a practice consisting of a whole series of postures (*asanas*) and breathing exercises (*pranayama*), as understood in a more comprehensive philosophical and religious system associated with Hinduism. In modern conceptions of yoga, it is quite often health that is promoted as its key value—reaching a state of well-being means achieving and maintaining good health.

Thus, yoga and health are very closely linked, and it is not just its followers who say so. Indeed, it is because of this aspect that WHO began to take an interest in yoga and, as we will see, it is also this factor that has attracted people to it. Yoga has gradually begun to be considered as a practice that can help heal or manage a disease in many societies.

According to WHO's definition, yoga can be considered a complementary health care system. India too—where the situation is almost similar—has adopted this view. The health guidelines espoused by the government show a serious interest in this issue for three main reasons. On the one hand, the Indian government already gives importance to so-called traditional health care systems (Ayurveda, Unani, Siddha, but also yoga) by providing a budget for research and for training competent staff. On the other hand, the re-emergence of this 'traditional knowledge' was reinforced at the end of the 1990s and the turn of the century with the 'cultural' line adopted by the BJP government.

Indeed, the Vajpayee government strove to rationalize the religious and Vedic corpus through a project aimed at strengthening 'Vedic Sciences'. The aim was to do an in-depth analysis of several disciplines of Vedic origin and present them as pillars of science: mathematics, astrology and yoga, among others. The strategy consisted of gathering experts from different religious and scientific fields together so that they could pool their knowledge and finally publish works for as wide a readership as possible as well as for schools.[8] The rationalization of knowledge of religious and philosophical origin thus took place through the intrusion of 'science' in the formulation of theories. But in fact, the rationalization was just a label and led to several cases of abuse on the part of certain theoreticians with strong political leanings.

Hence, favourable grounds exist in India for the emergence of yoga as a complementary course of therapy. With increasing research on yoga, the term 'yoga therapy' has emerged—a concept that blends health and religion, although this is nothing new if you look at some enduring Indian experiments, such as, for instance, those of the Lonavla[9] research centre.

In the case of yoga, the rationalization process was based on increasingly closer contacts with the medical field, leading to the 'healthism' of its definition.[10] Yoga is thus often understood as a beneficial and useful practice for good physical and mental health, keeping cultural and religious aspects in the background.

Finally, NGOs—often of Western origin—which have been showing a growing interest in the issue of complementary medicines, came to India to carry out more detailed research on this type of health care as well as the conditions of its adaptability to comprehensive health care systems.

INSTITUTIONALIZATION IN THE WEST

Outside India, the relationship established between yoga and health in the 1970s is not promoted in the same way in different countries where yoga is practised. Thus, in France, the authorities barely give any emphasis to this issue, unlike Great Britain, where the government views the issue of yoga as a complementary medicine more easily.

From the political perspective, yoga seems to be much more institutionalized in Great Britain,[11] so much so that its inclusion in the therapeutic field is much more evident than in France. In fact, in 2000, the British government launched a vast research programme on complementary and alternative medicines. Noting the growing importance of such systems in Western countries,[12] the British government wished to implement regulatory policies, with five main objectives: protecting the public from conmen, setting up appropriate facilities for patients, encouraging research on therapeutic efficiency (and developing tools and methods to do so), monitoring health professionals to keep a check on bad quality treatment and helping health professionals to incorporate training in complementary medicines in their curriculum.

The study undertaken in Great Britain made it possible to update statistics, which reinforced the idea that complementary medicines should be incorporated in Britain's health system. It revealed that in 1999, 20 per cent of the population had taken recourse to complementary medicines and that, of this population, 34 per cent of individuals had used yoga and meditation techniques.

Outside Europe, similar policies have been implemented in other countries, including the United States in particular. Statistics reveal a similar situation: between 1990 and 1997, researchers noted an increase of about 50 per cent visits to practitioners specializing in a complementary medicine system.[13] Table 3.1 shows the distribution of complementary medicine use in the United States:

TABLE 3.1: DISTRIBUTION OF COMPLEMENTARY MEDICINE USE IN UNITED STATES

	1990 (Of a total of 1,539 Persons) (%)	1997 (Of a total of 2,055 Persons) (%)
Use of CAM in the 12 preceding months	33.8	42.1
Including:		
Relaxation Techniques	13.1	16.3
Herbal Medicine	2.5	12.1
Massages	6.9	11.1
Chiropractics	10.1	11.0
Spiritual Healing	4.2	7.0
Homoeopathy	0.7	3.4
Acupuncture	0.4	1.0

Source: Report on Complementary and Alternative Medicine, English Parliament, House of Lords, 1999–2000 Session.

Consequently, the recourse to complementary medicines is on the rise all over the world, especially in the West, as well as in their country of origin, at the same time. This situation is the outcome of a feedback phenomenon between different societies witnessed since the 1950s. Indeed, the popularization of complementary medicines such as yoga in an ever-increasing number of countries seems to have 'revived' so-called 'traditional' systems in India. Their re-emergence is the result of the growing institutionalization of complementary medicines within the non-indigenous treatment system (in Great Britain, the USA), leading also to the reformulation of Indian identity orchestrated by politicians. Before dwelling on this sensitive issue, let us see what form the health aspects of yoga have taken in the centres where it is practised.

Yoga Therapy: Different Aspects

Following the analysis of these extensive studies in the West, the reader is entitled to wonder how individuals steer themselves toward complementary medicines. In the case of yoga, the health aspect has been given wide coverage, as we have seen, and is coupled with other considerations which are specific to each person's cultural environment. In fact, many people who do yoga are particularly drawn towards its philosophical system, which associates religion, spirituality, body and psyche. Further, these are systems that attract people because of their 'culturally creative' aspect and the fact that they are viewed as a 'transforming experience'. To understand who and what yoga is supposed to treat, I conducted several field studies in India and France.[14]

YOGA IN INDIA

Yoga is practised in India by a majority of women,[15] which is quite unique in the Indian social context, though it is understandable when you learn that the women who are drawn to it are basically from India's well-off so-called 'upwardly-mobile' classes,[16] who have considerably more freedom.

On the whole, yoga also attracts students (15 per cent) who have reached at least secondary school level, civil servants (14 per cent), retired persons (12.5 per cent) and businessmen (8 per cent). The remaining percentage is divided between professionals and health professionals.

As far as the caste is concerned, 53.3 per cent of those who practice yoga are Brahmins, while the others belong to other Forward Castes (FCs),[17] with local dominant castes imitating these practices. For instance, some castes in Tamil Nadu or in Maharashtra are castes whose activities have made it possible for them to achieve a certain level of economic or technological development in certain areas. They have attained a socio-professional status that allows them to claim a way of life that is close to that of intellectually dominant castes, i.e. a Brahmanic way of life, a phenomenon that the sociologist Srinivas[18] calls 'Sanskritisation'.

Thus, yoga followers are for the most part composed of the working population belonging to the middle and upper classes, women and higher-education students. They are the elite in the economic sector (given their professional category), social sector (mostly privileged castes) and intellectual sphere (well-read, educated people). Most are 'urban'—born and bred in the urban milieu.[19]

Health is their primary reason for adopting yoga (Table 3.2). However, spiritual motivations are also superimposed on health concerns, also leading to health-related notions (notion of well-being, mental relaxation, and so on).

These surveys were conducted among individuals who practice yoga regularly, without it being their main activity. The path followed by

TABLE 3.2: REASON FOR RECOURSE TO YOGA

Reason for recourse to yoga		No. of persons	Share (%)	No. of persons	Share (%)
Physical Health	For treating a disease	126	59.4	191	90.1
	To keep in good health	53	25.0		
	For post-operative recovery	4	1.9		
	To avoid taking too many medicines	3	1.4		
	To avoid an operation	3	1.4		
	To reduce stress	2	0.9		
Spiritual reasons	Out of interest in spirituality	21	9.9	35	16.5
	For lifestyle reasons	10	4.7		
	For peace of mind	3	1.4		
	To learn *pranayama*	1	0.5		
Psychological reasons	For mental relaxation	8	3.8	13	6.1
	To enhance concentration capacity	4	1.9		
	For psychological reasons	1	0.5		
Other reasons	For exercise	11	5.2	22	10.4
	To accompany a close relative or friend	3	1.4		
	No specific reason	3	1.4		
	To lose weight	3	1.4		
	For suppleness	1	0.5		
	Out of curiosity	1	0.5		
Total Obs.		261		261	123.1

Source: Personal surveys in three yoga centres in India, 2000–1.

their teachers—often the outcome of several years of 'maturing'—is interesting in itself. In fact, it has been observed that among yoga teachers, the starting point of their relationship with yoga was a health problem. In other words, I learnt from the interviews they gave me that at that they had all begun to practice yoga as a therapy in response to a fairly serious physical or mental health problem or even a combination of the both (multiple sclerosis, chronic malaise, chronic migraines). Consequently, their teachings and discourses also focus on treatment-related questions raised by their disciples.

This was borne out clearly in the statistics of some centres, as shown in Table 3.3.

Hence, health plays an important role in yoga courses, whether for those practising it (as their interest in yoga is often motivated by a health problem) or for yoga centres, who place a lot of emphasis on the health of those who go there. Thus, in many yoga centres, anyone who comes to register has to present his or her medical file first and meet the centre's doctor. The latter then gives directions about the type of *asanas* (postures) the person is allowed or not allowed to do (some *asanas* can be dangerous, especially from the articular point of view).

Thus, yoga centres are turning into therapy centres and we have even noticed a shift in yoga teaching towards a therapeutic vocabulary: yoga teachers become 'doctors', students become 'patients' and *asanas* 'prescriptions'.

YOGA IN FRANCE

France has a large number of yoga centres which are affiliated to Indian yoga centres. I interviewed about a hundred yoga students in Rouen and they presented the same socio-economic profile overall as the Indians. Rouen's *yogis* belong to the urban middle and upper classes, mainly (working) women and professionals, or people working in national education or other public sector fields. Their motivations are similar to those I identified in the Indian context, with physical and psychological health topping the list (Table 3.4).

TABLE 3.3: HEALTH PROBLEMS

Diseases	Men	Women	Total
1. Backache	11	22	33
2. Sinusitis	8	12	20
3. Knee problems	4	14	18
4. Gynaecological problems	0	17	17
5. Migraines	6	10	16
6. Obesity	4	12	16
7. Essential hypertension	8	6	14
8. Diabetes	5	6	11
9. Gastric problems	4	7	11

Sources: Krishnamacharya Yoga Mandiram, 2002.

TABLE 3.4: REASONS FOR RECOURSE TO YOGA IN FRANCE

	Centre A	Centre B	Centre C	Total
In search of relaxation	33	18	31	83
To add physical exercise to mental techniques	28	18	26	72
To remedy a health problem	16	9	18	43
Including:				
Back problems	*5*	*5*	*3*	*13*
Stress	*5*	*3*	*2*	*10*
Migraines	*1*	*1*	*1*	*3*
Others	*1*	*1*	*1*	*3*
Loss of range of motion	*1*	*0*	*1*	*2*
Depression	*1*	*1*	*0*	*2*
Existential suffering	*2*	*0*	*0*	*2*
Essential hypertension	*1*	*1*	*0*	*2*
Renal problems	*2*	*0*	*0*	*2*
For psychological help	16	12	14	42
For the experience	11	11	13	35
On a doctor's advice	5	5	9	19
To learn about the tradition of yoga	2	9	5	16
Others	6	2	2	10
No response	0	0	2	2

Source: Personal surveys in three yoga centres in France, 2000–1.

The search for ways to relax—a primary motivation—shows that those who practice yoga essentially do so with the intention of improving their well-being. The state of 'well-being' is supposed to be achieved by regularly working the body and emotions. Thus, students arrive with a 'malaise' that needs to be taken care of—a more or less subjective state that they may have been suffering for some time, according to what emerged from the interviews I conducted with some yoga followers. Today, social science research as well as medical science research tend to support the fact that good health is not just the absence of illness, but also an individual perception that is specific to each person's own environment.

YOGA AND WELL-BEING

According to WHO's definition, health revolves around the notion of 'well-being', a field that makes it necessary to refer to several implicit theories. In fact, a state of well-being is above all a matter of individual perception. Indeed, the diffidence of public health policies in this regard has left the field wide open for a host of definitions. Consequently, defining well-being today depends on how society and public policies see individual preoccupations within the framework of extremely different cultural, social and religious contexts.

Public health seems quite distant and defenceless when faced with the notion of well-being, not only because it is specific to the patient but also because there are no 'miracle solutions' governing well-being. Rather, it is complementary therapies such as yoga (which rarely have anything to do with the public sector) that lay claim to promoting well-being. These systems, which can be described as 'traditional' and/or spiritual are often based on considerations that are alien to Western thought processes, which makes it all the more complex to study them.

Thinking of well-being from the individual's perspective calls upon physiological, physical, psychological and spiritual concerns. The number of yoga centres responding to these concerns is thus rising continuously, along with growing discourses on health, inevitably tinged with cultural references.

Thus, to understand well-being today—a term that is used a bit too systematically—it is easier to examine its opposite—'bad-being'. The students at the centres come with 'bad-being', to be taken care of. It could be a physical or psychological state that may have developed in the form of different sociopathies or a negative perception of the environment in which they live (precarious living conditions, industrial pollution, noise pollution and so on). To make up for this state of 'bad-being', these students visit spaces corresponding to an ideal that is as close as possible to well-being—spaces caught up in the dynamics of globalization, with all the cultural consequences that this implies.

GLOBALIZATION OF YOGA: LARGER ISSUES

As we have seen so far, there are a number of discourses on yoga today. They may all begin with health as the starting point, but its interpretations are as varied as are societal and cultural conditions in the world. When health creeps into individual perceptions, it has several ramifications and therefore involves the subtlest of notions (cultural, psychological and so on).

These aspects have been studied in-depth by several authors, such as Sudhir Kakar to give an example among the Indians or Wilbert Gesler among Europeans,[20] and have to be taken into consideration while observing the spaces produced or reproduced. These spaces belong to the macro level (that of the world) as well as to the micro level (that of the individual). They are indissociable and lead to quite interesting conjunctions of circumstances.

INTERNATIONAL PERSPECTIVES: TRANSNATIONAL YOGA NETWORKS

India's health care system also includes a spiritual and religious component, which is still a common practice. This particular aspect has been exported to or transplanted in the West over the last few decades. Thus, this is the right time to bring to light an original phenomenon of dissemination in which it is no longer a Western system of medicine that is being transplanted elsewhere, but an aspect of Indian health care that is being incorporated into the dominant health systems of the West.

The long years of intercultural relations between India and the rest of the world led to the strengthening of certain individual links and, consequently, played a role in strengthening a network of inter-dependence. In fact, these networks interact with each other on a continuous basis—a phenomenon further promoted by the use of modern means of communication (Internet, etc.) and the growing institutionalization in all countries. In fact, yoga has entered a phase of administrative construction, with the setting up of federations (at national level), confederations (at regional level—Europe, North America, etc.) or even confederations of federations (at a pan-regional level). By forming associations based on their interest in yoga, individuals are playing a role in creating a worldwide space characterized by places, links, the circulation of ideas and people, thereby leading to the establishment of a sort of 'community of yogis'.[21]

MODES OF PRODUCTION: IDENTITIES AND POLICIES

The links that have been established within these networks are not fortuitous. They go beyond mere understandings between individuals to project themselves with the objective of pooling fairly specific identity-related resources. Thus, as mentioned earlier, yoga has been propelled to the international scene on the 'pretext' of health. But beyond this, some saw it as an opportunity to prove that yoga—an element of Hindu identity—could be placed at the service of the West. Thus, by identifying the possibility of reversing conventional hegemonic trends (i.e. cultural domination of the West in India), Hindu nationalists seized the opportunity to reinforce the Hindu identity.

Following India's Independence, yoga has been the subject of several 'publicity' campaigns promoting India's identity: television, stamps, tourism, etc. The emergence of this idea thus played on the reinterpretation of cultural values in India. I have often heard my interlocutors speak of yoga with a certain patriotic pride during my interviews in India. But it must be stressed that these people are not the ones responsible for nationalist discourses. Politicians implement strategies based on the instrumentalization of a growing number of *yogis*—a significant demographic and electoral pool that is playing a role in this situation.[22]

However, identity-related resources associated with the practice of yoga are not at all the same in the West. A European or an American is drawn by yoga first and foremost because of individual health concerns and the cultural or rather exotic aspects of practising a new discipline are only of secondary importance. Thus, quite often, Western *yogis* have a special sensibility *vis-à-vis* India (they dream of visiting it, they love the idea of India, etc.) and retranscribe it into attitudes of intellectual and/or cultural openness to the world, by participating, directly or indirectly in building the identity of 'world citizens'. This can be seen in their political positioning: I met French people (in France) and many Westerners (in India), who described themselves as environmental activists of the left. In the Western scenario, values based on a strong criticism of the rationalist way of thinking and the promotion of lifestyles influenced by multi-cultural elements are promoted, with a strong back-to-nature streak.

This political paradox is eminently interesting because the two extremes need each other to flourish: Indian Hindutva activists promote their ideas through highly anti-establishment groups, and Westerners—far removed from the conservatism of pro-Hindu nationalist parties—develop their discourse based more on an imaginary India rather than its existing political realities.

In fact, each of the parties conceals a fraction of the message. For instance, Western *yogis* are unable to perceive the sometimes polemical nature of the stand adopted by certain yoga centres (both in India and in the West). Thus, Westerners are often ignorant about India's socio-political conditions and are therefore not in a position to understand the fact that in some conceptions of health and the body, lines of the Hindu civic code, which was developed by extreme-right Hindu theoreticians during India's struggle for independence, are reinterpreted and romanticized (Strauss, 1997).

IDENTITY-RELATED AND CULTURAL LANDSCAPES OF GLOBAL DIMENSIONS

When yoga practices are extended to such a varied and malleable range of identity-related practices, they reinforce the theoretical and conceptual tools used in social sciences. The study of the spread of yoga is not just the reflection of a unique phenomenon but is also part and parcel of the formulation of methodologies and great ideas. In fact, yoga can be interpreted in a host of different ways, depending on the group promoting it. Thus, it enters a more global framework, calling for the observation of the forms it takes in the individual and collective imagination specific to the context of globalization.

In geographic terms, globalization provides yoga with a cultural, political economic, and other frameworks, giving birth to specific therapeutic landscapes (Gesler, 1992). In the broader sense of the term, these landscapes are composed of places that have gained the reputation of being able to offer treatment based on a spiritual, mental and physical reading, over a period of time. The concept is also based on temporal and spatial links, interactions between the natural characteristics of a place and the human constructions that have taken shape. In the semantic field stemming from the patronization and recognition of therapeutic landscapes, we repeatedly find the idea of 'warmth', 'identity', 'taking root', 'authenticity', the re-emergence of the myth of healing and of popular beliefs and the development of behaviours and lifestyles—all in an atmosphere in which cultural differences and social inequalities are at their minimum.

Thus, therapeutic landscapes can be associated with yoga, which incites us to look into the question of a 'sense of place' and 'topophilia'. All the places where yoga is practised are attached to specific lifestyles, often recalling Hindu thought—or at least a hybrid interpretation of it. The 'sense of place' here is largely dependent on well-being, which we discussed earlier—a well-being that is based on the perception of the place. Such a perception would be formed on the basis of the interpretation of material and symbolic ideals, which would then play on individual emotions, themselves 'classified' along lines shared by several individuals: the community or the group.

These 'well-being landscapes', produced and interpreted by different groups, are also projected in the cultural imagination examined by anthropologists—the famous 'ethnoscapes', to use the neologism coined by Arjun Appadurai (1996). According to him, these 'ethnoscapes' stem from 'transnational culturalist movements' in which you can clearly measure 'changes in social, territorial and cultural production of the group's identity', as for instance in the case of the spread of cricket, the game he studied, or yoga, as we have just seen.

Finally, the factors that play a part in yoga's area of action take on different shapes in different societies: a therapeutic identity-related political, cultural or spiritual form, depending on the groups and individuals concerned.

Conclusion

For geographers, identity-related landscapes, which are recreated by groups of individuals in a socio-spatial environment differing from the original environment are highly revealing of the meaning assumed by space and time in the post-modern era.

Yoga is broadly perceived as a link in the therapeutic itineraries of several countries. It is still difficult to find these therapeutic assets within the framework of medical research and the WHO's work today. But the moment the issue of the definition of the relationship between yoga and health is resolved, we can certainly expect it to emerge in increasingly institutionalized forms in health systems.

However, since the cultural, political and religious dimensions involved are very dense, we cannot merely restrict yoga to the 'official' frameworks within which it may be placed. This was evident when we raised the issues of identity-related reappropriation within the framework of the production of yoga and the use of the tools of modernity to reinvent traditions, but we also saw it when we studied its economic aspects and those related to land, tourism and others fields. The combination of the various conjunctions of circumstances is highly interesting, because it raises the complex problematics linking health with cultural and/or religious identities. This paves the way for a much larger number of research avenues, as suggested by a few seminal geographers in their recent studies (Asthana et al., 2002): the study of health, in particular complementary treatments, thus becomes the starting point for the formulation of new methodological approaches in fields as varied as health, social sciences and, in particular, geography.

NOTES

1. 'Tinkering with' refers here to an attitude of 'pick and choose'. Michel de Certeau spoke of 'everyday tinkering' ('bricolage quotidien') in 1980 (in Arts de Faire, Paris, Union Générale d'Editions, p. 374), but I am using the expression 'tinker with' here, in relation to Mary André's theory, according to which contemporary practices of belief are the outcome of 'tinkering' by individuals (Mary André, 'Bricolage afro-brésilien et bris-collage moderne', in Philippe Laburthe-Tolra (ed.), Roger Bastide ou le « réjouissement de l'abîme » : échos du colloque tenu à Cerisy-la-Salle du 7 au 14 septembre 1992. Paris: L'Harmattan, 1994, pp. 85–98).
2. The biographical work by the Frenchman Romain Rolland (Romain Rolland, La vie de Vivekananda et l'évangile universel, Paris: Stock, 1978), the German Max Muller and the Ramakrishna Missions and Monasteries' publication division in Belur (Kolkata) or elsewhere are some examples. For a more critical approach, see Robert D. Baird, (ed.), *Religion in Modern India*, 4th rev. edn., New Delhi: Manohar, 2001, p. 626.
3. A number of publications on this subject are available among the Theosophical Society's publications (Helena P. Blavatsky, *The Secret Doctrine: The Synthesis of Science, Religion and Philosophy*, 2 vols., London–New York–Madras: Theosophical Publishing Company, 1888, rpt. Pasadena: Theosophical University Press, 1988; Helena P. Blavatsky, *What Theosophy is*, Bombay: Theosophy Company, rpt. 1992. There is also a critical counterpoint among certain social science researchers, such as the work by M.P. Kamerkar ('The Theosophy Movement in India, with Special Reference to Maharashtra', in S.P. Sen, *Social Content of Indian Religious Reform Movements*, Calcutta: Institute of Historical Studies, 1978, pp. 399–410) or of Mark Bevir, 'Theosophy as a Political Movement', in Anthony Copley (ed.), *Gurus and Their Followers: New Religious Reform Movements*, New Delhi: Oxford University Press, 2000, pp. 159–79, 235.
4. See Carl G. Jung, *Ma vie. Souvenirs, rêves et pensées*, ed. Gallimard, Coll. Folio, 1973.
5. See a debate on the appellation 'traditional medicines' in Craig R. Janes, 'The Health Transition, Global Modernity and the Crisis of Traditional Medicine: The Tibetan Case', in *Social Science and Medicine*, vol. 12, June 1999, pp. 1803–20.

6. This can be seen in the WHO report as well as in the increasing number of articles devoted to the relationship between yoga and health in online world forums on the Internet.
7. See Jean Benoist, 1996, *Soigner au Pluriel, Essais sur le pluralisme médical*, Paris: Karthala, Frédéric Bourdier, *Système de soins et bilan de santé. Etude de cas en milieu rural, Inde du Sud*, Cahiers Géos no. 28, 1994, Jean Benoist, Raymond Massé, *Convocations Thérapeutiques du Sacré*, Paris: Karthala.
8. This measure provoked an outcry in India; in 2002 and 2003, a commission decided to initiate a rewriting of India's history in school textbooks from the primary to the secondary classes.
9. The Lonavla Centre, also called Kaivalyadhama Yoga Ashram, was set up 1924.
10. The expression 'healthism' was put forward by Claudine Herzlich, 'Représentations sociales de la santé et de la maladie et leur dynamique dans le champ social', in Doise W., Palmonari A. (eds), *L'étude des représentations sociales*, Neuchatel-Paris, Delachaux et Niéstlé, 1986, pp. 157–70.
11. See Report on Complementary and Alternative Medicine, English Parliament, House of Lords, Session 1999–2000.
12. In GB: 50,000 doctors belong to the Complementary and Alternative Medicines' (CAM) category, including 10,000 listed professionals, 5 million patients and a growing number of patients and practitioners.
13. The figure seems to have risen from 427 million to 629 million; i.e. higher than visits to general practitioners; estimated expenditure: US$ 27 billion.
14. Surveys were conducted between 2000 and 2002 in three yoga centres in Rouen (88 individuals), two centres in Pune and one in Chennai (212 individuals). At the same time, a number of interviews and observations in several other Indian cities, including Rishikesh, considered to be the 'world yoga capital', contributed to these studies.
15. Women accounted for 52 per cent of the total number of individuals in Indian centres. Of them, it emerged that 34 per cent were housewives, 44.30 per cent working women, 16.40 per cent students and 4.80 per cent unemployed or retired.
16. 67 per cent of the total number had an income of more than Rs. 10,000 per month. International criteria estimate that the poverty line is Rs. 1,500 per month, but this does not have the same significance, depending on whether you live in the city or a rural area. Thus, life in Chennai is believed to be viable with Rs. 6,000 per month for a family of 4 persons.
17. FC = Forward Castes, the most 'forward' castes as per the value system associated with the caste system.
18. The reader can refer to two main articles: M.N. Srinivas, 'A Note on Sanskritisation and Westernisation', *Far Eastern Quarterly*, 15, 1956, pp. 481–96 and M.N. Srinivas, 1967, 'The Cohesive Role of Sanskritisation', in Philip Mason, *India and Ceylon: Unity and Diversity*, London: Oxford University Press, 1967.

19. The sample includes barely any villagers, who probably migrated to the city.
20. See S. Kakar, *Shamans, Mystics and Doctors: A Psychological Inquiry into India and its Healing Traditions*, New Delhi: Oxford University Press, 1986 [1982], p. 306; Wilbert M. Gesler, 'Aspects Culturels des systèmes de soins de santé', *Bulletin de la Société Neuchâteloise de Géographie*, no. 39, 1995, pp. 155–62.
21. See the contextualization of this situation in Ulf Hannerz, *Transnational Connexions: Culture, People, Places*, New York: Routledge, 1997, and details on the creation of transnational communities in Benedict Anderson *Imagined Communities, Reflections on the Origin and Spread of Nationalism*, London: Verso, 1991, p. 224.
22. In this regard, see Christophe Jaffrelot, *The Hindu Nationalist Movement and Indian Politics: 1925 to the 1990s: Strategies of Identity-building, Implantation and Mobilisation (with Special Reference to Central India)*, London: Hurst, 1996, p. 592, or Peter Van der Veer, *Religious Nationalism: Hindus and Muslims in India*, Delhi: Oxford India Paperbacks, 1998, p. 247.

REFERENCES

Anderson, Benedict, *Imagined Communities: Reflections on the Origin and Spread of Nationalism*, London: Verso, 1991.

Appadurai, A., *Modernity at Large: Cultural Dimensions of Globalisation*, Minneapolis: University of Minnesota Press, 1996.

Asthana, Sheena, Sarah Curtis, Craig Duncan and Myles Gould, 'Themes in British Health Geography at the End of the Century: A Review of Published Research 1998–2000', *Social Sciences and Medicine*, 55, 2002, pp. 167–73.

De Certeau, Michel, *Arts de Faire*, Paris: Union Générale d'Editions, 1980.

Gesler, Wilbert, 'Therapeutic Landscapes: Medical Issues in Light of the New Cultural Geography', *Social Sciences and Medicine*, vol. 34, no. 7, 1992, pp. 735–46.

Hannerz, Ulf, *Transnational Connexions: Culture, People, Places*, New York: Routledge, 1997.

Jaffrelot, Christophe, *The Hindu Nationalist Movement and Indian Politics: 1925 to the 1990s: Strategies of Identity-building, Implantation and Mobilisation (with Special Reference to Central India)*, London: Hurst, 1996.

Kearns, Robin A. and Wilbert M. Gesler, *Putting Health into Place: Landscape, Identity and Well-Being*, Syracuse-New York: Syracuse University Press, 1998.

Parr, Hester, 'Medical Geography: Critical Medical and Health Geography?', *Progress in Human Geography*, vol. 28, issue 2, 2004, April, pp. 246–57.

Sen, S.P., *Social Content of Indian Religious Reform Movements*, Calcutta: Institute of Historical Studies, 1978.

Strauss, Sarah, 'Re-orienting Yoga: Transnational Flows from an Indian Centre', Ph.D. dissertation in anthropology presented to the Faculties of the University of Pennsylvania, 1997.

Strauss, Sarah, ' "Adapt, Adjust, Accommodate": The Production of Yoga in a Transnational World', *History and Anthropology*, vol. 13, issue 3, 2002, pp. 231–51.

Tuan, Yi-Fu, *Topophilia: A Study of Environmental Perception, Attitudes and Values*, New York: Columbia University Press, 1974.

Van der Veer, Peter, *Religious Nationalism: Hindus and Muslims in India*, Delhi: Oxford India Paperbacks, 1998.

World Health Organisation, *WHO Strategy for Traditional Medicine 2002–5*, Geneva, 2002.

PART I

EMERGING HEALTH LANDSCAPES

B. Towards Landscapes of Globalization

CHAPTER 4

'Bringing World-class Health Care to India': The Rise of Corporate Hospitals

BERTRAND LEFEBVRE

In 1983, Prathap C. Reddy created the first Indian corporate hospital in Chennai. Corporate hospitals can be defined as private for-profit hospitals (as opposed to charitable hospitals) offering general or specialist tertiary level care (e.g. cardiac care). They are different from other hospitals because of their private corporate limited status. The corporatization of health care and hospital sector occurred previously in the United States in the late 1960s. Under the Nixon and Reagan administration, the hospital sector was 'rationalized' and marketized mainly to the benefit of newly formed corporate hospitals (Salmon, 1990). This corporatization affected also the rest of the hospital sector which was constituted of not-for-profit facilities (voluntary and public hospitals). Some became the targets of corporate hospitals and entered in the large hospital chains created by companies like Hospital Corporation of America. Some hospitals simply mimicked the profit-led management of the corporate hospitals. Finally many public hospitals simply closed down. US hospital chains later entered the United Kingdom following reforms initiated by Prime Minister Margaret Thatcher (Salmon, 1990). The model of corporate hospital spread in Europe, Latin America, South-East Asia and Middle East. In many countries the corporatization of the hospital sector followed economic reforms and the liberalization of local economies. Some are prompted to denunciate this development as a negative outcome of globalization.

Following the liberalization and economic reforms of 1991, we may suppose that corporate hospitals mushroomed all over India. Such hospitals are expanding rapidly in number especially in the metropolises such as Delhi, Kolkata, Bangalore and Hyderabad. But more than ten years after economic reforms, they hardly tap 7 per cent of the total spendings in private health care (CII-McKinsey, 2002). Because of their for-profit orientation and certain misuses of public subsidies their expansion has become controversial in a country where public hospitals and primary care facilities are in such a bad shape. With the best medical teams and the wealthiest patients fleeing from public hospitals to these institutions reserved for elite, the gap in the delivery of quality care has surely increased. But who is responsible for this situation? The World Bank and the International Monetary Fund and their Structural Adjustment Policy? The national and local political elites who followed the prescriptions of the international agencies? The corporate hospitals and the economic powers behind these hospitals? The NRIs who came back to India with new concepts of care?

In this paper we would like to offer a different angle on the emergence of corporate hospitals in India. If globalization has a lot to explain about the emergence of corporate hospitals, we would like to remind of and analyse the complexity that prevailed during the birth and the development of this innovation. The interactions between local and global forces were numerous and took different channels. The birth and expansion of corporate hospitals are embedded in those channels. In the first part, we will analyse the roots of corporate hospitals. Then we will assess the present corporatization of the hospital sector in India. Finally we would like to present how the Indian corporate hospitals are now going global with various objectives.

Introducing Corporate Hospitals

In the 1970s the public sector was the main provider of health care in India. The hospital sector was broadly divided between government hospitals, charitable hospitals and a growing number of small private nursing homes. At the start of the 1970s, the private health care sector underwent significant development. In the districts and states that had benefitted from the positive effects of the Green Revolution, part of the profits gained from agriculture were reinvested in small-scale industries and service sector (Omvedt, 1981). Landlords, cultivators, traders, especially those from south India, encouraged their children to study, sometimes abroad. After completing their medical studies, some children opened nursing homes that allowed their families to diversify their activities (Baru, 1998).

The story of Dr Prathap C. Reddy, the founder of the first Indian corporate hospital, is a good example of such a trend. His father was a plantation owner from Chitoor district in Andhra Pradesh. Dr Reddy completed his medical studies in Chennai and left for the United States in 1958 on a medical fellowship. He worked there until 1970–1 when he returned to Chennai. After starting his own practice, Dr Reddy invested in a cardiology clinic. Because the import duty on medical equipment was high he could not import the necessary equipment for certain therapies (Loveman, O'Connell, 1995). He was therefore forced to send some of his patients to the United States for treatment. When one of his patients died because he could not afford to travel to the US, Dr Reddy decided to start a hospital. At that time, he was not allowed to receive loans from governmental financial institutions. After a three-year long lobbying, Dr Reddy obtained a one-time exemption from Prime Minister Indira Gandhi. He made several visits to the US, met one the founders of Hospital Corporation of America, Thomas Frizt Jr., and some Non-Resident Indian (NRI) doctors, and succeeded in rasing $ 4.6 million in 1983. Forty per cent of the shares of the hospital were in the hands of NRI doctors from the United States (Loveman and O'Connell, 1995). From the 1980s, NRI doctors, particularly from the US, played a pioneering role in different parts of India to set-up or to finance corporate hospitals. In Hyderabad, Medwin Banjara Hospital and Susruth Hospital had NRI involvement from the start (Baru, 1998). In 1995, Dr Kamal K. Dutta created the Ruby General Hospital, the first hospital founded by a NRI in Kolkata. This sudden interest in Indian health care was facilitated by a change in the Indian health policy.

The early 1980s have been a turning point in the Indian political economy. With public debt crisis in sight, India initiated economic openness and began the process of relaxing investment rules. For the first time, the National Health Policy of 1982 recognized the role played by the private sector in health care. The Sixth Plan (1980–5) followed a similar agenda. The government not only recognized its failures in providing health care to the Indian population but also acknowledged the growth of the private sector. According to the 42nd NSSO Round (1986–7), over 70 per cent of the population was using private health care. It was also around this time that the State's disengagement had begun to be more obvious in health. The share of health expenditure in different Five-Year Plans had gradually fallen from 3.30 per cent in the mid-1950s to 1.80 per cent at the end of the 1970s (Rihouey, 1997). In the 1980s, the health care sector underwent further changes. In 1986, at the special request of Dr Reddy, Prime Minister Rajiv Gandhi recognized the hospital sector as an industry, allowing easier access to financing from public financial institutions like Industrial Development Bank of India. Some special concessions were also given to NRIs and on the import duties on high-technology medical equipment (Baru, 1998). The availability of loans at favourable rates and cuts in customs duties for imports of high-technology medical equipment played an important role in promoting the development of new private hospitals.

In the spring of 1991, India took recourse to loans from the International Monetary Fund, the World Bank and the Asian Development Bank. A Structural Adjustment Policy aimed at reimbursing the public debt was launched. The World Bank itself acknowledged that these adjustments would result in the irremediable reduction in public expenditure on health (World Bank, 1993: 45): 'Because cuts in government spending are usually central to an adjustment program, health spending is likely to be reduced.' With decentralization as the pretext, the structural adjustment process shifted the financial burden from the centre to the lower administrative levels. While central government investments in health remained at around 1.30 per cent of the total budget, investments by the states fell from 7 to 5.50 per cent (Ministry of Health and Family Welfare, 2002). The poorest states suffered the most, since they were constrained to mobilize their own resources to pay salaries and to reduce their investment in infrastructure (Selvaraju and Anniger, 2001).

To compensate for the reduction in public investment, different state governments encouraged the private sector. This policy fitted well with the World Bank's vision, which saw the private sector and the market forces as more effective and efficient due to competition (World Bank, 1993: 131). In its World Development Report (1993), the World Bank recommended certain adjustments for the developing countries like cut-back on tertiary care in the public sector and limit the financing of essential clinical services to the poor section of the population. At each administrative level, the authorities developed incentives for the private sector. Tax exemptions were increased. Land was given free to private hospitals. The authorities went as far as to obtain shares in the new hospitals. For instance, the Government of Delhi owns about 26 per cent of the Indraprastha Apollo Hospital. In compensation, the new private hospitals had to reserve a certain number of beds for the underprivileged or organize health camps in slums or villages. Thus, this was public-private partnership at its peak, which was supposed to place the efficiency and competence of private hospitals at the service of public health, under the aegis of the World Bank. It is now well documented that this policy has not yielded the desired results, mainly because the private hospitals have not respected their commitments (see Purohit, 2001, Public Account Committee, 2005).

The World Bank has also been instrumental in directly financing the development of new corporate hospitals. While granting a loan of $ 134 million to the state of Maharashtra, it imposed the condition that 5 per cent ($ 7 million) of this amount be allocated for the construction of a tertiary private hospital in Mumbai, to be governed by a private hospital group (Yamey, 2001). Over the past ten years, the International Finance Corporation (IFC), the private sector arm of the World Bank, has been regularly involved in the funding of corporate hospital projects. IFC finances private sector investments in the developing countries. Many corporate hospitals have received financial support from the IFC through loans or equity, accounting for 20 to 30 per cent of the total cost of the project (Table 4.1).

Corporatization of the Indian Hospital Sector

After 1991, the increasingly favourable investment climate drew new actors to this sector. The increased life expectancy and the development of the middle-class are elements that also attract newcomers in the health care sector. According to the Confederation of Private Sector Initiatives in the Health Sector, 3,000 beds for specialized health care were created in 2001, while actually 60,000 are needed every year to meet demand (Purohit, 2001). But gradually, the pioneering days when doctors founded ultramodern hospitals with the support of their relatives (Baru, 1998) came to an end. Henceforth, mainly industrial or financial

TABLE 4.1: IFC LOANS TO HOSPITAL PROJECTS IN INDIA

Project	Project Cost ($ Million)	IFC Contribution ($ Million)
Duncan-Gleneagles	29.40	7 (24%)
Artemis	40.00	10 (25%)
Max Healthcare	84.00	18 (21%)
Apollo Hospitals	70.00	20 (29%)

Source: www.ifc.org

groups invested in this sector. Prior to the 1990s, big business families had created charitable hospitals for the welfare of all the population. Sometime following tragic familial events, the Tatas and the Hindujas in Mumbai, the Naidus in Coimbatore and the Nandas in Faridabad established hospitals as trusts and thus received tax exemptions. Nowadays, local and national business families (e.g. Kanwars from Apollo Tyres, Singhs from Ranbaxy) are entering into health care market with big investment plans to secure comfortable profits in the long term. For certain groups, diversification into the health sector is part of a complete change in strategy. In 1999, Analjit Singh (Max India) sold part of his telecom activity. After commissioning a report to decide his future investments, he selected the services sector (IT, insurance and health) to nurture his group's future growth. Certain groups are not complete outsiders to the health sector. Pharmaceutical groups like Ranbaxy and Wockhardt developed their own hospital branches, like Ranbaxy's Fortis.

The corporatization of the hospital sector has taken different forms. Some of the newcomers are taking the control of charitable hospitals, on the basis of management contract. The land and the hospital remain the property of the trust society but the management falls in the hands of corporations (e.g. Fortis Jessa Ram Hospital and Max Devki Devi in Delhi). Some trusts and charitable hospitals are even transformed into corporations. One of the most controversial operations has been the transformation of the Escorts Heart Institute and Research Centre (EHIRC). Following the death of his father in 2000, Rajan Nanda decided to change EHIRC from a charitable trust to a private limited company. The reason was apparently to build a partnership with an international health care company (Ahmed, 2005). Because of its status, the trust's income was exempt from tax. After ten years, the EHIRC had reserves of almost Rs. 110 crore out of which Rs. 95 crore was tax-free surplus. The trust's assets and profits could not be distributed for non-charitable purposes. A corporate society by the name of Escorts Heart Institute and Research Centre was registered in Chandigarh. Six months later a merger between the Delhi-registered EHIRC and the Chandigarh-registered EHIRC was organized. All the assets and profits of the Delhi EHIRC were transferred to the Chandigarh one. The Delhi EHIRC disappeared and so the limitations linked to its charitable trust's status. Later the new EHIRC became a limited liability company with Rajan Nanda holding the majority of the shares.

The last ten years have witnessed a rapid development of private hospital groups. While these actors are competitors in the Indian market, they also form an effective and powerful lobby through the Indian Healthcare Federation. Incorporated into the health services branch of the Confederation of Indian Industry, they have used their weight to influence the national health policy in their favour. Exemptions and government assistance are important to ensure their fragile profits. The hospital sector can eventually be financially viable only in the long term. Apart from Apollo Hospitals, very few groups from the 1980s have been able to grow out of their hometown. But what is perhaps much more important is that the corporate hospital groups will have to win the battle of ideas in order to take the Indian health system in the direction in which it would work in their interest. The 2002 CII-McKinsey report is symptomatic of this desire to impose their views. This report makes it possible to bombard the media with figures and ideas legitimizing the stand taken by private hospital groups. In interviews to the press, the McKinsey report is often cited in support of the arguments put forward by private hospital owners. The then central government (BJP) itself used this report to reshape its health-sector budget (2003–4). Thus, private hospitals benefitted from new tax exemptions on long-term investments. The exemption would also be applicable for financial institutions investing in hospitals with more than 100 beds (Sankar and Kathuria, 2003). It was of course the private tertiary sector that benefitted the most from this. More recently, the medical tourism fever reached India on the recommendations of this report. The CII's assumed objective is to see the development of a privatized health system in India in which the public sector would only take care of non-solvent population and limit itself to providing primary health care. Some of the managers from corporate hospitals go even further. They believe that in fifteen years' time, only a few groups will dominate health services and secondary-level private nursing homes (less than 50 beds) will have disappeared or will have been incorporated in franchizing systems. For the moment, the reality of the Indian health care market is such that private health care is still dispersed, undervalued and unregulated.

Nevertheless, a lot of changes have happened since 2004. The hospital sector has entered into a concentration phase. Some groups that diversified into the hospital sector in the 1990s are undertaking a reality check. Promoters are facing financial problems. Profits are meagre. It takes long time to find the proper formula in a business where the first asset is your reputation, the quality of your staff and your equipment.

Because of their limited funds some groups cannot expand and create hospital chains to generate more profits. On the other side, groups like Apollo Hospitals, Wockhardt or Fortis, with strong financial back-up, are looking at every opportunity to expand their network. Through mergers and acquisitions, greenfield (new hospitals) and brownfield projects (take-over of existing hospitals), these groups wish to become national players. The metropolitan areas are thus turning into battlefields. In 2002, Apollo bought the share of the Goenkas in the Duncan-Gleneagles Hospital in Kolkata that was rechristened Apollo-Gleneagles. More recently, because of debt burden, Rajan Nanda wanted to sell EHIRC. Apollo, Fortis and a foreign hospital chain were in the race to buy the chain. Finally Fortis, bought Rajan Nanda's shares for Rs. 585 crore. With this acquisition, Fortis became the leading player in Delhi and the second largest hospital chain in India, after Apollo but ahead of Wockhardt. Interestingly we can spot some difference between Fortis and Wockhardt in the expansion of their network (Figure 4.1). Both groups target metropolises. While Wockhardt expanded its network across India (Bangalore, Mumbai, Hyderabad, Nagpur), Fortis particularly after the Escorts acquisition, has centred its development in Delhi and north India (Chandigarh, Amritsar). After opening a new hospital in Rajkot, Wockhardt is planning to open a hospital in Delhi. Meanwhile Fortis is looking at new opportunities in other metropolises (e.g. Mumbai, Bangalore, Chennai) after securing its position in north India.

Another way for corporate hospitals to expand their activity is to develop a network of secondary and primary health care facilities. Building and managing a hospital is a huge task that requires years of efforts and a lot of funds. Large sections of the upper and middle class living in secondary towns or big metropolises still remain out of reach for the corporate hospitals. Instead of building hospitals in those towns, the corporate hospitals are developing a network of referring centres, based on a hub and spokes model. In Delhi, Max Healthcare first opened primary and secondary care infrastructure before establishing tertiary care hospital. Apollo Hospitals put the model at its peak with a franchise named 'The Apollo Clinic'. Relying on the reputation of Apollo Hospitals, these centres offer out-patient care with all the necessary diagnostic equipments. Thank to telemedicine, specialists from Apollo Hospitals (e.g. from Delhi) can be consulted by each Apollo Clinic. In case of surgery, a patient from the Apollo Clinic can be sent directly to any Apollo hospital. In four years, fifty Apollo Clinic franchises opened mainly in north, east and west India where Apollo Hospitals' presence

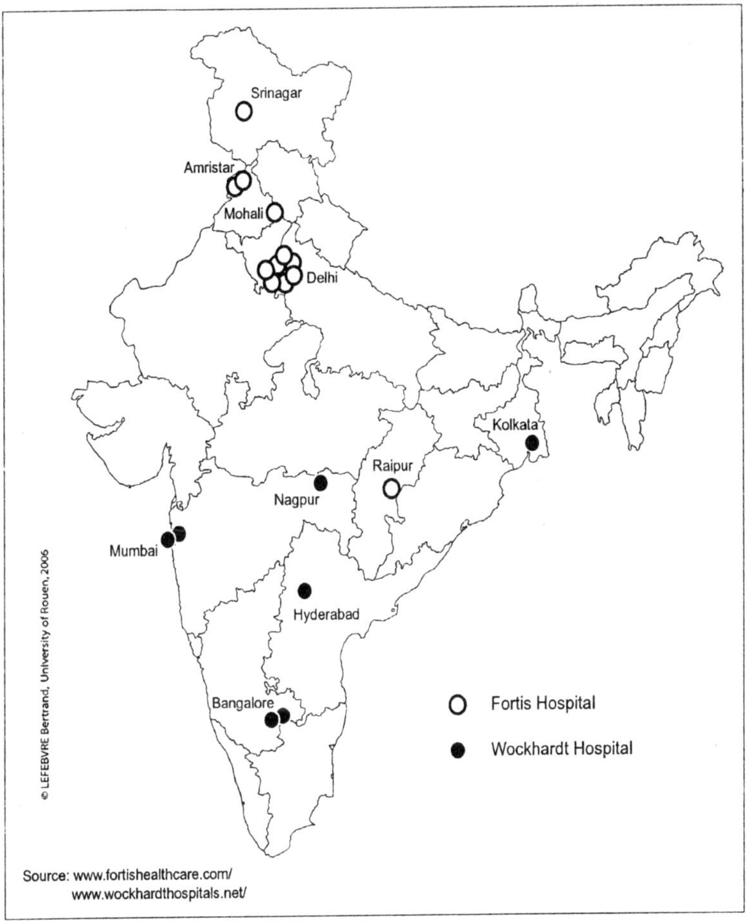

FIGURE 4.1: FORTIS AND WOCKHARDT HOSPITAL NETWORKS IN INDIA (2006)

is rather weak compared to the South (Figure 4.2). Franchises in metropolises are expected to act as satellite clinics to the main Apollo Hospitals (e.g. in Delhi and in Kolkata). Escorts developed a similar network of referring centres in north India (Patna, Udaipur and Delhi suburbs).

This hub and spokes model is also part of a diversification strategy. Inspired again by the US experience, the objective of some groups is to become a health maintenance organization (HMO). More than

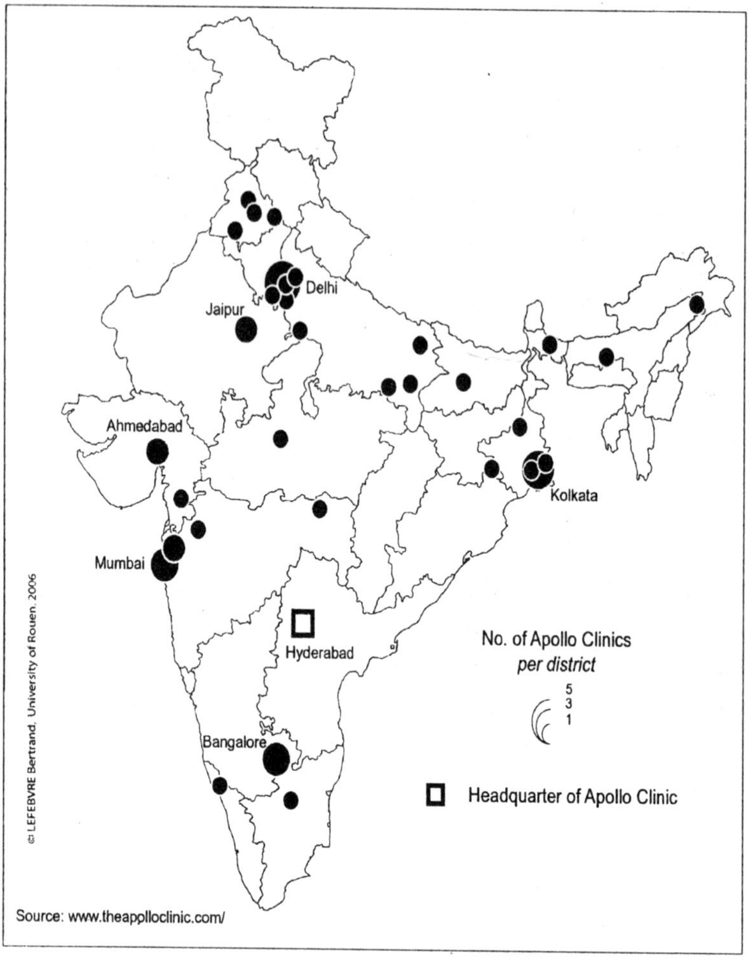

FIGURE 4.2: APOLLO CLINIC NETWORK IN INDIA (2006)

80 per cent of the health expenditure in India is out-of-pocket expenditure. The recent development of invasive surgery that requires top-end medical equipment and the hiring of the best medical team come at a cost in corporate hospitals. The development of health insurance is then a major issue that would allow the corporate hospitals to expand their patient base. The health insurance sector has been very recently liberalized (1999) and some corporate hospitals have stepped and are

now offering health insurance scheme to their patients or to corporations. It is then of primary importance for corporate hospitals to build an integrated health service. Prevention (diagnostic, health checks) is thus be as important, and as profitable, as curing. In addition to its clinics, Apollo Hospitals has launched a network of pharmacies across the country. Fortis and Ranbaxy through a joint venture launched HealthWorld (now called 'Religare Wellness'), where people can purchase medicines and go for laboratory tests.

Back to the Global: Indian Hospitals Worldwide?

The very idea of running a hospital as a corporate organization and some organizational models (like the hubs and spoke, HMO) came to India from abroad through various channels. The Indian corporate hospitals are now in search of global partnership for various reasons. As already mentioned, many NRIs were at the start of the corporate hospital, most notably through funding. Between 1991 and 1997, the Foreign Investment Promotion Board approved FDI worth almost $100 million in the health sector (Pundit, 2001). In 2004, Fortis unveiled an investment plan of Rs. 1,100 crore over five years. Max Healthcare needs Rs. 400 crore for its expansion plans. These investment plans can be fuelled through loan but more often through equity. With its recent consistent economic growth, India is now an appealing economy for private international investment funds. Warburg Pincus (US) invested Rs. 200 crore in Max group and part of this will be invested in health care. In June 2005 Temasek, a Singaporean investment fund, invested in a branch of Apollo Hospitals. Sixty-two foreign institutional investors, mostly from the United States and Mauritius, are now shareholders of Apollo Hospitals' capital equity, accounting for 43 per cent of the total shares.

Indian corporate hospitals are also looking for technical partnerships. Some new hospitals are modelled and designed after the US Cleveland Clinic or the Mayo Clinic. Apollo Hospitals has entered into an agreement with Johns Hopkins Medicine International for collaboration in numerous clinical departments. Wockhardt is associated with Harvard Medical International, which gives them access to some of the best hospitals in the US for knowledge and research. Apollo Hospital in Delhi, for instance, is affiliated to the American Heart Association,

Galvin Heart Centre (Illinois), St. Vincent's Hospital (Portland), Pomona Valley Hospital (California) and so on. Philips and Artemis, who has opened a hospital in Gurgaon in 2007, signed a partnership for the provision of medical equipment and for joint medical imaging research. General Electric signed a similar agreement with Dr Naresh Trehan for his Medicity project in Gurgaon. These agreements are important to establish the quality of new hospitals. In a business where reputation is your first asset, Indian corporate hospital groups have been constantly seeking legitimization from the US and other countries. With the recent development of medical tourism, Indian corporate hospitals are looking to receive international accreditation, like from the US Joint Commission International (JCI). Wockhardt Mumbai was the first in India to receive the JCI accreditation. After hiring a US manager for two years, Indraprastha Apollo has received the accreditation. More accredited hospitals are about to come up in India.

Interestingly, more and more foreign hospital chains are eying the Indian health sector. Through joint venture, Singaporean Gleneagles opened a hospital in Kolkata. In 2005, Columbia Asia from US opened a 65-bed infrastructure in Bangalore. In 2006, Parkways from Singapore signed an agreement with the Heart Institute in Mumbai to open a new hospital. Thai Bumrungrad Hospital is said to be looking at opportunities in India. Most of these newcomers are indeed looking for local partners. For the moment everybody seems to be a gainer. The foreign groups rely on the local health care providers to penetrate the Indian market and thus expand their global presence. The Indian hospital groups, with their new allies, are able to fund their expansion all over the country and have access to technical and managerial knowledge.

Indian corporate hospitals are themselves foraying into foreign markets. International markets appeared as golden opportunities from them. Having unquestionably drawn inspiration from their own experience in the Indian market, which nonetheless remains a developing country, they are able to replicate these models in other countries. Thus, from the position of a receiver India has become the distributor of private biomedical model of care. Sometimes at the request of local governments, they build technical and consulting partnerships in Middle East, Africa and in Central and South Asia. Indian corporate hospitals are training local medical and management staff. They also help in designing hospital and supervising the building and the management of the infrastructure. South Asia has become the backyard for the expansion of Indian private hospital groups. Apollo Hospitals was indeed the first Indian hospital group to open a hospital in a foreign country. In 1997 they built a hospital in Colombo (Sri Lanka) in a joint venture with local investors. The large number of NRIs and the economic development of the region make the Gulf States an appealing market. They recently signed an agreement with a Yemenite hospital. In 2005 an Apollo Clinic franchise opened in Qatar and more are supposed to come in Middle East and Bangladesh. Escorts opened referral centres in Uzbekistan, Nepal, Bangladesh and Afghanistan. Apollo Hospitals with the support of investment funds is now looking at opportunities in the United Kingdom, Eastern Europe and South-East Asia. But managing an activity in a foreign environment is not an easy task. In 2006, Apollo Hospitals sold the shares of its Colombo hospital after a hostile bid from a local business group led by Harry Jayawardene. They later signed an agreement that makes Apollo Hospitals the manager of the facility for the next five years.

Some groups have also specialized in subcontracting services to American health professionals. Indeed, this sector is not just limited to health care actors, but is also open to groups specializing in Business Process Outsourcing (BPO). While medical transcription is currently stagnating, medical imaging and diagnostic and legal services offer new prospects for profits. Apollo Hospitals created a branch called Apollo Health Street dedicated to medical BPO services US hospitals. In order to expand rapidly in the US, this branch recently took the control of Armanti Financial Services for $31 million. Indeed, to continue with the outsourcing perspective, and making the most of the General Agreement on Trade in Services (GATS), hospital groups have begun to think of providing medical services. In fact, this practice already exists. Thus, Escorts might send teams to the Middle East for a few days to conduct operations there. There is a requirement for medical staff (nurses, etc.) in North America and especially Europe. The ageing of the population would undoubtedly enhance this demand. Apollo has considered finding employment for nurses in Western hospitals, after providing them with training and charging a licence fee ($4,000 to 5,000 per nurse). The entry of corporate would completely change the face of this sector. Many Indian nurses after getting their degrees are going to work in the Middle East. After spending a few years there, the best of them clear new exams to be able to go and work in the US or

Europe. Representatives from certain European countries such as Germany even go to the Gulf countries to recruit such manpower. But the recent crisis faced by 16,000 NRI doctors in UK due the changes in European Union immigration laws, shows that the future of this sector is very much dependent upon immigration laws. Workforce is not yet as mobile as funds or ideas. But the patients are.

Over the past five years, corporate hospital groups are founding their hopes on medical tourism. After the CII-McKinsey report was published, which estimated a turnover of $2.1 billion in 2012 for this activity, the major actors have begun to position themselves in this market. In the 1990s there had already been movements from the Middle East or NRIs from North America coming to India. But India (175,000 patients) still lags behind Singapore and the number one, Thailand (1.4 million patients last year). For the moment, most of the medical tourists are either NRIs visiting their family or patients from neighbouring states (Bangladesh, Afghanistan and Nepal). Indian private hospital groups hope to enhance their profits by leveraging more competitive prices and reputed medical teams and by concluding agreements with American insurance companies. As previously described, Indian hospitals are doing their best to get international accreditations. Hospital managers have made several trips to the UK, Middle East and South-East Asia (2003–4) under the CII banner to present their services. Apollo Hospitals opened an office in London recently. The opening of referring centres (Escorts in Uzbekistan, Nepal) or OPD structures (Apollo Clinic in Qatar), should also help in attracting more foreign patients. The CII would like to use health professionals of Indian origin in US or UK as ambassadors. All sorts of agreements between hospital groups, tourist agencies and airlines are in the making. Corporate hospitals are receiving full support from the central government, with for example, the recent implementation of a medical visa. Some states like Kerala and Tamil Nadu are also putting a lot of efforts to market a new image of India as a healing centre in order to attract foreign patients. Some states like Haryana and West Bengal are supporting through incentives the creation of large hospital campuses that will offer full range of treatments and leisure to medical tourists in a preserved environment. By making patients with high purchasing power come to India under the banner of medical tourism, a certain level of profitability can be ensured for corporate hospitals. With the internationalization of their strategies, we may wonder what place is left for the Indian patients, even rich ones.

Conclusion

The emergence and expansion of corporate hospitals in India tell us a great deal about the complex relations between global and local scales. There is no simple determinism in the emergence of corporate hospitals. Actually, more than ten years before the 1991 Structural Adjustment Policy, Dr Reddy had the idea to run a hospital on a corporate basis. It took him three years of lobbying before receiving a loan from a public financial institution. The determination of this man and other NRIs has been probably more important in the creation of corporate hospitals than the macro-economic and political changes. The 1990s have surely been a deciding period for the expansion of corporate hospitals. While many private hospitals were stagnating in the late 1980s, the economic reforms gave a new impulse to the sector. Surprisingly, the reforms did not imply a laissez-faire policy or a disengagement of the State in favour of market forces. On the contrary, State and international organizations supported the development of corporate hospitals through loans, tax exemption and free land. Thank to this decisive support, the corporate hospitals have not only been able to survive but also to expand. We may well agree with Mukherjee-Reed when she wrote (2003: 24):

> Contrary to the principal neo-liberal claim that reforms bring about a separation between state and business, what emerges as a critical structural characteristic of the post-interventionist era in India is the positive association between corporate growth and increased state support. This continuity with the interventionist era is rather striking. Indeed, it is manifest in the way public resources continue to be deployed in an otherwise 'liberalised' regime: through state-led demand management programmes, through increased disbursement from financial institutions, through increased state spending on infrastructure, through sacrifices in the state's revenue incomes as a result of tax concessions and so on.

In fact, the State's support attracted many newcomers to the hospital sector. Some business families with strong local and national political connection created hospitals without any idea of what were the requirements of the health care business. As Kapil Sibal, Minister for Science and Technology, reminded during the CII Health Summit 2004, 40 per cent of private hospitals are losing money. Contrary to these speculation-led investments, groups like Max Healthcare or Fortis entered this market with a long-term vision and enough funds to reshape their development strategies. The nexus between political and economic elite can be seen from the continuous unanimous support from politicians in favour of corporate hospitals. From Indira Gandhi to

Rajiv Gandhi, Narasimha Rao, and later the BJP-led government, corporate hospitals received support from all the political class. Even in West Bengal, the Communist Party of India (Marxist) is supporting the creation of a medicity. The same way economic reforms were not as inevitable as it has been said, corporatization of the Indian hospital sector has not so much to do with external forces. The World Bank surely came in time to support the corporate hospitals and to give argument in their defence, but it has been a local political decision or non-decision. The emergence of corporate hospitals is probably symptomatic of the lack of interest of the Indian political elite in public health and health policy. While it has been long documented that few corporate hospitals were implementing the reservation of free beds or free treatments, no serious action has been undertaken against the responsible hospitals. Ironically, it is now the corporate hospitals which are pushing the public authorities to implement a national accreditation system to better assess and control the quality of hospital care. If the CII-McKinsey report is entitled 'Healthcare in India: The Road Ahead', we may wonder who is eventually behind the wheel.

REFERENCES

Ahmed, F., 'The Battleground', *Business World*, 24 October 2005, New Delhi.

Baru R., *Private Healthcare in India: Social Characteristics and Trends*, New Delhi: Sage, 1998.

CII-McKinsey, *Healthcare in India: The Road Ahead*, New Delhi: CII-McKinsey, 2002.

Government of India (GOI), *National Health Policy—2002*, online document at URL http://mohfw.nic.in/np2002.htm [accessed on 14 November 2006].

Loveman, G. and J. O'Connell, *Apollo Hospitals of India*, Borton: Harvard Business School, 1995.

Mukherjee-Reed, A., 'Conceptualising Corporate Capitalism in Contemporary South Asia: Conventional Wisdoms and South Asian Realities' in Mukherjee-Reed, A. (ed.), *Corporate Capitalism in Contemporary South Asia: Conventional Wisdoms and South Asian Realities*, London: Palgrave MacMillan, 2003, pp. 1–34.

Omvedt, G., 'Capitalist Agriculture and Rural Class in India', *Economic and Political Weekly*, 1981, 16(52), pp. 140–53.

Public Account Committee, 'Allotment Land to Private Hospital and Dispensaries by Delhi Development Authority', Lok Sabha, 2005, New Delhi.

Purohit, B., 'Private Initiatives and Policy Options: Recent Health System Experience in India', *Health Policy and Planning*, 2001, 16 (3), pp. 87–97.

Rihouey, F., 'L'émergence de nouveaux réseaux de soins en Inde. Hyderabad, un centre d'innovation', *Espace, Populations, Sociétés*, 1997, 2–3, pp. 265–78.

Salmon, J., *The Corporate Transformation of Health Care: Issues and Directions*, Amity Ville: Baywood Publications, 1990.

Sankar, D. and V. Kathuria 'Health Sector in 2003–4 Budget', *Economic and Political Weekly*, 2003, online document at URL http://www.epw.org.in/articles/2003/04/5686.html [accessed on 14 November 2006].

Selvaraju, V. and V.B. Anniger, *Trends in Public Spending on Health in India*, New Delhi: Indian Council for Research on International Economic Relations, 2001.

World Bank, *World Development Report 1993: Investing in Health*, New York: World Bank, 1993.

Yamey, G., 'World Bank Funds Private Hospitals in India', *British Medical Journal*, 2001, 32 (3), Online document at URL http://www.bmj.com/cgi/content/full/322/7281/257/a [accessed on 14 November 2006].

CHAPTER 5

Delhi: Towards a Healthy City

SURINDER AGGARWAL*

BACKGROUND

At the turn of the century, nearly half of the world's population lives in cities and this urban population continues to grow across space and time (United Nations, 2002). A large share of new urban growth shall be borne by developing countries like India and China. Ecological imbalance and environmental degradation created due to abuse and overuse of environmental services by the rising population, social disorganization and continuing poverty in the city are posing new threats to human health in the urbanizing economies. Mega cities are at greater risk through this global urbanization process (Kraas, 2003: 10).

The city in the developing countries is subjected to congestion and high density of population living in poor sanitary conditions, uncontrolled demand on the immediate resources of the urban region and exploitation beyond their carrying capacity. Hyper-urbanization thus leads to 'insecure environments' and health risks (Krafft, Aggarwal and Wolf, 2003). Globalization, with liberalization of economies and structural adjustment programmes underway in many developing countries has reduced hopes for more investment in social sectors, including health.

Therefore, a major question for the future is how to ensure that health and environment are not damaged by economic progress and growing urbanization trends. The argument here is not to justify anti-urbanism, but to bring about a balance between the two. It further aims at encouraging the stakeholders to be the actors and motivating as well as enabling them to develop lifestyles and environments that support positive health. The concerns which are addressed in this paper with particular reference to Delhi are:

* In writing this chapter, the author has used material and ideas while preparing two studies for WHO-SEARO on (a) Strengthening Healty Cities in South-East Asia and (b) Evaluation of Healthy Cities Programme in South-East Asia.

- What are the challenges to health in Delhi?
- How can the city power be strengthened to create and promote positive health in the future?
- How to empower individuals and communities for promoting positive health in the city?
- What are the initiatives towards promotion of healthy environments?

Interventions and actions at various stages of environmental pressure, state of environment, human exposures and vulnerabilities to such states are keys to promote health in hyper-urbanizing situations.

Challenges to Health in Delhi: Hyper-Urbanization and Health Risk

In Delhi, land, air and water environments are under stress due to the pressures of intense urbanization, indiscriminate industrialization, inefficient transport system, unplanned land use changes, and in-migrating poor people. Delhi's urban area has grown from 182 km^2 in 1969 to more than 900 km^2 in 2000 (Government of India and Government of NCT, 2001). The current population of Delhi is about 15 million (13.8 million in 2001) and is estimated to rise to 22.42 million by 2021 (TERI, 2001).[1] It is among the fastest growing megacity of India with decadal growth ranging from 26.42 per cent in 1961 to 39.09 per cent during 1991–2001 (Census of India, 2001).[2] Despite a slight decline in the growth rate, the annual absolute increase of about one-half million to Delhi's population is alarming. High economic proficiency and employment opportunities have perhaps manifested themselves as the root cause of the city's serious environmental problems. Furthermore, the distribution of population is becoming uneven in general and denser in low income and old city areas in particular. This process of population redistribution facilitates the spread of diseases, largely in low-income squatter settlements. New migrants, who contribute close to one-half of Delhi's population growth and economy also harbour diseases from their native places and facilitate their spread and hence add to the existing disease burden. The above demographic situation scares and warns us because these trends are contrary to growth in social and environmental infrastructure and enhance health risks.

The Environmental Challenge to Health

Environmental challenge includes degraded environments mainly caused by air, water, land, noise pollution, overcrowding in the built environment, inadequate urban services and housing. Due to poor dispersion and disposal mechanisms, non-availability of low-cost technologies, biological, chemical and physical pollutants have become new threats to human life. Excessive concentration of heavy metals such as lead, and automobile and industrial pollutants such as hydrocarbons, suspended particulate matter (SPM), oxides of nitrogen and carbon monoxide will increasingly pollute the ambient air. Discussed below briefly is the state of Delhi's environment as influenced by various economic and service sectors and their linkage towards deteriorating health conditions. These sectors, of course, produce economic opportunities but also produce externalities that impinge on human health.

AIR POLLUTION AND HEALTH RISKS

Ambient Air Quality Status in Delhi

Delhi has been labelled as one of the most polluted cities and also the asthmatic capital of the world. The sources and major driving forces of air pollution load in Delhi remain emissions from vehicles (67 per cent), industries and thermal power plants (25 per cent) and domestic sources (8 per cent) (Government of India and Government of NCT, 2001). The major gaseous pollutants from all these sources include sulfur oxide (SO_2), nitrogen oxides (NOX), and carbon monoxide (CO). Other major pollutants associated with vehicular emissions include lead (Pb), benzene, and CO. The ambient air quality levels for most pollutants (CO, SPM, respirable suspended particulate matter (RSPM) and lead) remained higher than the permissible limits during the 1980s, however their present reduced levels is an encouraging trend (Table 5.1). The ambient air quality data from 1989 to the present indicates that SPM remains the most critical pollutant of Delhi's environment (Government of India 2000, 2001, 2002) and the World Bank estimates huge health damage cost due to SPM pollution alone. Recent high health risk values of RSPM reflect contribution of man-made sources such as roadside settled dust, auto exhaust and coal combustion. Benzene concentrations have increased in the ambient air after the introduction of unleaded petrol (TERI, 2001). Pollution load estimates exhibit a

TABLE 5.1: TRENDS IN AMBIENT AIR QUALITY IN DELHI

Pollutants	Permissible limit (Res.) Annual	1994	1996	1998	2000	2001 (January–June)
CO ($\mu g/m^3$)	2.0.00	33.43	55.87	54.50	46.86	30.69
SO_2 ($\mu g/m^3$)	60.00	42.00	35.00	25.00	18.00	16.00
NO_x ($\mu g/m^3$)	80.00	66.00	75.00	63.00	59.00	–
Pb (mg/m^3)	0.75	0.408	0.312	0.136	0.101	–
SPM ($\mu g/m^3$)	140.00	–	377.00	370.00		
RPM ($\mu g/m^3$)	60.00	–	–	200.00	191.00	163.00

Source: Government of India, CPCB, Annual Reports, 2000–1, 2002 and Government of India 2001.

consistent increase from 2,400 mt in 1994 to 3,000 tons in 1998 (Government of India and Government of NCT 2001).

The vehicular and industrial pollution load has been controlled over a medium-term timeframe because of stringent regulation on use of fuel quality (coal with low ash content, unleaded petrol), improved vehicular technology for both cars and two-wheelers, withdrawal of old vehicles, emphasis on gradual fuel shift to natural gas and shifting of polluting industries from non-conforming areas. Most thermal plants operate now with electrostatic precipitators. Furthermore, stringent regulatory regime facilitated by judicial intervention and involvement of civil society with respect to awareness and advocacy for clean air has made the real difference. Impact of Delhi Metro, introduced in a phased manner since 2005, on air quality is difficult to assess at this stage, nevertheless it may stabilize or reduce the present trends.

The situation is yet not completely comfortable as the number of automobiles keep increasing in Delhi without commensurate growth in road length and width. Still, ambient and indoor air pollution remain great health risks to large vulnerable population groups living in slums, working and living close to polluting industries and commuting long distances to work on congested roads. What is different now than a few years back is that pollution levels have declined or stabilized whereas the exposure levels have intensified and exposure to new pollutants such as benzene, ozone and RPM has increased.

Indoor Air Pollution

Indoor air pollution levels are not monitored in Delhi by any agency, except a few research studies on health impacts conducted by independent researchers. It is, therefore, difficult to give accurate levels and trends of indoor air pollution, except the findings of some research studies. Apart from ambient pollution, indoor air pollution due to the use of unclean biomass-based fuels such as wood and dung and kerosene used in squatter and other low-income settlements (nearly 1,200 slum clusters and 4 million people) is becoming a significant source of health problem in Delhi. Biomass smoke contains thousands of substances, many of which damage human health. Most important are particulates, carbon monoxide, nitrous oxides, sulphur oxides (more with coal), formaldehyde, and polycyclic organic matter which include carcinogens such as benzo[a]pyrene (DeKoning et al., 1985). Small particles of diameter less than 10 microns (termed PM_{10}), and in particular those less than 2.5 microns ($PM_{2.5}$), are able to penetrate deep into the lungs and appear to have the greatest health-damaging potential (United States Environmental Protection Agency, 1997).

Air Pollution and Health Risks

Health risks affected by air pollution are well recognized. Pollutants like CO, NO_2, SO_2, RSPM, HC, lead, benzene and ozone pose a serious threat to human health. A World Bank (1996) study estimates that the number of people dying in urban India due to deteriorating air quality is rising every year (United States Environmental Protection Agency, 1997). An astounding 51,779 people were estimated to have died prematurely in 36 Indian cities due to air pollution in 1995 as against 40,351 in 1991–2. Kolkata, Delhi, Mumbai, Kanpur and Ahmedabad account for 66 per cent of such premature deaths. Delhi alone accounts for 7,500 preventable deaths. Cost for such preventable deaths, hospital admissions and minor sickness were estimated to be around half a billion US dollars. RPM and sulfur dioxide are responsible for more than 95 per cent of the health impact damages. The number of air pollution related ailments requiring medical treatment and hospital admissions has also increased to 25 million cases.

Many studies by individual researchers and medical experts (Aggarwal and Davgun, 1994; WHO 1997; World Resources et al., 1998–9; CSE 1997) clearly establish strong health risks linked to long exposure of pollutants to different vulnerable groups like children, women, traffic policemen and other occupational groups. According to a recent study of Indian Council for Medical Research (ICMR) alarming levels of heavy metals such as lead and cadmium were found in several placental tissues of Delhi women. In another study in Delhi, more than 40 per cent of children going to school out of a sample of 200 had lead levels much higher than the safe limit of 10 mg/dl. The All India Institute of Medical Sciences (AIIMS) also carried out a study in 1991 on the effects of road traffic pollution on the health of Delhi traffic policemen. Traffic policemen posted at intersections and road sides faced high risk. The study revealed that 18 per cent of the exposed group suffered from lung disorders such as tuberculosis and 98 per cent had excessive COHb (Carboxyhaemoglobin) which results in lower oxygen carrying capacity of blood. Another study done by CPCB and AIIMS in Delhi in the year 2000 indicated that CO levels in blood among smokers, factory workers and petrol pump workers are higher and symptoms related to adverse impact of respiratory, cardio-vascular and nervous system were observed.

Indoor air pollution can be particularly hazardous to health because it is released in close proximity to people. The 'rule of 1000' states that a pollutant released indoor is 1,000 times more likely to reach people's lungs than a pollutant released outdoors. Indoor air pollution contributes significantly to acute lower respiratory infections, chronic lung diseases, lung cancer, asthma, low birth weight, blindness and heart diseases. Epidemiological studies (De Koning et al., 1985) in developing countries have linked exposure to indoor air pollution from dirty fuels with at least four major categories of illnesses: acute respiratory infections (ARI) in children; chronic obstructive lung diseases such as asthma and chronic bronchitis; lung cancer; and stillbirths and other problems at birth. Of these, ARI appears to have the greatest health impact in terms of the number of people affected and the time lost due to illness, especially in children younger than age five. Many respiratory infections in the developing world result in death, and evidence shows that exposure to cook stove smoke may contribute to higher mortality rates. Overall, studies indicate that exposure to wood smoke from cooking fires in poorly ventilated conditions may increase the risk of a young child contracting a serious respiratory infection from two to six times.

Not much epidemiological research is found on Delhi's vulnerable population including those living in squatter settlement without a title or affordability to own a safe fuel like LPG. More than one-fourth of

Delhi population living in such settlements is at greater risk to indoor air pollution than outdoor air pollution. Children and women who stay longer at such hazardous settings are exposed more than men. An epidemiological study on 642 children in two Delhi slums concluded that fuel wood and kerosene oil use in indoor environment causes incidence of acute lower respiratory infection (ALRI). Higher incidence of ALRI was reported, however, from children living with households using kerosene oil. Bronchiolitis was reported in 22.5 per cent of the wood group and 27.1 per cent of the kerosene group (Sharma et al., 1998). Exposure to high indoor smoke levels has also been linked with pregnancy related problems like stillbirths and low birth weight.

Solid and Hazardous Waste

The shift in the land use pattern, changing consumer habits with increasing prevalence 'use and throw' goods along with rising per capita income have intensified the problem of waste disposal in Delhi. Current municipal-waste generation in the National Capital Territory is 7,000 tonnes per day. Per capita generation of waste is still very low in Indian mega cities as compared to industrial counterparts. However, mismanagement of its collection, transportation and disposal is a major challenge. Per capita generation of 500 gm of waste is still low. The value is one-tenth of many mega cities of the industrial world. Its inefficient and unsafe disposal, nevertheless, has become a serious environmental degradation cause with accompanied ecological and human health risks. The problem of disposal and health risks shall be substantial in the coming years as the expected range of waste generated by 2021 is 17,000 to 25,000 tonnes per day (TERI, 2001).

Some of the important issues related to the management of solid waste include: inadequate present and future disposal sites; lack of coverage of poor communities; deficiency in the infrastructure network; non-segregation of hazardous and medical waste; inappropriate equipment, and suspicion of the private sector in waste management (Tulika, 2004 and Koberlein, 2003). Even if reasonable waste-reduction measures (i.e. segregation and composting) are followed, the landfill requirement for solid waste will be 8,000,000 m^2 by 2021. Incineration is 10 times more expensive than landfill disposal and does not appear to be a cost-effective alternative (TERI, 2001). Space availability for landfills will remain a major concern in land-starved Delhi in the coming years.

Hazardous Waste

Hazardous waste in Delhi includes sludge from treatment plants, acid/ alkaline slurry, heavy metals, waste oil, and hospital waste. Although biomedical waste forms only a small share in total solid-waste generation (less than 2 per cent), its unsafe collection and transportation methods, along with its disposal in the common municipal landfill sites, makes it a health hazard. Of the total hospital waste, nearly one-half is biomedical or infectious waste. Delhi produces approximately 60 metric tones of biomedical waste every day, and only a small portion is disposed of in incinerators, which are themselves badly operated (Agarwal, 2001 and Government of India, Ministry of Environment and Forest & NCT of Delhi, 2001). Even though the share of medical waste is small in total waste generation, however, its non-segregation and unsafe disposal has produced wider exposure and high greater health risks as illustrated below:

- The human anatomical waste, body fluid, blood, fluid waste from laboratory cultures, or those containing infectious or contagious pathogens are not being destroyed at the required temperatures in most hospital or nursing home incinerators. Unsafe waste from such incinerators later becomes part of the other solid waste.
- Most of the disposable equipment and other material like syringes, catheters, blood bags, bandages and cotton get back in circulation either after a simple wash or many times without it.
- Segregation of medical waste is not being undertaken at source, it does happen at the bin of a waste dealer (*kabari*) or wholesale market level for further circulation at a health cost.
- Safe practices in handling medical waste are often limited to health professionals and the top tier of the sanitation team and the lower level workers in medical establishments are often ignored.
- Besides, most health care facilities use various hazardous chemicals in processes such as disinfection, radiotherapy, and X-ray film processing. The wastes generated from such activities are invariably discharged into sewer drains.
- Uncontrolled hospital waste management outside the hospital premises is yet another problem. Almost two-thirds of the waste that leaves the hospitals daily are picked up by ragpickers. They come in close contact with hazardous waste and are the worst affected group.
- Unsegregated medical waste dumped in the unlined landfill sites of

Delhi gets leached into the ground water. The poor settlements close to such sites are being exposed to heavy dose of contaminated water or wind blown pathogens or through vectors like flies, rats and cockroaches. There is weak conclusive statement on this exposure as scientific studies lack on this topic.

From a survey of hospitals in Delhi (Agarwal, 2001), an epidemiological study in Kolkata and other studies (Koberlein, 2003) we find the ragpickers, hospital patients, lower-level health workers, and low-income residents in peripheral urban settlements are the most vulnerable groups of health hazards related to medical waste disposal. In a recent study on Delhi's largest Bhalaswa landfill site (Figure 5.1), Aggarwal and Tulika (2004) determined general health risks to the surrounding communities with continuous exposure to contaminated water, polluted air and diffusion of disease organisms through carriers like rodents, flies and mosquitoes. The authors found the incidence of skin, respiratory, ear, eyes, malaria and water-borne diseases influenced by living close to the waste site (Table 5.2).

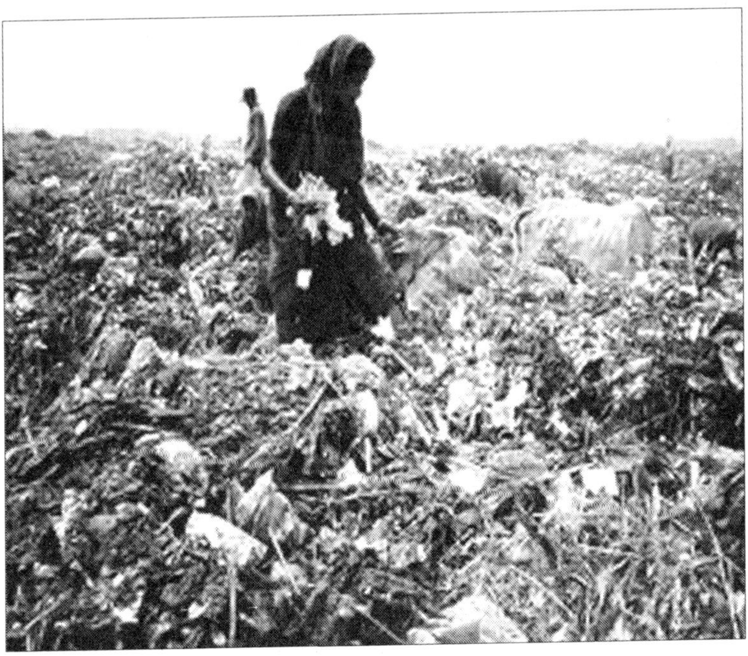

FIGURE 5.1: BHALASWA LANDFILL SITE

TABLE 5.2: HEALTH RISKS OF BHALASWA LANDFILL SITE

Zones/Diseases	A	B	C	D
Dysentery	44	44	42	44
Gastroenteritis	26	28	22	20
Jaundice	14	19	26	22
Hookworm	8	5	–	6
Typhoid	2	2	4	8
Polio	6	2	6	–
Total	100	100	100	100

WATER STRESS: QUANTITY AND QUALITY CRISIS

Stress on Water Sources and Health Risks

Inadequate infrastructure, rapid population growth and an increasing water demand per capita have put pressure on the water resources and water supply system in Delhi. Drinking water sources, surface and ground, within the NCR quite limited and excessive water demands are met to a large degree through agreements with neighbouring states and Delhi's share in the Yamuna and Ganges river systems. With increasing demand from the competing agriculture sector, the neighbouring states are not in a position to meet excessive demand and that has resulted into growing water conflicts. The two river systems supply 87 per cent of the total water requirements and their share in the total water supply is on the decline. Depleting ground sources including rainy wells meet rest of the 13 per cent demand. Although Delhi's deep underground strata is not suitable for being tapped on account of unacceptable quality of water, still the quantity of groundwater abstracted over the years is on a rise and has caused a decline in water table to the extent of 6-30 m in several blocks of Alipur, Kanjhawla, Najafgarh and Mehrauli (Government of India, 1999). Both ground and surface water sources are hence threatened. Delhi is, thus, tapping distant river basins to augment extra water supplies with strong possible ecological footprints. Likewise the growing dependence on deep aquifers has exposed many communities in the above blocks to excessive does of nitrates, chlorides and fluorides. Health risks are serious in such areas with prolonged consumption of water without adequate treatment.

Unequal Distribution of Water and Health Risks

According to Delhi Jal Board (DJB), water supply in 1999 was 2,645 mld while the demand for it was 4,765 mld, based on the Master Plan Delhi 2001 norm of 363 litres per capita per day for urban population and 100 litres per capita per day for rural population. There was hence a shortage of 2,120 mld (45 per cent shortage). In 2001 this gap increased to 47 per cent and is likely to increase further to 57 per cent by 2021 (TERI, 2001 and MPD, 2007). Delhi loses as much as 40 per cent of water as unaccounted for water (UFW) in the form of leakage, theft by illegal connections, meter under-registration, meter reading errors and other malpractices. If such losses can be reduced to half by good water management practices, the gap can be overcome without much stress on the distant river basins.

Major problem of water supply in Delhi is linked with its unequal distribution largely influenced by location, legal status of settlements and inefficiency in water services. North and central areas of Delhi receive around 5–10 times the levels in large areas of south Delhi. Most low income, unauthorized, resettlement and peripheral colonies are at a higher disadvantage. A recent report shows that people in Mehrauli and Narela receive only 29 and 31 litres per person per day respectively, while those in the Cantonment Board get 509 litres and residents of Lutyens' Delhi 462 litres. Erratic supply limited to a few hours further accentuates the stress situation. Better-off communities in water stress areas resort to alternate sources of water supply such as water tankers from DJB, bottled water, neighbour's hand pumps and private water tankers to augment minimum water need for hygiene, cooking and washing. Residents in low-income resettlement colonies and *Jhuggi-Jhonpri* (JJ) Clusters on the contrary suffer more and are at greater health risk as the water supply from market mechanisms is unaffordable. This compels the residents to obtain water from the unsafe sources like hand pumps which are painted red symbolizing water quality not safe for drinking or inexpensive private vendors whose water is unsafe. Lack of storage capacity also leads to unhygienic practices of handling and usage of water. Selected studies indicate high incidence of water-borne diseases like cholera, typhoid, amoebiases, diarrhoea, and gastroenteritis in such settlements when compared with other locations with regular and sufficient water supply. Water conflicts, particularly during summer months, are also quite common in low-income settlements due to the erratic and inadequate water supply.

Women and children who have to reschedule their leisure time are found most vulnerable to health risks.

Water Quality and Health Risks

Water quality related environmental issues in mega cities have direct health links within and outside (downstream) city boundaries. If not managed comprehensively, the entire region is likely to suffer health risks that are easily avoidable.

Water quality issues in Delhi are linked to inefficient water supply and sewerage systems. Delhi suffers from both aspects. Drinking and waste water infrastructure is largely old and also inaccessible to repairs in old and densely populated areas. In such areas, which cover more than 25 per cent of Delhi's population, the sewage and drinking water pipes are not safely distanced and hence mixing of sewer water with drinking water is quite common, at least in summer months and in areas of erratic water supply. Outbreak of water-borne diseases (gastro-enteritis, hepatitis, cholera, typhoid) is a regular phenomenon in summer and monsoon months. Likewise, in urban villages and low-income peripheral settlements where water supplies are highly inadequate, DJB supplies ground water through a network of surface water pipes. In such areas, the author found leaky water pipes cross over open waste water drains and mixing of waste water with drinking water is seen as a new and emerging water-related health risk to large communities.

Risks to health also arise from the unsafe disposal of waste water from point and area sources. Many illegal industries operating in non-conforming areas discharge effluents into open drains and water bodies. Residents of unauthorized settlements, dependent on such industries for employment, are found to be exposed to the effluents indirectly through use of shallow hand pump waters and directly through contaminated water during the monsoon months or other flooding situations (Kataria, Aggarwal and Bentinck, 1997). In Delhi a large number of illegal colony residents also lives close to waste water bodies like drains, ponds, water depressions and contaminated Yamuna river bed. No scientific study is available to estimate the health risks of such population groups, though the expected outcomes are quite obvious. Area sources like waste disposal sites in Delhi threaten health to surrounding communities through leachate contamination of ground water. Recent study by Aggarwal and Tulika (2004), as stated in a previous section, provide sufficient evidence to health risks at such locations.

Of the total population of Delhi, 70 per cent do not have access to water-borne sewage. The proportion is nearly 100 per cent in the unauthorized colonies and in many of the resettlement colonies and the new planning divisions, and is as high as 50 per cent in the walled city. Currently, of the 242 million litres of liquid waste that is generated daily, only 46 million litres receives full treatment and 72 million litres receives partial treatment before entering the Yamuna river. Unchecked domestic and industrial discharges of 211 tonnes/day (CPCB, 2000) into the Yamuna from different drains have led to the complete depletion of dissolved oxygen levels in the Yamuna river stretch in Delhi. The faecal coliform content in this stretch of the river is as high as 0.135 million, rendering the water unfit for any domestic use. Similarly, other parameters such as pH, COD (chemical oxygen demand), and TDS (total dissolved solids) have also deteriorated drastically in the city river stretch as compared to upstream of Delhi. In fact, the general opinion is that only sewage water flows in the Yamuna during the summer months because 17 drains bring large quantities of untreated or partially treated water to it whereas the river dilution capacity is almost nil. Health impact of heavily polluted water on downstream communities has become a serious public health research and political debate between Delhi and neighbouring states on the question of dumping city externalities on the peripheral zones.

Challenges to the Health Sector

With a massive disease burden of communicable and non-communicable diseases the public health care system is overburdened and private health care fills the gap, at least for those who can afford it. Still the poor and other lower middle income groups depend on the public health care system that suffers from inequality in distribution, bad governance, physical inaccessibility, and unconcerned attitude towards patients. Health care facilities in the national capital territory of Delhi are provided by multiple agencies, each operating a number of hospitals, dispensaries, special clinics and nursing homes. Locational disadvantages of distribution include clustering in the central city and low availability in the peripheral areas where most poor live. The greatest challenge to the health sector is how to strengthen intra-agency coordination, promote demand driven new public health approach, improve health services distribution in under-served areas, and introduce governance approach rather administration to improve the efficiency of existing services.

This is achievable with a healthy city type approach as we notice in later sections.

SOCIO-ECONOMIC CHALLENGES TO HEALTH

Social support system in Delhi is getting weak. There are tendencies towards disorganization of the extended family system, which provided social and economic support to the elderly and those without jobs. With the withdrawal of social support to the elderly, their health care needs and costs are going to rise. Furthermore, nuclear families in the emerging global cities like Delhi are going to be under tremendous mental stress to cope with the growing work culture and intense mobility. Consequently, there will be more incidences of mental health disorders and non-communicable diseases of cancer and the circulatory system with growing lifestyle changes among young rich. Social diseases like AIDS may result from high mobility behaviours and lifestyle changes. Alienation of the youth arising from growing unemployment and withdrawal of social support system may lead to more substance abuse and alcoholism. The poor will face high health risks resulting from inequalities, deprivation and marginalization.

The above account on environmental degradation and social pathology of diseases illustrates with certainty that disease burden in Delhi is largely attributed to deficiency of environmental infrastructure and unhealthy lifestyles. Most disease burden is avoidable with intervention of preventive and health promotive approaches. Sections below illustrate how a healthy city approach can be helpful in promoting health without much financial commitment.

A Possible Framework for Intervention: A Healthy City Approach

DETERMINANTS OF FUTURE HEALTHY CITIES

The challenges stated above are by no means insurmountable. These are expected to result from the current trend of hyper-urbanization and under the influence of growing globalization. If governments in the developing countries realize the inevitability of urbanization and its resultant health implications and analyse the causes as indicated in Figure 5.2 there is no reason that future cities will not be healthy.

A close examination of the determinants of future healthy city (Figure 5.2) suggests that not much financial investment on health

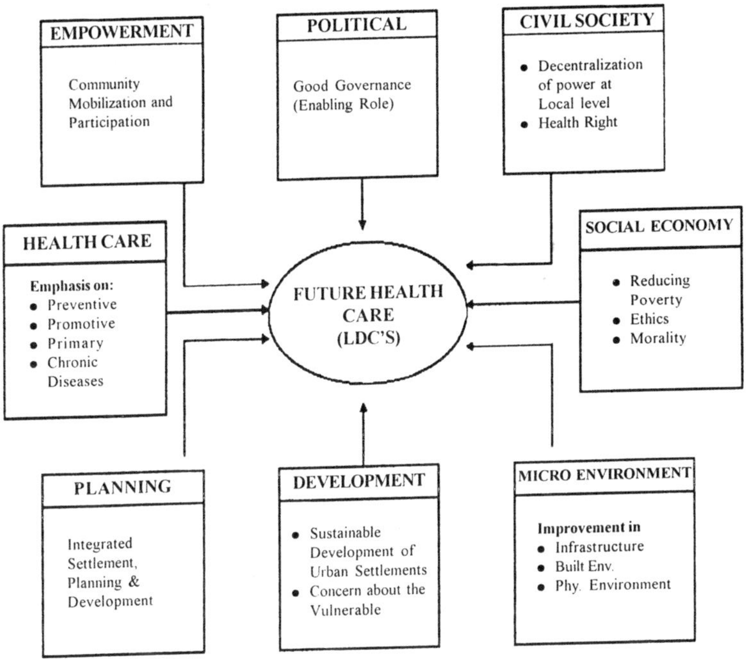

FIGURE 5.2: DETERMINANTS OF FUTURE HEALTHY CITIES

systems is required to promote healthy city. Only a few attitudinal changes in the governance of cities, political will, preventive and promotive health care, strong community participation and improvement in social economy will produce considerable impact on future health scenario within present and future mega cities like Delhi.

Healthy City Concept of WHO

Solutions to some of the concerns and challenges raised above are available in the Healthy City (HC) concept developed by WHO in 1986. 'A Healthy City is one that is continually creating and improving those physical and social environments and expanding those community resources which enable people to mutually support each other in performing all the functions of life and in developing to their maximum potential' (Goldstein and Kickbusch, 1996). Achieving healthy cities basically means building on each city's own resources and on the skills and managerial capacities of its people and formal and informal institutions. A Healthy City/Town/Village/Setting is defined in terms of the process and not just the output and ultimate outcome like reducing infant mortality rate or cardiovascular diseases. A 'healthy city' is one that has developed a keen awareness of health (in the holistic sense) and is striving to improve and promote it. Therefore, any city, community or setting could be part of the HC movement regardless of its current health status. What is called for is a commitment to health, the well-being of the community and a sustainable process for continuous health improvement.

Basically, community participation, inter-sectoral collaboration, decentralization of governance and holistic nature of health have been the most admired components of healthy cities approach to improve health in urban settings. The concept also patronises health public policy with micro level emphasis. Unfortunately, the 'settings' approach, backbone of HCP, has not been mentioned at all as its major strength and that raises our concern of its utility and applicability to the regional countries (Aggarwal, 2000).

Need for a Healthy City Concept

The healthy city concept, therefore, seeks to build a strong case for public health at the local level and to put health issues on to the local agenda for urban policy makers. It demonstrates how various interrelated factors influence a society's health and well-being (quality of life) within a given urban setting such as a community, school, workplace, and so on. The concept is based on the realization that the bio-medical approach alone is not enough to solve human health problems. In fact, a holistic view of health is needed considering the interaction of social, economic and environmental domains of our settlements for promoting improved health. Public health experts broadly accept that only limited disease burden of the world can be taken care of by curative medicines. Further, the state alone cannot provide adequate health care and we need to involve non-governmental actors such as NGOs, community-based organizations (religious organizations), schools, the private sector and the recipient population as partners in promoting healthy cities. 'Creating health' is best possible through synergistic actions of many interested partners (stakeholders). Health is now a major concern of all sectors and not just the health sector alone. This is precisely the message given by the healthy city concept as it has evolved over the years from the experiences gained mainly from the health, environment and urban sectors.

Practice of HC Concept in Cities across the World and its Relevance for the Developing Countries

The basic concept of HC has been practised in more than 800 cities in developed countries in a variety of ways and settings and is being promoted in the developing countries. In the latter countries many big cities are facing serious public health problems related to degraded environments and rapid socio-economic transformations. Such situations have been produced in the last two decades by the globalization forces and other local and regional challenges of economic development. The HC approach is being applied in such cities to improve the environmental health conditions by involving communities and empowering the cities for better governance practices. Nevertheless, it will take time to practice it on a large scale and to refine and tune it to suit regional and local conditions.

RELEVANCE OF HC CONCEPT IN A DEVELOPING COUNTRY LIKE INDIA

- adapted to new public health thinking where community rather than individual health is more important
- promotes proactive approach to health
- supports preventive and promotive view of health rather than expensive curative approach
- considers strong linkage between degraded environment and health
- facilitates reduction of environmental health related disease burden with community participation approach
- promotes urban governance and intersectorality towards health issues
- places health on the political agenda
- addresses the equity, accessibility and other social justice concerns in the health sector
- encourages ownership and pride for the city/settings
- incorporates sustainable development thinking to solve health and urban development problems at least in the fast growing cities.

HOW TO BUILD A HEALTHY CITY?

The aim of a properly functioning HC programme is to institute a HC process which facilitates community participation and develops action plans which cover major health and development issues. A well functioning HC programme generates change in the way health and development issues are addressed at the local level. It also implies a commitment to participatory local governance based on the principle of partnership among government departments and agencies (inter-sectorality), NGOs and the private sector. The following approaches and processes can facilitate in developing a healthy city project.

1. *Settings Approach*

The strength of the concept is that it can be applied in a variety of settings. In making the environment 'supportive for health', health authorities and NGOs must do more than merely look for the hazards and risk factors that damage health. Rather the emphasis of the HCP is on improvements and support for the 'settings' where health is maintained, promoted and indeed created. The idea of a supportive environment and the 'settings' approach has turned out to be a powerful and valuable one for the promotion of health in many countries. The home, the village, the workplace, the neighbourhood, the school, the city are the places where people live and work. These and many more settings are where health may be maintained and indeed created by engaging all participants and authorities that operate in the settings, in activities to create a supportive environment for health (WHO, 1995). The health status is determined more by the living conditions in these settings than by the health care facilities that we can provide. Settings are major social structures that provide channels and mechanisms of influence for reaching defined populations (Werna, 1998).

Success of a HCP, if other conditions are fulfilled, depends on the selection of setting where it is to be launched. Site selection is important considering the resource constraints and the magnitude and nature of health hazards present in the setting. In developing societies, priorities may go for under privileged communities living in environmentally degraded situations. Respondents in the survey preferred commercial areas (markets, hotels, motor garages) and institutional settings (schools, colleges, hospitals) and residential settings, municipal wards, neighbourhood slums, homes, clustered settlements) and workplaces (offices).

2. *Engagement of Civil Society to Create Healthy Cities*

Individuals can contribute towards promotion of health in a variety of ways including participation in community activities towards improved environment, change in lifestyles, promotion of simple life, developing habits of physical exercise, yoga, meditation and sports, and self-empowerment through education and training in public health. In the developing countries community participation in the social sector has been limited and such functions are expected to be performed by the city or the state government. There are in fact contextual issues involved in the concept of community participation. Community involvement for a common good like environmental improvement is strong in developed industrial societies. In the developing societies like India, on the contrary, community or neighbourhood participation is strong for social ends such as marriage and religious functions. At the moment, due to the financial limitations of the various levels of government, communities have to be educated to be actively involved in such issues. This can be achieved, for example, by relating health issues with folklore, politicizing health as an election agenda, introducing health campaigns, networking with other neighbourhoods, involving religious leaders, leading professionals, administrators and teachers. The national and state governments need to decentralize power at the local level to enable local bodies to make their own decisions to raise tax base, hold elections and perform functions which are expected from them by the communities. Ill health in the urban settlement of developing countries is largely produced by the inability of the local government to provide basic health infrastructure. Strengthening the governance and the capacity can go a long way in promoting health in the future cities. This can be achieved, if most national governments adopt local Agenda 21 and implement the recent recommendation of the Habitat II Conference.

3. *Institutionalization of Intersectoral Action for Health (IAH)*

Considering the complexity and multidimensional nature of urban health problems, WHO has been propagating the need for IAH strategy ever since Health for All (HFA) declaration in 1977. It got diluted over time and again became an important vehicle of action after the Ottawa Charter Declaration on Health Promotion and the WHO is now strongly promoting the renewal of HFA. An acceptable definition or meaning of the term is desirable for its effective application in the regional context. At the 1997 Halifax Conference on Intersectoral Action for Health the participants consented to the following definition: 'a recognised relationship between part or parts of the health sector with part or parts of another sector which has been formed to take action on an issue to achieve health outcomes, (or intermediate health outcomes) in a way that is more effective, efficient or sustainable than could be achieved by health sector acting alone'.

In the opinion survey respondents in South-East Asia understood IAH to mean:

- coordinated action by all city stakeholders
- collaboration and cooperation among government departments
- combined action by various sectoral agencies in a city
- health awareness among various sectors
- partnership between health and environmental sectors and association with other sectors as appropriate
- integration of initiatives/actions under different sectors leading to improvement of health
- solving problems and implementing development activities by different related sectors in the city through coordination and participation.

In the view of the respondents, health can be produced more effectively, efficiently and synergistically by joint actions between different sectors. All respondents agreed to a strong need for IAH to promote health in the SEAR countries and most expressed optimism about its feasibility and success in using intersectoral approach, even considering watertight segregated functions of health-related sectors. The message is clear that IAH works, is possible and effective.

4. *Capacity Building*

Health promotion programmes include activities that can be described as 'capacity building', i.e. giving other people resources to enable them to promote health. Capacity building implies empowerment of local authorities, the community and other stakeholders to effectuate and implement policies and take ownership of projects that are going to improve the quality of life of the citizens. Empowerment further implies a redistribution of power from those who possess it to those who do not. It needs to be asked what empowerment means in a culture that continues to look to experts to solve problems. The process of capacity building is found to be a fundamental and key instrument to bring about change and also to sustain such a change in quality of life parameters like health and environment. Capacity building for HCP should be done at two levels: municipal and community.

Strengthening of local bodies with respect to resource generation; upgrading the skills and sensitizing the staff to health needs; study visits; preparing action plans; developing pilot projects and involving the private sector and NGOs in decision-making processes are among the most important suggested measures. The empowerment of the community was found to be equally essential to involve them and for seeking their cooperation in civic activities like HCP. It can be largely achieved through health awareness and motivation campaigns, networking with other neighbourhoods, incentives and public forums.

5. *New Town and City Planning Approach*

Historically, city planning in Europe and other industrial countries was introduced basically to improve the health conditions of the people by providing safe drinking water, efficient disposal of human waste and land use controls and zoning of residential, industrial, commercial and recreational areas. City planning played a pivotal role in preventing diseases and promoting health largely through the land use planning approach. The principles and practices of city planning got diffused into the colonial countries and contributed towards improved living conditions in the administrative cities and benefitted mainly the middle and higher income communities. With the growing forces of urbanization and industrialization, land use approach of town planning could not resolve many social conflicts, inequalities in provision of services, emergence of slums and rising environmental degradation which had a strong bearing on health. Social, economic, environmental and health concerns need to be integrated in new town planning if the latter has to play a significant role in improving the quality of living conditions in the city. New town planning approach should also include elements of participatory planning, planning for new poor migrants, health and environment impact assessment and training to produce health plans along with land use plans. For example, a new plan for Chittagong has recently been prepared. It has accepted the approach of flexible planning that incorporates the above concerns.

6. *Decentralisation of Power*

Centralization of power in simple words implies the concentration of decision-making process in a few individuals or institutions. The process discourages people or communities to participate in development-related activities. The individual is unable to exercise his full potential or right to effectuate change in his own life conditions or in the immediate environment where he lives or works. Poverty, ignorance, population pressures, hierarchical decision-making processes continued from colonial administration, and strong bureaucracy hinder the decentralization process. Decentralization of power is, therefore, an essential condition for and an instrument to improve quality of living conditions in a particular setting in a sustained manner. Only recently the demand for decentralization of power at the local level has emerged.

Local governments in the region are generally at the mercy of their higher level governments and have very little resource revenue generation power and are heavily burdened by strong bureaucracy. Since the healthy city approach is heavily inter-sectoral, centralization of authority and resources produces constraints in its effective operation. Autonomy to local bodies, capacity building efforts, legislative changes and reforms in decision-making process can go a long way in the decentralization of power. In the developing countries there is no real effort by various levels of government to decentralize the decision-making process. Some countries like India, Nepal and Indonesia have recently taken initiatives directed towards decentralization and devolution of responsibilities to the local level. The 74th constitutional amendment of the Government of India to empower local bodies is a classic example of that effort. Emergence of environmental NGOs, growing public-private partnerships in selected urban services and housing activities are positive steps in this direction.

7. *Urban Governance*

'Governance is the system through which society organises and manages the affairs of sectors and partners in order to achieve the expectations of the people.' New theories and models are emerging about the nature of relationship between and within nation-states. At the national, regional and local levels, governments are struggling to define what they do best. In many countries, this examination of roles and responsibilities has also extended to the private sector and the voluntary or civic sector. A central aspect of this rethinking includes articulating what governments need to ensure to promote long-term, sustainable improvements in economic and social well-being, including health, for all citizens. Urban governance basically includes efficient, effective and ethical municipal government keen on improving the quality of living conditions of the civil society. Decentralization of power, capacity building, transparent and accountable administration, sound financial management and intersectorality are among the key elements of urban governance.

Unfortunately in case of the SEAR countries and other less developed countries urban governance is not only pathetically low, centralization of power, strong bureaucracy, corrupt officials, lack of work culture, ad-hoc decisions, and limited scope for community participation in decision-making has led to the inefficient provision and delivery of basic services and amenities. The resource-hungry local bodies with little efforts to mobilize resources don't show much optimism to improve quality of living condition in the near future. Massive migration to large cities is further producing chaotic conditions and growing inequality in urban basic services. Since environmental health linked with environment-infrastructure is a basic issue in most big cities of the region, urban governance has a significant role to play in promoting healthy city conditions. In our opinion survey, the respondents suggested actions to improve urban governance in their city or country. The most common suggestions included: ensured participation of stakeholders like private sector, NGOs, CBOs in municipal activities and planning decisions; entrust administrative and executive powers to mayors; increased use of information technology (database management) in decision-making process; more autonomy in decision-making at lower levels of administrative hierarchy; training of municipal staff and task force persons in technical and managerial aspects of health projects; transparency and accountability in administration and resource mobilization at the city level.

Building Delhi into a Healthy City

Delhi with a population of around 15 million is among the fastest growing mega cities of India. It suffers from typical mega city problems such as overcrowding, high population growth, inadequate urban services in low-income squatter settlements, growing air, water and noise pollution, rise in accidents and crime, hazardous working conditions in factories and overburdened transport system. WHO has already declared Delhi among the four most polluted cities of the world. Against this background of environment degradation and social pathology the healthy city programme was initiated in 1997 with WHO-SEARO assistance and the commitment of the state government towards improved health conditions in Delhi. An inter-sectoral approach has been followed in pursuing the project. The major objectives of the project were to create healthy physical environment, health promoting behaviour, health promoting mechanisms and mass awareness of healthy city concept. Community participation was encouraged through schools, market associations, social-welfare associations, group-housing societies, and voluntary agencies.

The major proposed activities included:

- access to basic health services
- health education
- mass immunization of the children through campaigns
- prevention and control of communicable diseases
- safe water supply and sanitation in selected squatter settlements
- water quality surveillance
- solid waste management including hospital waste, prevention and control of pollution
- accidents and crime prevention.

PILOT STUDY: TRANS-YAMUNA AREA

On the award of seed money by WHO-SEARO, that Trans-Yamuna Area (TYA) was selected by the Delhi Government as a pilot study for implementing the healthy city project in a limited way. The area was chosen considering the concentration of low income settlements that lack basic services, high population density of migrant population, flood-prone conditions causing a large number of deaths due to diarrhoea. (Every year from 1991 to 1998, more than 700 children have died due to diarrhoea.)

The main objectives of the project were to:

- make the environment clean and safe.
- make the eco-system stable and sustainable.
- provide access to optimum level of health services.
- introduce community participation in planning and implementation.
- improve the health of the community in the TYA of Delhi by raising awareness, mobilizing community participation, recognizing and acting upon serious health and social issues, and by improving the environmental conditions.
- create partnerships with local municipal agencies, NGOs and CBOs.

Actions and Achievements

Steering committees and working groups were formed for various actions identified while launching the project. Public campaigns, like Pulse Polio, immunizing children against communicable diseases and pollution control were launched. Community response was encouraging, at least for the Pulse Polio vaccination. Pollution control is considered responsibility of the municipal corporation and the communities were less responsive on this account.

Hoardings and kiosks with different health messages were placed at critical points in TYA and other vulnerable settings. A large share of the budget was allocated for this activity. *Nukkad nataks* (street plays) were performed for those who could not read the messages. This is a popular medium to spread ideas among low income communities and was used effectively. Posters and pamphlets related to healthy city ideas and engagement of civil society were distributed. AIDS control measures were advertised in daily newspapers including mobile health exhibitions in schools and slums, debate competitions on health and poster competitions. Community involvement and participation was ensured through the involvement of various social and commercial groups like parent-teacher associations, market associations, women's organizations, residential welfare associations, Rotary and Lion's clubs, environmental groups and the Institute of Indian Town Planners.

Efforts were also made to improve the availability of safe water in the selected slums by checking the quality of water periodically. Steps for reducing incidences of diseases, included spraying of insecticides, cleaning of water coolers, public awareness campaigns to wear full sleeved clothes and filling waste-water collection pits. Health campaigns for TB control, Hepatitis B vaccination, immunization, cancer detection and non-smoking were launched in critical settings like slums, government schools and among women. To decrease the maternal mortality rate, campaigns were conducted for active promotion of safe motherhood practices and reduction in early pregnancy and closely spaced births. Public campaigns were also conducted for promotion of breastfeeding, prevention of vitamin A deficiency among children and disorders from iodine deficiency. Iodine testing kits were distributed to students and patients. Pollution prevention was done through planting of trees in schools and in different areas. Competitions were held for Healthy Schools and Healthy Markets. A workshop was held involving women's organizations and NGOs on the 'social and emotional health of women'.

Among the few achievements that will make some difference through institutionalization process was the preparation of a Healthy City Plan for TYA which has been approved for implementation by the National Capital Territory Government. A new sewerage system was implanted through HCP. The municipal corporation engage vehicles to transport garbage.

Evaluation of Healthy city Initiative

Evaluation was carried out by the author on behalf of WHO-SEARO, including other healthy cities in the region, largely focusing on process indicators. Methods used in the evaluation include stakeholders' analysis, evaluation of workshops and training programmes, document analysis and responses of experts and prominent stakeholders. Some of the findings are stated below.

1. inter-sector collaboration

Inter-sectoral collaboration was found common for activities like healthy schools, healthy markets, food adulteration, traffic and police. Such project activities crossed traditional sector boundaries and are implemented in an integrated manner. Influence of local and national policies was limited to selected activities like pollution control. Structure for collaboration needs to be established. There are no institutional mechanisms where education, health and city planning departments address the impact of one sector on another. Rather there is a tendency to blame other sectors for the existing problems.

2. community participation

The primary stakeholders in this area were citizens, students and customers. The secondary stakeholders were the Government of NCT, political leaders, professional associations, school teachers, market officials, environmental groups, and NGOs. Women had low or average knowledge about the healthy city project. Knowledge about project management was variable, ranging from low to high. People were involved through steering committee meetings, community participation workshops and so on. It was learnt that since in India many women still do not work, the assistance of housewives can be taken for neighbourhood planning. The area was politically motivated and there was a strong mobilization of human resources in the area. The representation of city leadership on HCP committees and task forces was high, but their participation in HCP events was moderate. And their role in selection of WHO-HCP was perfect.

The mechanisms for targeting the poor were related to awareness activities including street plays by communities and announcement about subsidies. Involvement in various decision-making activities were done through community participation. It was good to see that when the project was trying to prioritize the needs of the poor, they knew exactly what they wanted. It was learnt that one should think of developing a network of local leaders to perform HCP activities.

In TYA selection of key healthy settings was done with people's advice. In fact, settings like markets and schools selected for HCP were mostly from the poor areas. All schools were run by the government and were located in the poor areas.

3. NETWORKING IN TYA

There was no contact with other healthy cities both within the region and elsewhere, and hence human, technical or financial flows through creation of networks was absent. The sustainability of a project is maintained if such networking is strong and thereby the experiences, limitations, strengths of each can be shared. Networking also provides new ideas to get better results without much financial costs. Need for better interaction at various levels—line, interdepartmental, local-state government, inter-city exchanges—is needed.

4. CAPACITY BUILDING AND SUSTAINABILITY IN TYA

WHO provided a consultant in the initial years of the project. But very few seminars were held to provide exposure to decision makers about the healthy cities policies. Nonetheless, facilitators benefitted from such seminars. No examples of institutional capacity building were provided.

Some efforts were made to bring about social, environmental and cultural integration. But there were no economic gains unless one considers the economic valuation/productivity resulting from healthy or good quality of life. No direct cost recovery procedures existed.

In the Trans-Yamuna Area, the state government and WHO provided financial support for the project and Lal Bahadur Shastri Hospital, which was the facilitator, provided technical support. The ruling political party in the form of advocacy, public speaking, election manifesto, etc., ensured political support. Department of Health Services (NCT) provided administrative support. Financial support also came from the NCT Plan funds. WHO funds were only used as a catalyst. The NCT on the whole has adequate funds to implement the HCP policies.

Institutionalization of HCP policies has taken deeper roots in cities where Healthy City Action Plans were prepared and separate healthy city offices were established.

Conclusion

Based on healthy city literature and experience of cities where healthy city projects are in progress, including TYA in Delhi, we identified external finances, city resources, capacity building, urban governance, inter-sectoral governance, community participation and technical support as major driving forces that can advance and promote healthy cities. The importance and impact of these forces may vary from region to region and city to city, nevertheless the relative contribution of each towards healthy city development cannot be diluted. Despite this optimism, it is well known that intersectoral actions have not been much successful in the context of urban health, including in Delhi, except in countries where strong tradition of decentralization of power, weak bureaucracy, liberal democracy, and commitment to public cause is strong. In other situations it has been more of rhetoric and less action oriented. Research in intersectoral collaboration indicates that the existence of a formal framework does not guarantee collaboration and indeed, effective and successful collaboration is rare.

NOTES

1. See http://www.teriin.org/reports/rep09/rep091.htm
2. See http://www.censusindia.net

REFERENCES

Agarwal, Ravi, 'Medical Waste Management Still a Far Cry', *Indian Journal of Environmental Protection*, 21: 26, 2001, p. 549.

Aggarwal, Surinder and Tulika Sandhya, 'Exposure to Health Risks of a Solid Waste Site in North Delhi Squatter Settlement', *Journal of Regional Health*, 2004, 9, pp. 1–2.

Aggarwal, Surinder, *Strengthening Healthy Cities in the Southeast Asia Region: An Opinion Survey.* WHO-SEARO, 2000.

Aggarwal, Surinder and Satish Davgun, *Air Pollution and Healthy Delhi Proceedings*, IGU Commission on Health and Environment, Brno, Czech Republic, 1994, pp. 17–28.

Barton, H. and C. Tsourou, *Healthy Urban Planning: A WHO Guide to Planning for People*, London: Spon Press, 2000.

Census of India, *Series 8: Delhi Provisional Population Totals: Distribution of Workers and Non-Workers*, Paper-1 of 2001 NCT of Delhi, 2001.

Centre for Science and Environment, 'Slow Murder: The Deadly Story of Vehicular Pollution in India, Delhi', *State of the Environment*, 1996, Series 3.

———, 'Death is in the Air', *Down to Earth*, 6, 1997, 12.

De Koning, H.W., K.R. Smith and J.M. Last, 'Biomass Fuel Consumption and Health', *Bulletin of the World Health Organization*, 63, 1985, pp. 11–25.

Delhi Statistics Handbook, *Directorate of Economics and Statistics*, Delhi.

Goldstein, G. and I. Kickbush, 'A Healthy City is a Better City', *World Health*, 1, 1996, pp. 4–6.

Government of India, Central Pollution Control Board (CPCB), *Annual Report 2000–1.*

——— and Government of NCT of Delhi, *Delhi Urban Environment and Infrastructure Improvement Project (DUEIIP): Status Report for Delhi*, 2001, p. 21.

———, NCR Planning Board, *Delhi: A Fact Sheet*, 1999.

———, Central Pollution Control Board (CPCB), 2002, http://envfor.nic.in/cpcb/cpcb.html.

———, Central Pollution Control Board (CPCB), *Air Quality in Delhi (1989-2000): NAAQMS/17/2000-2001*, Delhi, 2001.

———, Ministry of Environment and Forests, *White Paper on Pollution in Delhi: With An Action Plan*, 1997, http://www.teriin.org/reports/rep09/rep091.htm, http://www.un.org/esa/population//publi-cations/wup2003/WUP2003Report.pdf.

Kataria, V., S. Aggarwal and J.V. Bentick, *Environmental and Health Implications of Industrialization in an Urban Village at Delhi's Fringe*, Paper presented at the International Seminar for the Promotion of Environmentally Sound and Healthy Cities, University of Delhi, Delhi, 1997.

Koberlein, Michael, *Living from Waste: Livelihood of the Actors Involved in Delhi's Informal Waste Recycling Economy*, Verllag fur Entwicklungspolitik Saarbrucken, 2003.

Kraas, Frauka, 'Mega Cities as Global Risk Areas', *Petermanns Geographische Mitteilungen*, 147, 4, 2003, pp. 6–15.

Krafft, T., S. Aggarwal and T. Wolf, 'Environmental Degradation and Health Risks in Delhi: The Price of Rapid Urbanization', *Newsletter of the International Human Dimensions Programme*, 03, 2003, pp. 11–13.

Krafft, Thomas, Tanja Wolf and Surinder Aggarwal, 'A New Urban Penalty? Environmental and Health Risks in Delhi'. *Petermanns Geographische Mitteilungen*, 147, 4, 2003, pp. 20–7.

Malik, Iqbal, 'Hospital Waste: A Dangerous Infusion', *Vatavaran*, 1996.

Master Plan for Delhi 2021, JBA Publishers, 2007.

Sassen, S., *Cities in a World Economy*, Thousand Oaks: Pine Forge Press, 2000.

Sharma, Sangeeta et al., 'Indoor Air Quality and Acute Lower Respiratory Infection in Indian Urban Slums'. *Environmental Health Perspective*, 106: 5, 1988, pp. 291–7.

Federal Register, *Standards for Particles Matter*, 18 July 1997, 62: 38651–701.

Tata Energy Research Institute, *State of Environment Report for Delhi 2001*, TERI, New Delhi, 2001.

Sandhya, Tulika, 'Impact of Solid Waste Disposal on Water Quality and Health: A Study of Bhalaswa Landfill Site in Delhi', M.Phil. Dissertation, University of Delhi, 2004.

United Nations, *World Urbanization Prospects: The 2001 Revision*, 2002.

United States Environmental Protection Agency, *Revision to the National Ambient Air*, 1997.

Werna, E., T. Harpham. I. Blue and G. Goldstein, *Healthy City Projects in Developing Countries, An International Approach to Local Problems*, London: Earthscan, 1998.

WHO, *Health and Environment in Sustainable Development*, Geneva: World Health Organization, 1997.

———, *Building a Healthy City: A Practitioner's Guide*, Geneva: World Health Organization, 1995.

———, *WHO Healthy Cities: A Programme Framework*, Geneva: World Health Organization, 1995.

———, *Healthy Cities in Action: 5 Case Studies from Africa, Asia, Middle East and Latin America*, Geneva: World Health Organization, 2000.

World Bank, *India's Environment: Taking Stock of Plans, Programmes and Priorities*, New Delhi Regional Office, 1996.

World Resources Institute, UNEP, UNDP, *World Resources 1998–99*, New Delhi: Oxford University Press, 1999.

PART I

EMERGING HEALTH LANDSCAPES

C. ALLOPATHIC LANDSCAPES UNDER GLOBAL COMPETITION

CHAPTER 6

India in the World of Pharmaceuticals: Dualities of a New Challenger

PIERRE CHAPELET

INTRODUCTION

Since 1996, India has been the most rapidly growing Asian economy after China. When people refer to the subcontinent's spectacular economic development and its emergence on the international trade scenario, primarily two sectors come to mind: information technology and the pharmaceutical industry. In this article, we propose that readers examine the second. While at the dawn of Independence, the subcontinent's entire drug market was in the hands of foreign multinationals (mainly British), fifty years later, the Indian allopathic pharmaceutical industry is the biggest and most advanced in what many people continue to call the 'developing world', generating almost 8 per cent of the world production of pharmaceutical products in volume (1.5 per cent in value). Thanks to a unique policy marked by the desire for economic and social independence, the subcontinent is now able to produce almost all types of medicines. By the same occasion, India has become an actor to be reckoned with at the international level, capable of offering both generic products and copies of drugs still under patent at prices that defeat all competition. The 2001 South African example in the case of anti-retroviral drugs is very explicit in this regard. However, while incorporating itself in increasingly global economic systems, India will have to gradually submit to WTO's rules, especially by integrating international intellectual property agreements (TRIPS) in its legislation as of 2005. This change of direction is engendering changes in the organization of India's pharmaceutical industry as well as in the commercial reasoning behind its development.

Hence, this article proposes to position itself within a conceptual framework that questions the distribution of and access to Indian pharmaceutical products against the background of economic and societal globalization. Economic analyses dealing with drugs often start with the assumption of their duality—considered as both public health goods and trade goods. These two visions correspond to two underlying but contrasting arguments: that of equity for the first and that of profitability and maximization of profits for the other. It may be interesting to look at the issue from a geographical viewpoint and examine the spatial objects ensuing from this duality. We would then find interactions between two types of entities: networks, on the one hand, consisting of pharmaceutical firms or distribution networks, for instance, and territories on the other, such as states on which public health or industrial regulation policies are based. Finally, access and distribution potential of a given drug in a given place are induced by the outcome of these interactions. In this framework, globalization may then be viewed as an evolving spatial system consisting of subsystems of interaction between networks and territories. Then, from the local to the more global scale, we can bring to light a multiplicity of interaction systems between these two entities—each of them with an unstable balance, resulting partly from the balance obtained by the systems at the other scales.

In this article, we will attempt to identify some of these systems and their interconnections. We shall also try to assess the repercussions of current developments on their dynamics and thereby assess their consequences for access to drugs. To do so, the analysis will be done on several scales. We shall first describe India's position in the pharmaceutical sector while highlighting the subcontinent's specificities at this scale. This will lead us to questions about local factors leading to the emergence of the current industrial profile, as well as about changes now taking place due to the signing of the intellectual property agreements. A detour in which we will briefly analyse developments in pharmaceutical imports and exports from or to India that will enable us to bring to light the strategies developed by Indian firms at the international level and emerging perspectives at this scale. Finally, we will compare these analyses to local realities of access to medicines in India.

The World Medicine Situation

Before specifically examining the Indian scenario, let us take a brief look at the international allopathic pharmaceutical 'landscape', as it will serve as the background for our study.

To get an idea of the size of the pharmaceutical sector at the international level, we may recall that according to the WHO, the trends observed between 1985 and 1999 indicate that the production value of medicines increased four times faster than the world's income.[1] Although it is difficult to assess the value of production in this market, most sources agree on a figure of USD 320 billion in 1999 (1.12 per cent of global growth domestic product, GDP). This makes it clear to everyone that the pharmaceutical sector is very lucrative—something everyone knows. Yet, inequities regarding access to health care and especially to drugs—subsist, whether it is at the local level, which means within state territories themselves (sub-state scale), or at the global level, that of the world states' mosaic.[2] With regard to pharmaceutical consumption, for instance, the population of 'developing countries', estimated at 83 per cent of the world's population, consumes just 15 per cent of the medicines produced in the world. Over 10 million people die every year of common chronic infections for which medicines are available.

Today, two main trends can be observed in the pharmaceutical sector: first, the desire to harmonize trade regulations between States and secondly, the transformation of the industry's profile in terms of its actors and, especially, the rise of the generic drugs' industry. We shall look more closely at these points, since they are at the heart of the problem of globalization of the pharmaceutical industry as applied to India.

Within the framework of the WTO's negotiation rounds in 1995, the Agreements on Trade-Related Aspects of Intellectual Property Rights (the TRIPS Agreements) were surely the ones that sparked off the most debates. In fact, they establish minimal standards in the field of intellectual property, which every member state has to respect by modifying its domestic laws if necessary. The difference between these agreements and pre-existing multilateral conventions, especially within the GATT framework, is the obligation of states to grant patent protection to inventions. For drugs, such patents have to be established for a 20-year period and grant exclusive commercial rights to the owner of the innovation during this period. Patent protection applies both to the innovation itself (the active pharmaceutical ingredient (API), or the pharmaceutical speciality formulation) and on its manufacturing process. Thus, this marks the inception of a supra-national regulation in the sense that it transcends the choices of each member country, whereas until now, intellectual property rights could vary from one state to another. At best, they were negotiated for each of the major world trading zones (Europe, NAFTA, etc.). The new legislation was incorporated in the WTO's Uruguay Round Programme at the initiative of the industrialized countries, following pressure from various lobbies (obviously including the pharmaceutical lobby). Public opinion, as well as a number of researchers, have expressed doubts about the consequences of these agreements on the fairness of access to medicines in the world. They fear a substantial increase in drug prices in countries that did not grant patents in the past and even greater difficulty in access in the case of the most deprived populations.

The second major trend in the pharmaceutical sector is obviously the emergence of the generic drugs' industry, with a growing number of patented drugs falling in the public domain. Patents on almost 40 American medicines expired in end 2002 (market estimated at USD 20 billion in 2000 and 40 billion in 2005, of a total market of USD 300 billion currently). Again in the United States, of the 100 most prescribed drugs in 1986, just 21 were still protected by patents in 1990. The generic drugs industry has the advantage of being able to mass produce a wide spectrum of medicines able to heal almost all diseases, and at a lower price than with patented ones. It is therefore a very interesting alternative for health systems looking for savings.[3]

Following the emergence of this new type of competition, the world of pharmaceutical multinationals is witnessing a number of mergers and acquisitions of subsidiaries, with each multinational trying to reinforce its position in the market. In the same way, most big pharmaceutical companies are directing their research at the development of profitable medicines, i.e. for solvent consumers. In 1996, the WHO already declared that of the USD 56 billion spent on R&D in the world, only 0.4 per cent was spent on pneumonia, diarrhoea and tuberculosis, which accounted for 18 per cent of the causes of morbidity in the world but essentially affected poor populations, in Africa or Asia in particular (research on these diseases is primarily done through public or military agencies).[4] This economic rationalization of production reached its climax with examples such as Eflornithine—a highly effective drug against sleeping sickness—whose production was stopped in 1995 because of non-profitability, only 15 years after it came on the market. The association Médecins Sans Frontières (MSF) and WHO, now the license owners, are still trying to find a manufacturer ready to ensure the long-term production of this drug.[5]

Finally, if a geographical qualifier had to be found to characterize drug networks and territories, it would be that of 'consolidation'. Firstly, the consolidation of actors (networks), since just ten pharmaceutical companies account for half of the world's sales (besides, this kind of consolidation has been increasing since 1987). Secondly, a consolidation of therapeutic segments and products: the ten best sold medicines account for 12 per cent of the value of the world pharmaceutical production. Finally, a consolidation of territories, with two-thirds of the value of world production coming from businesses headquartered in just five countries (USA, Japan, Germany, France and England). In 1997, North America (36.10 per cent), Europe (29 per cent) and Japan (19.10 per cent) alone accounted for 84 per cent of world drug production. There has also been a territorial consolidation of consumption, as mentioned earlier, as a majority of men and women in 'developing' or 'emerging' countries have little or no access to drugs.

This consolidation and the inequities it generates can easily be seen in Figure 6.1, which displays the level of development of the pharmaceutical industry per country. The world geography appearing clearly illustrates the phenomenon and is characteristic of the duality between industrialized and 'developing' countries.

The first group brings together ten countries classified as having a sophisticated pharmaceutical industry with substantial research facilities. Most West European countries, the United States and Japan can be found here. These ten countries are the main sources of pharmaceutical innovation in the world, through about ten multinationals that have their head offices there and, sometimes, through public sector funded research. Although they represent only around 15 per cent of the world's population, they sum up 80 per cent of world drug sales.

A second set brings together sixteen other countries, including India and China, which are characterized by a certain capacity for innovation, which means that at least one new molecule has been discovered and marketed by these countries between 1961 and 1990. Over the last decade, major changes have taken place in this group, which includes some of the biggest exporters, including India, as we are going to see.

Furthermore, ninety-seven countries have a domestic industry based on reproductive capabilities, producing either branded or non-branded generics. While a majority (84) produce end products from imported ingredients, thirteen (including Brazil, Egypt, Norway, Turkey and Indonesia) are considered to have an industry that produces both active substances and end products.

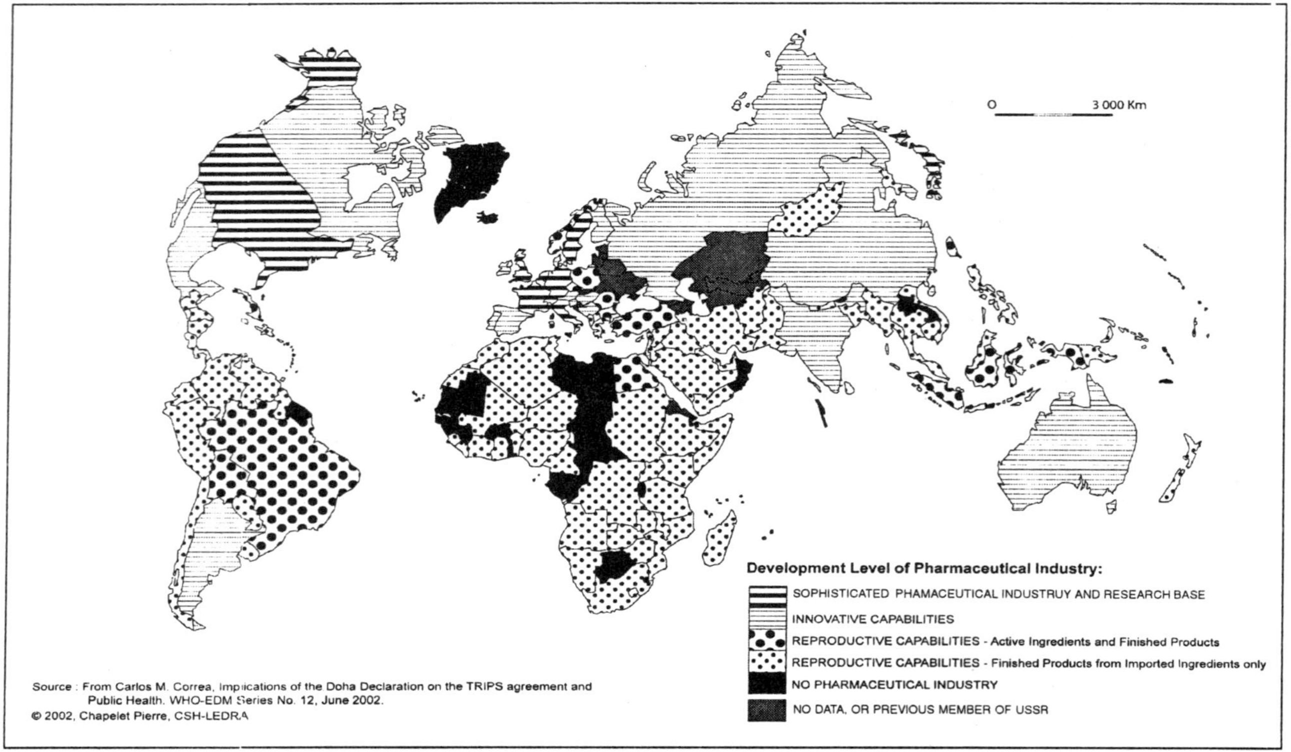

FIGURE 6.1: DEVELOPMENT LEVELS OF PHARMACEUTICAL INDUSTRY BY COUNTRY, 2002.

Finally, the last set (mostly found in Africa)—brings together countries with no production capacity, totally dependent on imports from foreign firms.

The polarities revealed by this map generate drug flows through distribution networks set up by pharmaceutical companies.

India's position in this typology—which may seem surprising at first, given the clichés that have long been transmitted by the media at the international level—is mainly due to the unique policy it adopted since its independence, which allowed it to develop an effective industrial sector. Before presenting the current situation and giving more details about the structure of this sector and its transformation, let us briefly examine the historic context and the unique policy choices that enabled its emergence. The pharmaceutical sector is a good illustration of India's 'non-alignment' policy and especially its desire for economic and societal independence through what is called the 'Indian way' or 'the third way', with reference to the Cold War era.

The Genesis of an Indian Pharmaceutical Industry: An Illustration of Non-alignment

While the genesis of the Indian pharmaceutical industry may be ascribed to the British, as the first factory was established in 1901 in Kolkata, its purpose was not production for the local market—which was almost non-existent at the time (at the time, allopathic medicine was used exclusively by the British)—but the processing of local raw materials for their export to England. Thus, this was a typical model of colonial exploitation.[6] At the time of India's Independence in 1947, while allopathic practice had begun to spread in the subcontinent, drug supplies were still marked by dependence. Foreign multinationals controlled 80 per cent of the market, and technology transfers and local investments were almost non-existent. According to UNICEF, the prices of allopathic drugs in India were among the highest in the world. This situation cannot but remind one of the current status in a number of African countries.

Faced with this situation, the government soon tried to improve people's access to drugs. The Indian government's desire to ensure the availability of inexpensive allopathic drugs went in step with the launch of major public health projects aimed at trying to improve the country's catastrophic health conditions at the time. It is against this background that the country developed strategies and methods advocated by the

WHO: creation of a hierarchical network of public health care centres, exemption from payment for such care, launching of vaccination campaigns and birth control policy through family planning. At the same time, the government gave official recognition to the traditional medicines still extensively used by the people. Until the 1970s, the development of the pharmaceutical industry was closely linked to the industrial planning policy instituted by the government. Thanks to the creation of public sector units with the help of WHO, UNICEF or the Soviet Union, such as Hindustan Antibiotic Limited (HAL) in 1956 or the Indian Drug and Pharmaceuticals Limited (IDPL) in 1961, the government was slowly able to reduce the prices of some essential drugs (up to almost 60 per cent for products such as penicillin and other anti-infectious drugs). But it soon became clear that in spite of all this, the public sector could not cater to local needs by itself. The market remained dominated by foreign multinationals and local companies produced less than 25 per cent of market needs (Lanjouw, 1997).

From the 1970s onwards, following the public sector's mixed results in the face of the dynamism of multinationals in the local market, the government adopted several original legislative schemes that would have a major impact on India's industrial profile.

The introduction of the Indian Patent Act, which came into force in 1972, is probably the main explanatory factor behind the dazzling growth of the Indian pharmaceutical industry. This text considerably weakened the legislation on intellectual property rights inherited from colonial times by not recognizing invention patents (product patents) for food and pharmaceutical products, but only patents on manufacturing processes (process patents) for a period of 5–7 years. Until then, India had a very strong intellectual property protection system. Towards the end of the 1960s, an expert committee (Ayyangar Committee) that favoured modifying the pre-existing system, noted that 80–90 per cent of patents were held by foreign firms as a means for the firms of erstwhile colonizers to retain total control of the market and thereby, to ensure dependence. Thus, the recognition of product patents had legally stopped India from importing medicinal drugs from more competitive sources. It is interesting to point out that Organisation for Economic Cooperation and Development (OECD) countries only introduced such patent systems when their economies reached a much higher level of development. For instance, Japan introduced drug patents in 1976,

Switzerland in 1977, Netherlands in 1978, Spain and Norway in 1992 (Subramanian, 2004).

This new law enabled Indian industry to take flight and develop new manufacturing processes (reverse engineering) for the active substances imported by multinationals. It therefore began to offer a competitive advantage to local industrialists who could sell a large spectrum of medicines while saving on the enormous research and development costs. This legislation helped in developing real knowhow in the field of chemical synthesis, which currently gives India a sizeable competitive advantage in the face of the recent mushrooming of 'generics manufacturers' in the world. For instance, this is how the Indian Institute of Chemical Technology developed AZT without reproducing the patent owner's (Burroughs-Wellcome) manufacturing process. The technique was then transferred to Cipla, the fourth-largest Indian player in the field. The process was then sold to a Brazilian producer. Another example: in 1996, seven years after the introduction of Ciproflaxine (under patent), 48 Indian businesses produced this drug in India.

In the same way, by raising considerable tariff barriers, the government limited imports of formulations and obliged industrialists to purchase a part of their raw materials from the local market. Within the framework of Foreign Exchange Regulation Act (FERA), multinationals had to limit their share in their Indian subsidiaries to 40 per cent. Finally, in 1962, strict drug price regulations were adopted Drug Price Control Order (DPCO), in particular for active substances essential to public health. The Indian market soon lost its attraction for foreign firms and several left the subcontinent at this time. Simultaneously price controls obliged firms to optimize their manufacturing costs.

Since 1991, the government has been gradually liberalizing the subcontinent's economy. Little by little, India's health system has adopted a more liberal model of 'managed care', carried forward by foreign firms in search of new markets, international institutions, and investments by the Indian diaspora.[7] The pharmaceutical sector too has followed this trend. Since 2001, foreign firms can once again open offices and units in India, holding 100 per cent of their shares, and on an equal footing with Indian firms with regard to legislations. In spite of these changes in the Indian legislative landscape and the renewal of interest on the part of foreign multinationals, the domestic industry continued to increase its market shares during the 1990s (Table 6.1). The market share of foreign companies decreased from 75 per cent in 1991 to 35 per cent currently (ICRA, 2002).

TABLE 6.1: ACTORS INVOLVED IN THE INDIAN PHARMACEUTICAL INDUSTRY (1970–93)

	1970	1982	1993
Multinationals	80	50	39
Indian Private Sector	10	48	60
Indian Public Sector	10	2	1

Source: H. Redwood, *New Horizons in India: The Consequences of Pharmaceutical Patent Protection*, Felixstowe: Oldwick Press, 1994.

Current Profile of the Indian Pharmaceutical Industry

The results of India's pharmaceutical policies are very convincing. Besides a decline in the number of multinationals present at the local level, India's domestic industry now meets about 90 per cent of the country's requirements in active pharmaceutical ingredients and almost the totality of its needs in formulations. In 2003, its turnover was estimated at USD 6 billion and at USD 25 billion in 2010. The sector employs close to 500,000 people and about 2.40 million indirectly (OPPI, 2002).

The Indian market is currently characterized by a marginal public sector (2 per cent of drugs sold) and a dynamic private sector consisting of a few large Indian groups (Ranbaxy, Cipla, Dr Reddy, Cadila, Lupin, Torrent, etc.), and foreign multinationals, surrounded by a dense network of small local enterprises whose number is currently estimated to be 17,000 (OPPI, 2004). However, this figure should be considered with caution. Most of these small enterprises make formulations, an activity that calls for very low investments and practically no major technological requirements. The government has long encouraged this sector through enterprise development assistance and exemptions of various taxes.[8] This probably explains the considerable rise in the number of these units. These production units essentially meet regional demands, on the one hand because their sales reasoning is often dependent on local networks (especially caste networks), and on the other hand because in any case, they can be competitive in price terms only at the local level, where they still manage to stimulate demand by offering substantial margins to dealers. It must be noted that some of these enterprises (the biggest) work on the basis of subcontracts for medium and large companies.

The large number of pharmaceutical companies can clearly be seen in Figure 6.2, which shows the geographical distribution of pharmaceutical industries per district. Several hubs can be identified. The main hub (in terms of the number of units) is located along the Gujarat coast, up to Mumbai. The location is far from surprising since the subcontinent's petrochemical activities are concentrated in this area. The presence of free zones, exempt of import taxes on raw materials and producer's goods in this area, has long enabled this nascent industry to obtain active pharmaceutical ingredient supplies. A second, spatially more diffused hub can be seen in the Delhi region. The industrial spread observed here illustrates the metropolization that is taking place in this area. Apart from these two main hubs, the remaining units have chosen to establish themselves in the subcontinent's main metros. Kolkata is probably a historic hub inherited from British times. But Hyderabad, Bangalore and, to a lesser degree, Chennai, are emerging pharmaceutical production hubs.

On the whole, in terms of the actors, a trend towards market concentration at the top of the hierarchy can be observed. Between 1995 and 2000, the share of the 20 main drug producers in the pharmaceutical sector's turnover rose from 28.6 per cent to 40.2 per cent. This trend can be explained by several factors. First of all, this dynamic illustrates the determination of big businesses to consolidate their activities through mergers and acquisitions. Secondly, many of them have turned toward the manufacture of formulations (more profitable than bulk drugs), and what is more, in the most profitable therapeutic segments (anti-diabetes, cardiovascular and central nervous system formulations). However, despite this, the fragmented nature (number of actors) of the industry makes the sector very competitive and partly explains the low prices prevailing. Indeed, the average price of a medicine in India stands at just 3 to 15 per cent of the price of the same medicine sold in the United States. In 2001, the price of one month's treatment of Hydrochlorothiazide was USD 0.17 in India, whereas it cost USD 11.65 in the United States (Lopert et al., 2002).

Implementation of the TRIPS Agreements in India

Given this background, and considering India's historic choices, we are better able to understand why the rollout of the TRIPS Agreements in India following its economic liberalization and its membership of the WTO has generated so much debate and polemics. Many view

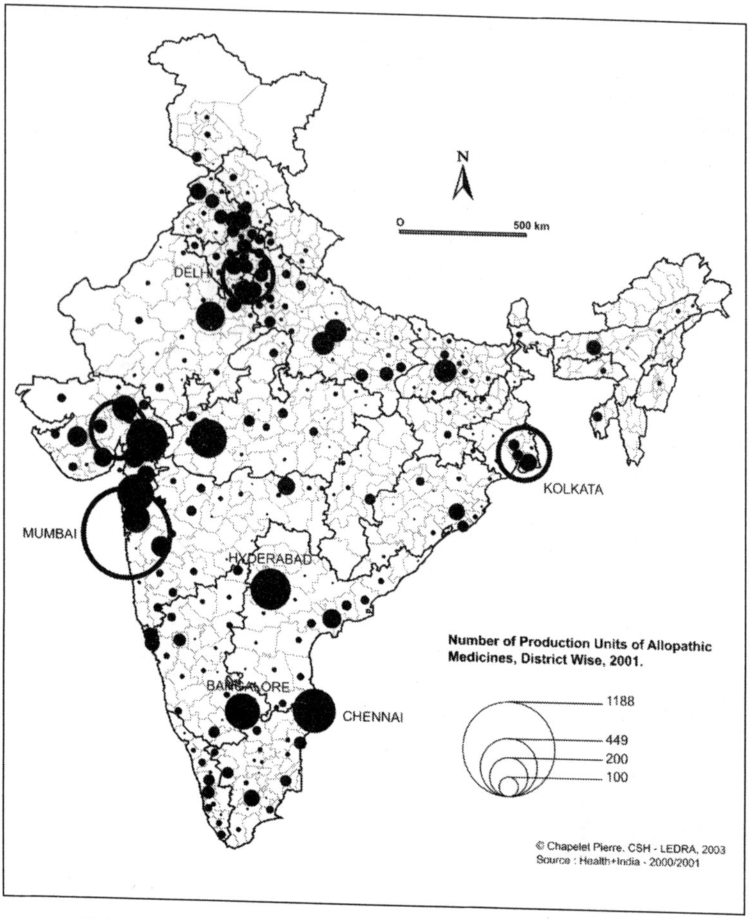

FIGURE 6.2: ALLOPATHIC PHARMACEUTICAL INDUSTRY PRODUCTION UNITS, 2001.

them as backtracking, with all the negative consequences suffered during the country's colonial and post-Independence history in terms of access to medicines.

Yet, by signing the TRIPS Agreements on 15 April 1994 and in spite of the strong opposition offered by fervent defenders of public health as well as by most Indian industrialists,[9] the reality is that India had until 2005 to fully implement the legislation on patents. From this date onwards, local industry is no longer able to copy any medicine without paying royalty to the patent owners. In order to comply with these rules, the Indian Parliament has already adopted three amendments to the 1970 Patent Act (in 2000, 2002 and 2005).[10]

In terms of the industrial landscape, multinationals and leading Indian industrialists believe that the pharmaceutical sector is mature enough now and that this change is necessary, so that the Indian industry moves toward R&D, rather than following the 'reverse engineering' model that it has in the past. The most optimistic scenario thus foresees an increase in multinational investments in research activities and clinical trials. And the same picture is painted by the specialized technical media, which regularly highlights India's potential in the field of biomedical and pharmaceutical research, explaining that the Indian model enabled it to develop adequate technical expertise, which very few developing countries can boast of (refer to Figure 6.1). At the same time, they underline the existence of a large pool of qualified scientific personnel and fairly low production costs, factors likely to convince industrialists to invest here.

It is true that there are some factors that support such a view. Some companies have already initiated such changes by beginning to develop research activities. Dr. Reddy's Laboratories was the first Indian company to set up a research programme in the early 1990s. It currently claims to spend 10 per cent of its income on R&D. Three molecules are currently in the clinical development phase. Other companies, such as Ranbaxy, Cipla, Wockhardt and Nicholas Piramal, claim to spend 5 per cent of their revenue on R&D. There is also a lot being said about collaborations between multinational and Indian companies in this field, such as the one between Ranbaxy and GlaxoSmithKline.

However, the extent of these activities remains very limited. First of all, only a very small section of Indian industrialists is concerned (less than ten or so). If the Indian pharmaceutical industry's overall revenue is taken into account, the share of R&D activities represents just 1.9 per cent. Faced with the 10 to 15 per cent spent by multinational companies, this is a very low figure. Furthermore, infrastructural problems remain (India lacks certain costly facilities) and some fields of expertise are insufficiently developed (such as molecular biology), which could dissuade foreign businesses from establishing themselves in India. Especially when other actors on the international stage, such as China, Singapore and Ireland are also trying to capture multinational R&D investments.

That is why many researchers tend to assert that multinational R&D or even production activities may remain marginal in India.[11] On the other hand, the opening of the market could well incite them to once again adopt import-based strategies, in particular by acquiring so far independent Indian businesses in order to take advantage of their distribution networks and thereby develop their presence in the Indian market (Malhotra and Lofgren, 2004). In any case, it is clear that these companies will try to consolidate their position. Let us not forget that in demographic terms, India potentially represents the biggest pharmaceutical market in the world (after China, at present).

Is India an Emerging Actor on the International Stage?

The formidable growth of the Indian pharmaceutical industry was accompanied by an increase in exports of Indian medicines. Currently, exports account for a large proportion of India's production. Close to half the income of the biggest firms—such as Ranbaxy, Dr. Reddy's or Cipla—comes from exports. India is trying to find a place for itself in the emerging international generics market. Indian industrialists hope to secure a share in this market by taking advantage of their lead with regard to capacity and production costs. However, as we will see, this sector is very competitive and India will have to face the advent of very dynamic new actors on the international stage, such as China.

The export growth curve shown in Figure 6.3 is impressive. Whereas in the early 1980s, there were barely any exports, they grew exponentially, with a net acceleration in the beginning of the 1990s. This acceleration can be partly explained by the export promotion policies implemented since the country's economic liberalization in 1991. The growth in export values has been 10 per cent per year for about ten years now (Economist Intelligence Unit, database 2003) and the trade balance has favoured exports since the 1990s.

Currently, exports essentially consist of formulations, although active pharmaceutical ingredients are catching up gradually. Overall, while India exports drugs from all the therapeutic segments, antibiotics represent a major share (27 per cent). Then come medicines for the treatment of respiratory diseases (particularly asthma) (8 per cent). Exports of analgesics and Non-steroidal Anti-inflammatory Drugs (NSAIDs) are both formulations and active substances, most based on old molecules (ibuprofen or paracetamol). The share of medicines for

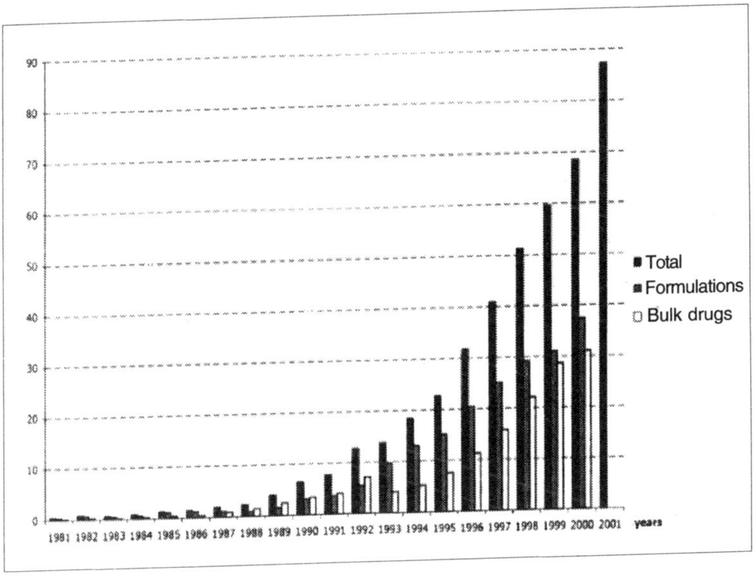

Source: Mittal (1993), OPPI (2001).

FIGURE 6.3: EVOLUTION OF EXPORTATIONS 1981–2000 (RS. MILLIONS)

the treatment of lifestyle related diseases (CVS, CNS, anti-diabetes) and of specialized medicines (cancer, AIDS) is fairly low and is solely directed towards developing countries in Asia and Africa. As several of the molecules used in these therapeutic segments are still under patent, margins are very high.

To better understand the situation of India's pharmaceutical industry within the world market, we have mapped country-wise growth in export volumes (in value terms) and the associated growth rates, from 1996 to 2004 (Figure 6.4). One of the main limitations of this set of maps is the absence of country-wise data before 1996, as it would have been even more interesting to be able to study these trends since the start of the 1980s. To summarize, until the mid-1980s, India exported its products rather diffidently to the former Soviet countries, as well as to South-East Asian, African and Latin American countries. Nevertheless, this set of maps gives us an idea of the situation over the last ten years and shows that the growth of Indian exports was due largely to a strengthening of flows towards the controlled markets of the major industrialized countries since the early 1990s. Thus, the United States

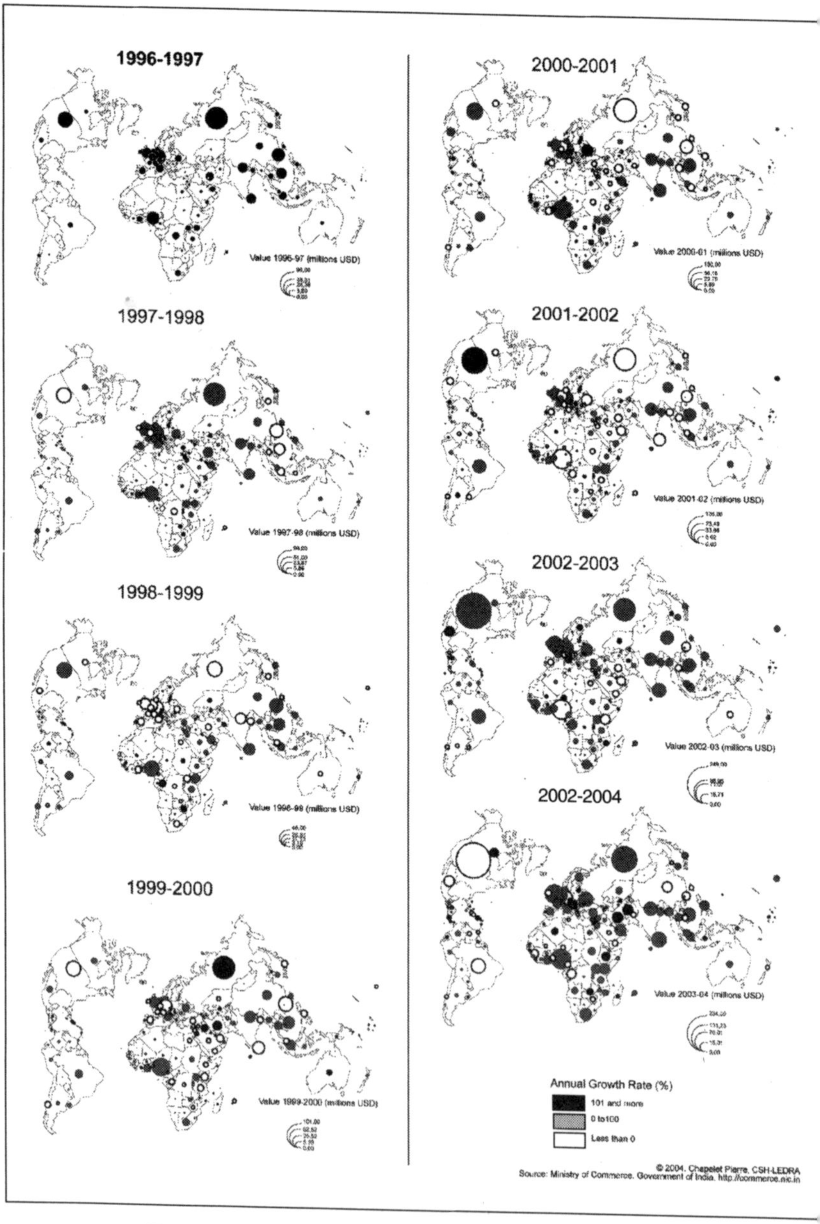

FIGURE 6.4: EVOLUTION OF INDIAN EXPORTS OF PHARMACEUTICALS 1996–2004

is presently the preferred destination for Indian exports. Exports to Europe are also strengthening, though less markedly. This can probably be explained by the desire of European Union countries to promote trade between member countries. Besides the impressive increase in volume during the period, for instance towards USA or Russia, it is interesting to note that Indian medicines are gradually being distributed in a growing number of countries. The conquest of the African continent from English-speaking countries such as Nigeria or South Africa is clearly unveiled, as well as the strengthering of Indian exports in Middle East and South America. Finally, the regional role India plays must also be noted, as it supplies medicines to Sri Lanka, Nepal, Bangladesh and even Pakistan.

Figure 6.5 summarizes these developments, showing the country-wise growth in exports between 1996 and 2004. Rather than merely mapping the growth rate, we preferred to compare the country-wise volume of exports between 1996 and 2004, with a linear adjustment between the values observed in these two years. This modelling has enabled us to highlight unexpected developments during the period, such as the fact that the United States is importing a much greater volume of Indian medicines presently than could be envisaged on the basis of the situation in 1996. On the other hand, although exports to Russia increased in absolute terms from 1996 to 2004, there has been a net slowdown. Hence, a rather interesting geography can be seen, one that reveals the strategy of Indian businesses at the international level.

One set of countries consists of those whose ties with Indian industrialists became more pronounced after 1996. North America, Brazil, Great Britain, Ukraine and Finland can be found at the forefront of this group. Then come a few African countries such as Nigeria, Algeria, South Africa and Ethiopia, as well as Turkey, the United Arab Emirates, Afghanistan, Myanmar and the Philippines.

On the other hand, a second set consists of countries whose observed exports in 2004 have been lower than the situation in 1996 would have led one to believe. Apart from Russia, two sub-sets can be seen in the map: on the one hand, some European countries (Germany, Netherlands, Switzerland, Italy and Belgium), and on the other hand, several South-East Asian countries (Hong Kong, which is increasingly relying on Chinese imports, Vietnam and Singapore).

Finally these documents clearly show to what extent India has been able to position itself as a generic manufacturer to be reckoned with on

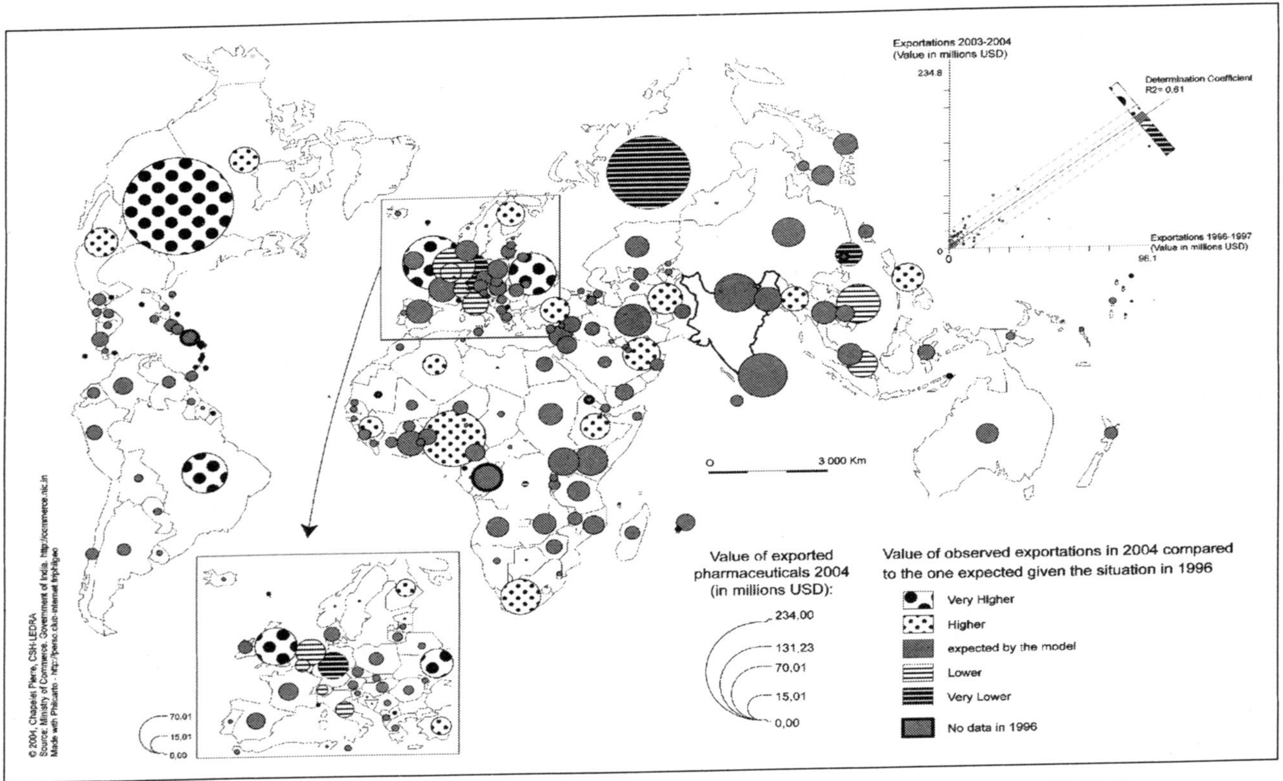

FIGURE 6.5: INDIAN EXPORTATIONS OF PHARMACEUTICALS BY COUNTRY VALUE IN 2004 AND TRENDS 1996–2004

the international stage, one that has also taken advantage of opportunities made available by the slow implementation of the TRIPS Agreements and the variety of State legislations. They also unveil the rising number of competitors on the international stage, who are slowing down the distribution of Indian medicines in some regions.

On the one hand, the subcontinent exports formulations as (non-patented) generic products to 'developed' countries. It thereby meets the demand of a number of countries with healthcare systems that are in search of savings. To do so, it relies on the fact that many of its factories are accredited by production monitoring bodies United States Food and Drugs Administration (USFDA) for the United States, United Kingdom Medicines Central Agency (UKMCA) for England. Thus, India is the country with the largest number of production units accredited by the USFDA, outside America. All this helps us better understand how Indian businesses succeeded in capturing close to 4 per cent of the American generics market, currently valued at USD 16 billion. For big Indian firms such as Ranbaxy, the American market constituted an opportunity that enabled it to globalize its activities, especially by counting on the revenue generated to diversify its activities to include R&D.[12] Several different strategies were adopted. Whereas firms like Ranbaxy created their own distribution network, others like Lupin or Wockhardt entered into the American market through joint ventures. Others, like Cipla, preferred to target the sale of active pharmaceutical ingredients to American firms. India is currently the country that submits the largest number of active pharmaceutical ingredients registration applications in the USA: today, a quarter of the applications for the sale of formulations in America come from Indian companies. However, some reservations were expressed lately on India's 'American pharmaceutical dream'.[13] Of course, the success of some of these firms is enviable and there are an increasing number of Indian players in the American market (particularly medium-scale firms working as sub-contractors for American firms). But, in the same way, it is possible that prices may fall and there is no warranty that the enormous sums invested by the precursors will be recovered in the long term, especially since competition is only increasing in the international generics market, as we will see.

Indian firms also export unbranded formulations against tenders from some African and Latin American countries, as well as branded formulations to relatively badly controlled markets such as Nigeria or East Europe. In Russia, for instance, the Prisolec marketed by

Dr. Reddy's is the drug with the highest sales for heartburn (acidity). Indian medicines are also present in Senegal's illegal market as well as in several West African countries. Their low price has led to parallel (illegal) distribution channels, through certain inter-state marketing networks. It is likely that medicines reach African countries that allow Indian medicine imports and are then re-exported through informal channels to countries whose laws disallow the import of these medicines. Nigeria has been identified as a major supply source for such networks in West Africa.

On the other hand, Indian industrialists are currently taking advantage of the differences in legislations in different countries and the slow implementation of the TRIPS Agreements within domestic laws to export their products. Thus, while India exports low priced generics to industrialized countries, it also offers copies of patented medicines or active substances to countries with low production capacities whose intellectual property laws are still somewhat nebulous or ineffective. Indian industrialists try to take advantage of the exclusion provisions still contained in the TRIPS Agreements and confirmed in Doha to export drugs for which they do not hold invention patents, in particular the principle of parallel imports and of compulsory licensing. In cases of 'national emergency' or public non-commercial use—terms that every country has to define precisely in its legislation—the former allows a country to import drugs from low-price sources such as India and to short-circuit the patent owner's exclusive marketing rights. The latter allows a country to set up low-priced local production facilities by allowing a private corporation or public organization to produce the drug, although it may be protected by a patent under normal circumstances. However, these clauses have to be explicitly specified in the laws and the diplomatic and commercial pressures exerted by patent-owning multinationals, through their governments, slow down their application considerably. The difficulties faced by the Brazilian government in setting up a local ARV drug production facility within the framework of its public anti-HIV/AIDS programme constitutes a striking example in this regard.[14] There is a similar example in South Africa, where Cipla had proposed a triple-therapy for USD 350 per person per year in 2001, whereas multinationals were offering the same at USD 10,000–12,000 (IDMA, 2004). Wanting to use its parallel import rights, the South African government immediately found itself facing a suit filed by the multinationals concerned. Despite all the pressure it had to face, the extensive coverage this occurrence was given in the media finally obliged the patent-owning firms to withdraw their suits in order to retain their credibility with the public. It also soon obliged them to lower their prices considerably.[15] Thus, several Indian companies started advocating the cause of access to medicines all over the world, asserting that they were able to produce pharmaceutical products that were still unaffordable in several developing countries in large volumes and to distribute them at very low prices. Conversely, one may wonder whether this discourse, however laudable, does not conceal obvious commercial interests in conquering new markets or strengthening trading positions. In fact, the cause of access to medicines enables Indian firms to strengthen their commercial ties or weave new ones with a number of countries, particularly African countries. Indian expertise is being increasingly used here for setting up production facilities. Again, Indian firms have promoted an image of the high quality of their products. However, a number of events have tarnished this image such as Ranbaxy's and Cipla's recent announcement that they were withdrawing several of their antiretroviral products from the world market following a WHO notice criticizing the validity of the bio-equivalence tests their products had undergone.[16]

While it may be clear that the TRIPS Agreements will shortly forbid Indian firms from exporting products for which they do not hold patents, it is nonetheless true that they have been able to position themselves in the international market by distributing their products all across the globe. Thus, with regard to the production of generic drugs, India undoubtedly stands out as a major producer on the international stage. However, the country's economic opening has complicated this situation and India will now have to face international competition in both the world and local markets.

Figure 6.6 shows the volume of drug imports in value terms in 2004. The same method that was adopted for the study of exports has been used here. Thus, the trends prevailing since 1996 can be seen. In the first place, if we compare the values observed with those of Figure 6.5 shows a very low level of imports *vis-à-vis* exports (in value terms). While they are increasing (22 per cent growth from 1991 to 2001), they remain far lower in absolute value. They essentially consist of organic compounds, biologic cultures (microorganism cultures), antibiotics, vaccines and vitamins. Active substances represent a major part of Indian imports (76 per cent).

Figure 6.5 reflects several phenomena. First of all, it highlights the activities of the multinationals present in the Indian market, which

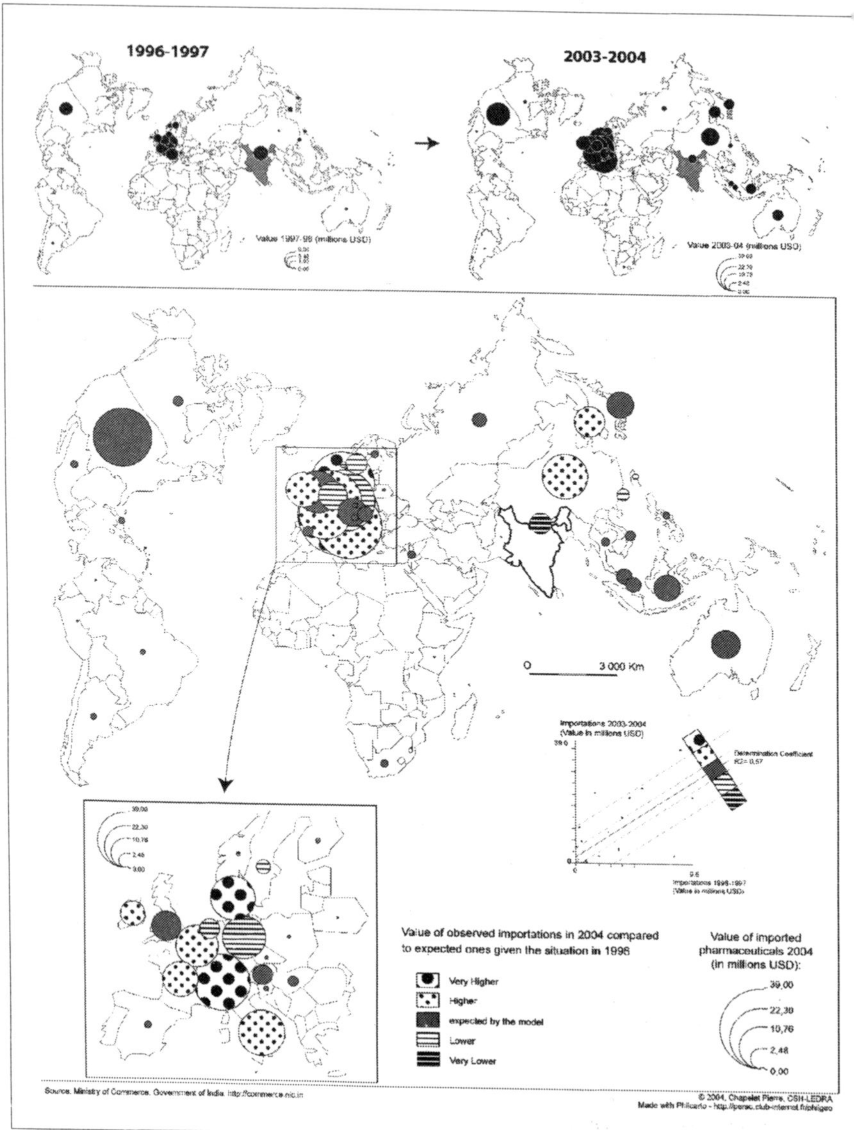

FIGURE 6.6: INDIAN IMPORTATIONS OF PHARMACEUTICALS BY COUNTRY VALUES AND TRENDS 1996–2004.

export their products mainly from Europe and the US (mainly antibiotics, vaccines and vitamins). A strengthening of flows from Europe can be observed, which tends to confirm that, at least at the moment, European multinationals prefer to increase drug exports to India rather than to set up production facilities there. Secondly it throws light on the growing role of countries like China and Korea in Indian supplies. These two actors are emerging on the international stage in the active pharmaceutical ingredients sector, where they are very competitive, to such an extent that Indian firms are themselves importing an increasing volume of products from these countries.

Finally, to return to the geographical problematic presented in the introduction, the preceding paragraphs have enabled us to give an account of the reconstruction of (pharmaceutical) networks currently underway, which develop on the basis of the opportunities offered by the territories in which they grow. More precisely, the changes in inter- and intra-State laws have a structural and functional impact on drug distribution networks (from the way production is organized to the distribution structure) and new polarities are developed in the world pharmaceutical system. Thus, India enjoys a unique position, essentially due to the ability it has displayed in managing to limit the activities of external networks and to promote its own networks in order to improve the access to drugs on its own soil. However, the opening of its economy and its concomitant incorporation into broader trade networks can no longer allow it to remain on the sidelines, but have obliged it to bring its domestic laws into compliance with international laws, such as the TRIPS Agreements. So it seems that the chapter that could be called the 'Indian Way' concerning drug production has come to an end. On the other hand, if India turns the page, the chapter it wrote has enabled its networks to occupy an increasingly important position internationally. Moreover, Indian networks were very clever at playing with the differences in the legislations of different countries and with the loopholes in the interpretation of the TRIPS Agreements in order to promote the distribution of their medicines all over the world. Despite all this, the pressure is increasing and many see the emergence of India's industry as increasingly disturbing and dangerous competition. Thus, the National Health Service—the powerful British health authority—filed a suit against Ranbaxy's English subsidiary and four other laboratories in June 2005, for abuse of dominant position, organized under-stocking, illegal price agreements and over-invoicing of products. The overall estimated value of the damage caused stood at USD 175 billion.[17]

The Realities of Access to Pharmaceuticals in India

The previous paragraphs showed India's formidable drug production capacity. Considering this situation, it seems obvious that these products should be easily available to its own people. But the reality is not as simple. In spite of its production and innovation capacities and despite the Central Government's extensive efforts to improve health care since Independence, only 35 per cent Indians currently have access to essential drugs (Swain et al., 2002). To understand this paradoxical situation, we now propose that the reader take a closer look at the local situation to better understand the modalities of access to drugs in India.

While many see an underlying concept of accessibility within the concept of access, accessibility does not capture the whole complexity of the modalities of drug use. Just because a pharmacy or a Primary Health Centre (PHC) can be found in a place does not mean that the use or recourse to medicines is necessarily effective there. Hence, our study will rely on a broader definition of access, based on the works of Thomas and Penchansky (1981). Although dating back to 1981, their work still offers the advantage of proposing a relevant conceptual framework for the analysis of access. They divide the concept into five dimensions: Availability, Accessibility, Accommodation (convenience), Affordability and Acceptability. Let us see how we can characterize each of these dimensions in India.

Analysed in terms of *accessibility*, i.e. ease of physical access to a drug-distributing infrastructure, it is true that access to medicines seems fairly easy in India. The large number of pharmacies in Indian cities well illustrates this.[18] In a city like Coimbatore (almost 1.5 million inhabitants in 2001), for instance, we were able to calculate an average service rate of 3,500 inhabitants per pharmacy in 1998, which is close to that of European countries like France. However, this number conceals a high level of intra-urban variations on the one hand and on the other, it is far from representative of the situation in rural areas. Despite all this, while the countryside may be less well covered than the cities, pharmacies cover Indian territory fairly well on the whole. This is perhaps due to the fact that they are often associated with a neighbourhood business, though one whose location is not controlled by the government, unlike the case in countries like France. In fact, it is rare for them to be absent in any marketplace, shopping area or communication hub. The choices made in the location of pharmacies are quite revealing of the commercial logic of cooperation underlying their activities. Figure 6.7 shows the location of health care infrastructure in a central area of the city of Coimbatore (Tamil Nadu). The first observation concerns the impressive number of pharmacies, with an obvious concentration along commercial arteries. Moreover, through the contiguities it reveals, Figure 6.7 clearly shows the relational connections between pharmacies and health care infrastructure. First of all, it may be seen that the clinics are established in the periphery, along major road arteries, and that few pharmacies are close by, as these establishments have their own pharmacies. On the other hand, it is astonishing to see to what extent the logic of cooperation between pharmacies and practitioners—whether general physicians or specialists—can be seen simply through their spatial proximity, for instance to the east of bus stand where there is nearly one pharmacy per physician. The same spatial configuration can be found in all the areas shown in the map. Their location close to the bus stand reinforces the idea of a desire to optimize potential customer uptake by positioning themselves close to areas with large population flows.

While it may be obvious that the absolute number of public infrastructure facilities is far lower than the number of pharmacies, the health coverage of public services is nonetheless very reasonable. Figure 6.8 compares the pharmacy establishment logic with, for instance, the public dispensary establishment logic in Gurgaon, in Delhi's periphery. These diagrams represent the establishment choices of these facilities on the basis of the land use of the city under study. In the case of pharmacies, the raised figures surveyed corroborate the preceding observations: 90 per cent of trading areas are less than 600 m away from a pharmacy, while industrial areas seem to be far more repulsive to such facilities. The choice of specific locations is clearly visible, in favour of certain types of land use urban fabric rather than others. If we now compare the pharmacy distribution graph with the one for dispensaries, we will note immediately that the curves are far closer, underlining a more homogeneous coverage by public infrastructure. However, although it does cover a majority of patients, notably the poorest, the public health care system is increasingly unable to meet their expectations. The shortage or absence of medicines, the lack of facilities or the absence of physicians who prefer consultations in their joint private clinics has long been noted.[19] It would appear that the public sector's acceptability rating is falling to the benefit of the private sector, which, with its current 13 per cent growth rate, is gradually

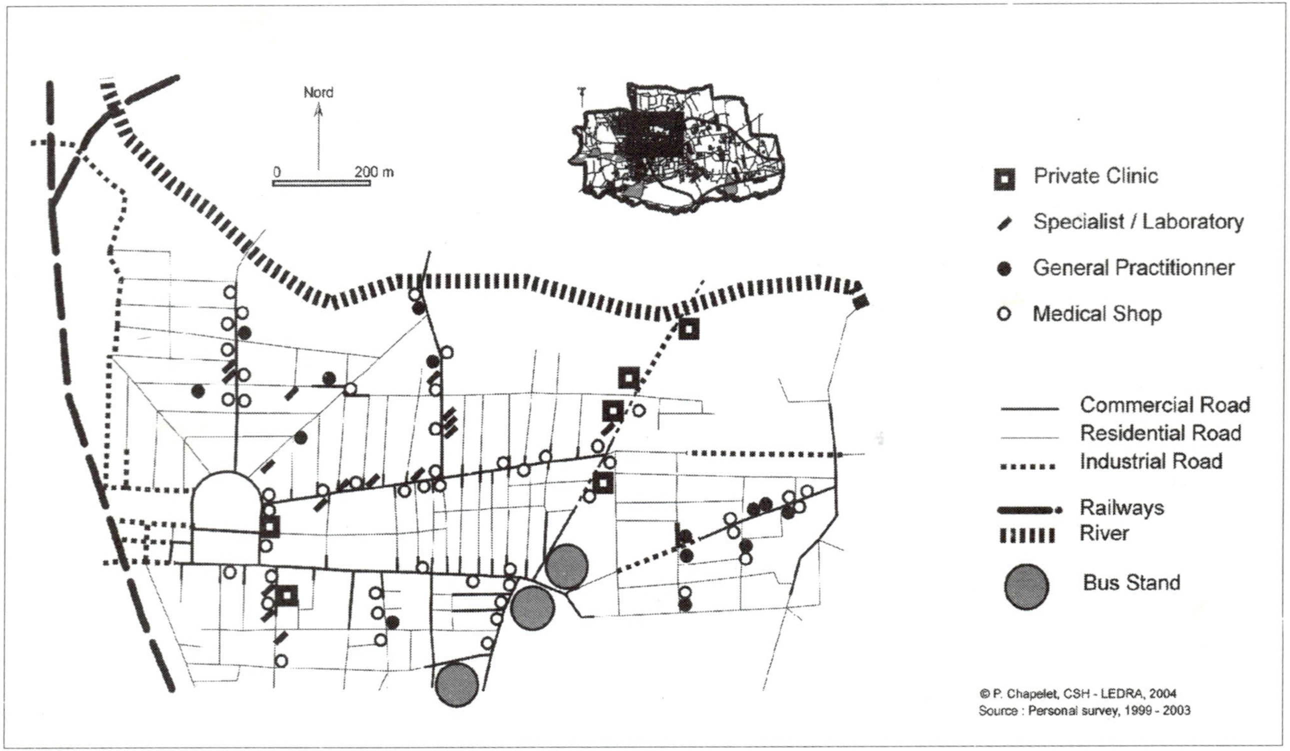

FIGURE 6.7: LOCATION STRATEGY OF HEALTH CARE INFRASTRUCTURES COIMBATORE (1999)—TAMIL NADU

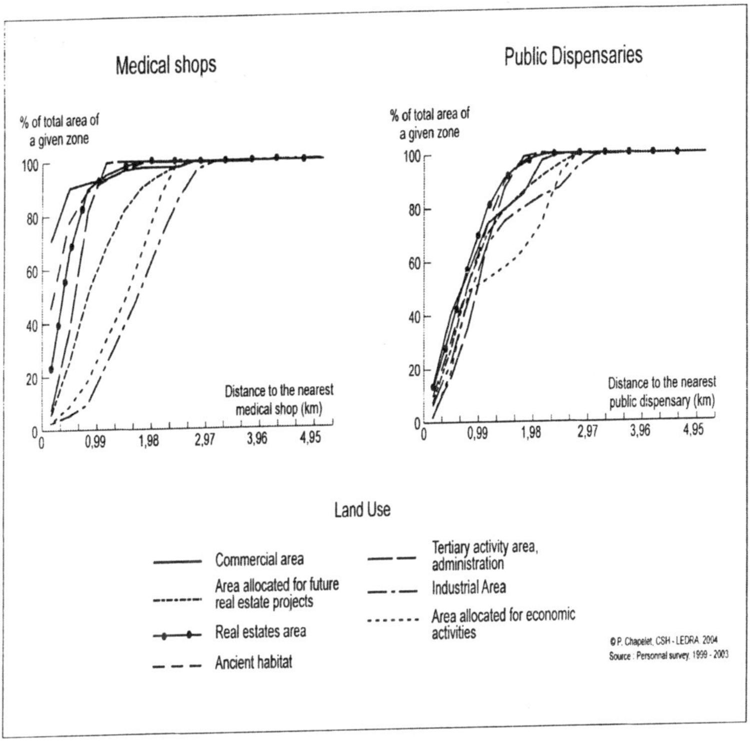

FIGURE 6.8: LOCATION OF MEDICAL SHOPS AND DISPENSARIES ACCORDING TO LAND USE (GURGAON, 2003)

gaining the upper hand.[20] Besides, it is this shortage of medicines, often decried by the media, which is evidently the reason behind the spatial proximity of private pharmacies to public health facilities.

This leads us to broach the issue of the *availability* of medicines in India and, as we will see, the picture immediately becomes a little more complex. Whereas the urban hierarchy serves as a framework for the spread of private facilities, certain 'islands of excellence' have also emerged in cities, to meet the demand of an emerging (essentially urban) middle class,[21] estimated at over 100 million inhabitants (for purposes of comparison, this equals 40 per cent of the American pharmaceutical market. Furthermore, the contours of this middle class are highly controversial. Following the emergence of the consumer society, pathological profiles vary considerably within society. Thus, while the Indian demographic giant still remains a badly controlled reservoir of infectious diseases (such as tuberculosis, AIDS, leprosy, acute respiratory infections, polio, rabies and viral hepatitis) and of deficiency diseases, today, stress overload and degeneration pathologies are increasingly being added (diabetes, cancers, cardiovascular diseases, etc.), along with a growing number of sociopathies. In the same way, in spite of the diversity of pathologies (which will, besides, ensure the sustainability of the pharmaceutical sector in India for a long time), the emergence of a sound demand tends to direct pharmaceutical production towards drugs that are increasingly focused on population groups that are ready to pay a high price for their health care. Thus, although anti-infectious drugs (penicillin, ampicillin) still largely dominate the market (26 per cent), their share is decreasing. On the contrary, the rate of introduction of products in the 'lifestyle drug' segment is very high—such as drugs to control diabetes, for the treatment of cardiovascular diseases or the central nervous system or for the treatment of respiratory problems. The most recent generations of antibiotics (cephalosporins) are also growing very fast,[22] and what is more, they are often prescribed for minor ailments. Indeed, many of the country's public health officials are appalled by this practice, as they understandably fear the emergence of greater resistance to such drugs and, therefore, their ineffectiveness in the future.

The aggressive trade practices of pharmaceutical corporation is supporting the extensive use of treatments that are often unjustified for a given ailment. Due to strong competition at the local level, these firms often adopt questionable marketing practices. Once again, the phenomenal growth of the private health care sector and the emergence of a solvent demand have turned drugs into a major commercial issue at the local level, one that the government still finds difficult to control. Whereas the marketing plans of pharmaceutical companies usually target doctors in countries like the United States or Europe, in India, the key role played by pharmacies in drug distribution leads firms to adopt doubtful marketing strategies to gain space on dealers' shelves and to increase their sales. An article published in the *Indian Express*[23] in September 2001 gave an account of the sales promotion techniques used by companies. The most popular of the rewards—the 'plan bonus'—offered one free tablet for about every 10 tablets ordered by the pharmacist. A survey carried out by Interlink Healthcare Consultancy showed that with the exception of one, India's primary 25 pharmaceutical companies offered this kind of transaction at least once a month.

Besides, close to half these offers were for antibiotics, which are already over-used or badly used.

It seems that finally, at least in the private sector, there is a tendency towards pharmaceutical over-availability. The large number of actors in the market leads to a large number of brands, and their competition results in the desire to sell at any price, whatever the means employed. That is why an increasing number of products containing irrational pharmaceutical combinations can be observed in the market. Thus, in an article, N. Lalitha (2002) wrote that according to a survey conducted in several firms in Gujarat, 86 per cent of the cough syrups sold were irrational formulations or that 85 per cent of anti-diarrhoea products were dubious pharmaceutical specialties with very limited effects. However, these medicines are proliferating. Indeed, monitoring authorities find it difficult to test all the medicines that regularly reach the market. Whereas 30,000 samples are tested every year by the health authorities, this number needs to be increased to 150,000 for these measures to be really effective (Gueniff, 2004; Lalitha, 2002). Besides, as production permits are handled at the level of the federation's states, some producers take advantage of differences in inter-state legislations to sell these products where their marketing is not yet prohibited. Another illustration of over-availability and the difficulty faced by the government in controlling these products is the presence in India of a number of medicines that are prohibited in several other countries and have been withdrawn from their market.[24]

The difficulties the government faces in controlling these products can also be seen in the development of a number of counterfeit drugs in the market. According to the WHO, 35 per cent of counterfeit medicines in the world come from India. It is estimated that close to 20 per cent of the medicines available in the country are fakes.[25]

These issues bring us to the aspect of *convenience* and we soon realize how easy it is to get medicines in India. Let us take another look at the case of pharmacies. These occupy a key position because of the imbalance in the health care system. Due to the public sector's weaknesses, which we will discuss further on, the poorest sections of the population are also turning towards the private sector. As they generally cannot afford to consult a physician due to their lack of means, they rationalize their intinerary in the health care system to such a point that it is often limited to consulting a pharmacist alone. However, pharmacy employees are often not qualified, especially—though not only—in rural areas. While according to the law, a pharmacist is obviously necessary in order to operate a pharmacy, in reality, one is often present only during rush hours, leaving the shop in the hands of less qualified employees the rest of the time. Thus, the choice of treatments is more often dictated by commercial rather than therapeutic rationality. It is often enough to simply go to a pharmacy and ask for antibiotics to get them, without even having to show a prescription. Besides, the antibiotics sold will often be of the latest generation or those for which firms are offering 'marketing' plans, whereas classical antibiotics would normally have sufficed. Even though this example may be somewhat of a caricature of the reality, where one fortunately does find conscientious pharmacists, irrational use of medicines often results from such a situation, with all its known consequences (increasing resistance). Indeed, that is why there has been a recent resurgence of tuberculosis. While it is true that this disease has re-emerged in association with the spread of HIV, it is nonetheless true that over- or under-consumption of treatments, caused by faulty observance, has led to the emergence of multi-resistant strains that current-day remedies are increasingly unable to control.

In terms of *financial capacity*, i.e. the relation between the price of medicines and the capacity of consumers to pay, it seems important to first emphasize the fact that while many say that medicine prices in India are among the lowest in the world, some researchers are less optimistic. They remind us that finally, only the drugs that are normally under patent outside the territory are less expensive. Thus, generic medicines, which as we may remember account for 80 per cent of the Indian market, are often more expensive than in other neighbouring developing countries such as Bangladesh or Sri Lanka (Ramachandran, 2002).

However, the government has always given a priority to drug price controls. With just 4 per cent of population currently covered by health insurance,[26] the majority have to cover health expenses through private financing. It was in 1962, within the framework of Sino-Indian tensions, that the Drug Price Control Order (DPCO) was set up to limit the rise in prices. Until 1966, producers had to obtain government authorization before increasing the prices of their preparations. In 1970, medicinal drugs were brought under the Essential Commodities Act. In the beginning, the producer decided on the price of his drug and in case of profits above 15 per cent of income, all surplus was due to the government. This was a minor intervention with few negative effects on the industry's growth, but on the other hand, it was fairly ineffective with regard to the dominance of multinationals in Indian territory. In 1979, the new DPCO, which had barely changed in the interim, fixed the price of certain active pharmaceutical ingredients and their formulations. But the choice of the drugs listed was the subject of a great deal of criticism. Some essential drugs were barely controlled whereas other more superfluous ones were tightly controlled. Under pressure from pharma firms and the liberalization of the economy, the government was gradually constrained to soften this law. In fact, the industry tended to stop production of the listed drugs and turn toward more lucrative products. That was in part the reason for the regular shortages of TB drugs, iodized salts or chloroquine for malaria that were observed. While the production of malarial drugs stagnated at 35 tonnes per year, imports rose from 52.8 to 166.3 tons between 1978 and 1982 (A. Vaguet, 2004). Under pressure from the pharmaceutical lobby, from 347 drugs at the start, the list was reduced to just 74 in 1995 and a mere 34 in 2002. In 2004, 80 per cent of the formulations were outside the DPCO's framework and prices of many drugs increased. Yet, in some cases, active pharmaceutical ingredients costs fell. In spite of everything, instead of carrying this decrease over to the prices patients had to pay, pharma firms often preferred to increase their trade margins.[27]

Considering this situation (difficulties in price control, irrational prescriptions or bad quality drugs), the central government tries its best to ensure the availability of appropriate medicines in the public health care network. The fact that health management is under the control of the federation's state governments seriously complicates the issue and very few of them have a clear, effective policy concerning pharmaceutical supplies. Nevertheless, little by little, within the framework of WHO's programme for the rational use of medicines (resulting from the Bamako Initiative and the encouraging results obtained in Guinea and Benin), several Indian states are now incorporating encouraging policies favouring the availability of medicines within the public health network. The first such policy began in 1994 in the state of Delhi.

It started with the observation made by the then Minister of Health and Social Affairs (Harsh Vardhan) that despite 30 to 35 per cent of the hospital budget being spent on drugs alone, shortages in essential medicines were chronic, whereas non-indispensable medicines were often over-available. Every hospital had its own list of medicines and until then, a number of products were purchased individually by each of the facilities, which obviously led to higher expenses. Thanks to the preparation of a list of essential medicines and the implementation of a pooled procurement system and an original 'double envelope' system guaranteeing both product quality and very low prices, this programme was an indubitable success for the Indian capital's public health sector. The results were striking, as now, in a hospital like the Aruna Asaf Ali Hospital, 98.3 per cent of prescriptions have to do with essential medicines alone and 97.3 per cent of them are available. For purposes of comparison, in some of the capital's hospitals that are not covered by this programme, only 5 per cent of the drugs prescribed are effectively delivered to the premises. In fact, regrettably, this programme is only operational for health facilities falling under the Delhi State Government for the meantime, whereas several other public actors provide extensive health care services in the capital. For instance, the All India Institute of Medical Sciences, which falls under the central government and is the city's biggest hospital, is not covered by this initiative. It is also interesting to take a look at the hospital's surrounding areas and note the number of private pharmacies that deliver drugs that are not available in the hospital itself. Another point to be underlined has to do with the way this programme was set up. In addition to the collaboration with the WHO, it gave birth to a NGO that now coordinates the project—the Delhi Society for Promotion of Rational Use of Drugs (DSPRUD). The latter acts as a link between the WHO and Indian federal authorities so that what is commonly called 'the Delhi model' can spread to India's other states. Currently, Rajasthan, Punjab, Himachal Pradesh, West Bengal, and Tamil Nadu are setting up this programme, with minor change.[28]

Through this rapid review of the various aspects of access, the local pharmaceutical situation seems paradoxical and it appears that despite the government's efforts, the trend favours the continuation of inequalities. It is true that there are a large number of medicines, and it is true that they are relatively inexpensive. However, a large number of medicines remain inaccessible or, when they are, their use is dictated more often by the patient's or seller's economic rationale rather than by any therapeutic rationale. Finally, the Indian example clearly illustrates the need to set up effective distribution control, which is unfortunately inadequate in our eyes. The over-availability of drugs does not necessarily mean their rational use and therefore the increased effectiveness of treatments—it is often the contrary. Further, we cannot finish this review on access to drugs in India without referring to the case of anti-retroviral drugs, which, better than any other, illustrates the entire paradox of the Indian drug situation. Indeed, whereas India is capable of providing the latest therapies in the international market, these are unfortunately barely accessible to the majority of patients.[29]

CONCLUSION

In this article, we wished to understand the complexity of the issue of access to medicines while trying to correlate the international dynamics involved with more local ones. After placing them in perspective using a geographical approach based on networks and territories interactions, an original situation has been revealed, proving that reconciling economic and health-related objectives is rarely an easy task. Thus, the situation depicted in the first part of this paper showed how Indian pharmaceutical industry networks were able to spread worldwide as well as in the Indian state, using opportunities given by differential territorial policies. However, we highlighted a contrasted situation at the local level where territories seem unable to efficiently regulate these networks, leading to a paradoxical situation of unsatisfactory access to pharmaceuticals in India.

In a WHO report of the 1980s entitled 'The World Pharmaceutical Situation', the authors summarized the Indian situation by concluding, 'India constitutes a paradoxical example where pharmaceutical over-production coexists with a shortage of essential medicines for the treatment of major diseases.' In the present circumstances, the term 'shortage' seems inappropriate. Above all, the dynamics of access to medicines in India and, especially, the rational use of drugs, now rests on the capacity of local actors to set up a regulation and control system in the distribution and sales sector. Finally, despite drafting a policy aimed at meeting the population's health requirements, economic priorities often overtake health priorities. The deregulation taking place could well reinforce this situation and stimulate the irrational use of pharmacopoeias.

NOTES

1. Expressed in constant prices to adjust to inflation, the average annual GDP growth was 3.6 per cent while that of the pharma industry was 14.9 per cent (between 1985 and 1999). WHO estimates.
2. With regard to the notion of equity in health, see A. Cattaneo, 'Equity' in *Health and Development: Focus on Health and the Market*, International Edition of *Cuamm Notizie*, January–April 1997, pp. 14–18.
3. Pharmaceutical markets grew substantially due to changes in consumer patterns in 'developed countries'. While the share of health expenditure in the GDP increased in most of these countries, with a higher rise in the case of

USA, it had also gone up over the previous twenty years in poor countries, although the percentage was lower and did not go beyond 3 per cent of the GDP in Sub-Saharan Africa for instance. It must be noted that while expenses on medicines generally increased, they were not directed at better meeting the need for essential drugs.

4. The situation has barely changed today, and WHO's last report on the pharmaceutical sector (2004) declared that just 10 per cent of R&D in the world was on health problems that constituted 90 per cent of the causes of morbidity. At the same time, as N. Wilbeaux noted, R&D funds were often spent on manufacturing new drugs that did not offer any benefits over and above those of already existing products (the so-called 'me too drugs'). In Switzerland, for instance, of the 300–500 new drugs registered each year, about 99 per cent were based on new formulations or new combinations of drugs already being used. Every year, just 2–8 substances offered real therapeutic benefits as compared to existing preparations. The main consequences of this strategy are that thousands of products are sold, while just a small number of them are necessary. (N. Wilbeaux, 2001, see http://users.skynet.be/gresea/nw_adpic_2_01.html)
5. For the next three years, laboratories that were producing Eflornithine (Aventis, Bristol Myers Squibb) until then, agreed to provide 60,000 doses of the product to *Medecins sans Frontières* as a donation. However, while selective production did restart, it was not because of the generosity or consideration of industrialists but essentially because they had recently discovered that the market for this product was not limited 'only' to the half-million or so people affected by sleeping sickness. In fact, the substance acts on the growth of facial hair and proved to be an interesting substance for depilatory creams! For more information, see in particular, www.msf.fr/site.nsf/pages/sommeiltraitement2.
6. For more clarifications on the profile of India's pharmaceutical industry during the Raj, refer to A. Kumar, 'The Indian Drug Industry Under the Raj, 1860–1920', in Pati et al. (ed.), *Health, Medecine and Empire: Perspectives on Colonial India*, Hyderabad: Orient Longman, pp. 356–85.
7. For more details on these dynamics and the emergence of the private health care sector in India, refer to R.V. Baru, *Private Health Care in India: Social Characteristics and Trends*, New Delhi: Sage Publications, p. 184.
8. Most of these small-scale companies continue to be governed by the 'Loan Licensing System'. Set up in the 1950s in order to take care of any possible production shortfalls in the bigger companies, it initially consisted of permitting the selected establishment of small production units, whose production costs were lower thanks to various reliefs and exemptions, given that they work on the basis of sub-contracts for big industries and thereby help maintain the national production level.
9. The pharmaceutical industry is represented through two organizations. The Indian Drug Manufacturers Association (IDMA) represents domestic firms,

mostly small-scale ones, and is rather adverse to the implementation of the TRIPS Agreements. On the other hand, the Organisation of Pharmaceutical Producers of India (OPPI) represents India's biggest pharmaceutical firms and foreign companies and is a fervent supporter of the strict application of the TRIPS Agreements.

10. For more details on the modalities of the implementation of these agreements, refer to the paper by J. Chaisse and S. Guennif in this volume.
11. While R&D activities may have remained marginal in India, the media is now highlighting India's potential as a platform for clinical trials by overseas firms. According to a report ('For Tough Regulation of Clinical Trials', *Economic Times*, 29 October 2004), 'The very attractiveness of India as a clinical trials destination lies in its huge population and prevalence of a large number of diseases, which makes enrolment of trials relatively easy. Unfortunately much of this recruitable universe is also very poor and ignorant. In a country where a patient loses a kidney while going under the knife for appendicitis, there is a serious risk of the gullible and often hapless masses being exploited.' Information taken from M.N. Kulkarni, 'Drug Makers, Providers and Users: Opportunities and Challenges in Pharma Sector', *Economic and Political Weekly*, vol. 39, no. 50, 11 December 2004.
12. Ranbaxy is currently the world's ninth biggest generics producer. According to a press report, three-quarters of the sales of a company like Ranbaxy are from abroad (and 48 per cent from exports to USA). In January 2004, Ranbaxy was the first Indian firm to set up business in France. J. Joly, 'Inde. Un Tigre dans la pharmacie', *L'Express*, 20 December 2004.
13. See, for instance, the article 'Is the Pharma Dream Over?', *Business World*, 1 November 2004.
14. In fact, the Brazilian government is providing free ARV cocktails within the framework of its anti-HIV/AIDS programme. Other than the recourse to Indian and Chinese imports, it has also found it possible to set up local production facilities in order to circumvent the prices demanded by multinationals, which are deemed excessive, by invoking the national emergency clause under the TRIPS Agreements. Brazil now produces 8 of the 15 products distributed under its programme and should soon be able to produce 5 more. Pressures from foreign pharmaceutical firms that were selling their products on Brazilian soil as well as from the American government had long delayed the establishment of this production facility, although the latter eventually withdrew its complaints in 2001. In relation to this subject, refer to the excellent website: http://www.cptech.org/ip/health/c/brazil. For relevant details about the implementation of the Brazilian programme, see F. Bourdier, 'Les illusions du grand partage', in I. Gobatto (ed.), *Les pratiques de santé dans un monde globalisé*, Karthala—MSHA, 2003, pp. 81–108.
15. For more information on this case, see in particular, http://www.cptech.org/ip/health/sa/

16. See the official WHO announcement: http://www.who.int/mediacentre/news/releases/2004/pr79/en/index.html
17. More recently, the World Health Organisation had officially questioned the actual effectiveness of 10 generic antiretrovirals produced by the company. The issue was crucial: all the credit given to the Indian laboratory could be destroyed. Ranbaxy gave itself less than two months to provide proof of its reliability.
18. The number of pharmacies in India was estimated at 550,000 in 2000. According to the Retail Druggists and Chemists Association, the number of pharmacies had therefore risen fivefold in 20 years. Anant Iyer, 'Rationalising Drug Distribution in India', 2001, http://www.domain-b.com
19. See reports such as O.P. Lathwal and A. Banerjee, 'Availability and Utilization of Major Equipment at District Hospital Gurgaon, Haryana', *Journal of the Academy of Hospital Administration*, vol. 13, no. 2, December 2001, Delhi: All India Institute of Medical Sciences, 2001, pp. 23–8.
20. To get a better idea of the public sector's acceptability, see for example, P. Mahapatra, S. Srilatha and P. Sridhar, 'A Patient Satisfaction Survey in Public Hospitals', *Journal of the Academy of Hospital Administration*, vol. 13, no. 2, December 2001, Delhi: All India Institute of Medical Sciences, pp. 11–15.
21. On this subject, see Chapter 4 in this volume.
22. Hence, of the 25 medicines launched in 2001–2, sixteen were antibiotics, two were drugs for cardiovascular diseases and one for diabetes. The others were for ulcers, asthma or pain relief, 'Return of the Bug-Busters', *The Economic Times*, New Delhi, 12 June 2002.
23. 'Safety on the Margins in Pharma Profits War', *Indian Express*, 2 September 2001.
24. Thus, Rofecoxib (used to treat arthritis) is still made by more than 20 Indian laboratories, although it has been prohibited by the Drug Controller General of India, following media pressure. In the same way, 11 other products, including Cisaprid, Furazolidon, Nimesulid and even Phenylpropanolamin, which were withdrawn from the market or permitted but only under certain conditions in North America, Europe and a number of Asian countries, continue to be sold in India. The regulatory authorities are increasingly being accused of laxity in this regard. See, G. Mudur, 'Indian Regulators are Accused of Laxity in not Banning Drugs', *British Medical Journal*, 2004. See http://bmj.bmjjournals.com/cgi/content/full/329/7471/878-f?ecoll
25. On this subject, see for instance the article 'Flood of Fake Medicines' by N. Bhanutej and Najmi Quaied that was published in the magazine, *The Week*: 18 May 2003. The authors show us how well organized fake drug production networks are, even able to spread their nets at the international level, with destinations like Russia, Uzbekistan, border countries like

Bangladesh or African countries like Nigeria. At a local level, the rural areas are the most targeted for the distribution of such counterfeit drugs.

26. On this subject, see A. Ranade, and R. Ahuja, 'Life Insurance in India: Emerging Issues', *EPW*, vol. 34, January 1999.
27. A recent study by the National Pharmaceutical Pricing Authority showed that consumers paid six to thirty-two times more than the pharmacist's negotiated price. This study is based on the case of three drugs: Nimesulid (anti-inflammatory drug), Omeprazole (gastric ulcer treatment) and Cetrizine (antihistamine). For more details, see S. Kumar, 'India to Extend Price Control on Drugs', *British Medical Journal*, 14 August 2004.
28. See www.dsprud.org for an updated list of activities conducted by DSPRUD in Indian states.
29. See Chapter 9 in this volume or S. Guennif, *AIDS in India: Public Health Related Aspects of Intellectual Property Rights Policies in a Developing Country*, Occasional Paper No. 8, New Delhi: Centre de Sciences Humaines, p. 179.

REFERENCES

Addlakha, R., 'Global-Local Dialectic in Medico-Administrative Practice', *Economic and Political Weekly*, vol. XXXV, nos. 8 & 9, 2000, pp. 676–83.

Addlakha, R. and A. Grover, 'User Configuration and Perspective: Hepatitis B Introductory Trial in East Delhi', *Economic and Political Weekly*, vol. XXXV, nos. 8 & 9, 2000, pp. 736–744.

Agrawal, P. and P. Saibaba, 'TRIPS and India's Pharmaceutical Industry', *Economic and Political Weekly*, vol. 36, no. 39, 29 September–5 October 2001.

Arora, P., R.K. Jain and U. Vasudeva, 'A New Paradigm in Health Care Services in Public Sector Units (PSUs) in India', *Journal of the Academy of Hospital Administration*, vol. 13, no. 1, 2001, pp. 37–41.

Baggchi, S., 'What Happened at Doha', *Economic and Political Weekly*, vol. XXXVI, no. 52, 2001, pp. 4782–5.

Baru, R., *Private Health Care in India: Social Characteristics and Trends*, New Delhi: Sage, 1998.

———, 'Health-Sector Reform: The Indian Experience', in Twaddle (ed.), *Health Care Reform Around the World*, Westport: Auburn House (Greenwood Publishers), 2002, pp. 267–81.

Bennett, S., J. Quick and G. Velasquez, 'Rôles des secteurs public et privé dans le domaine pharmaceutique. Incidence sur l'équité en matière d'accès et sur l'usage rationnel des médicaments'. *Economie de la santé et médicaments series*, no. 5, 1997, WHO.

Bourdier, F., *Sickness and Health in the Village: An Assessment of Health Conditions in South India (Coimbatore District)*, Pondy Papers in Social Sciences, Institut Français de Pondichery, 1995.

Brudon-Jakobwicz, P., *La situation pharmaceutique dans le monde. Programme d'action pour les médicaments essentiels*, 1990, WHO.

Centre for Energy, Environment & Technology, *The Indian Pharmaceutical Industry*, Report, World Bank, 2000.

Cadene, P. and D. Vidal (eds.), *Webs of Trade: Dynamics of Business Communities in Western India*, Delhi: CSH and Manohar, 1997.

Carsten, F., *How Stronger Patent Protection in India Might Affect the Behavior of Transnational Pharmaceutical Industries?*, Working Paper, World Bank, 1999.

Cattaneo, A., 'Equity', in *Health and Development: Focus on Health and the Market*. International Edition of 'CUAMM Notizie', January–April 1997, pp. 14–18.

Chapelet, P., *Le géographe et le médicament: une approche en milieu urbain, Coimbatore, Inde du Sud*, Geography Master's dissertation, University of Rouen, 1998, p. 170.

Chaudhuri, S., 'TRIPS Agreement and Amendment of Patents Act in India', *Economic and Political Weekly*, vol. 37, no. 32, 2002, pp. 3354–60.

Debroy, B., *Beyond the Uruguay Round: The Indian Perspective on GATT*, New Delhi: Sage, 1996, p. 225.

Djurfeldt, G. and S. Lindberg, *Pills Against Poverty: A Study of the Introduction of Western Medicine in a Tamil Village*. Lund: Student Litteratur and London: Curzon Press, 1975, p. 232.

Ferreiro, A., *Private Health Insurance in India: Would its Implementation Affect the Poor?*, Seminar on Introduction of Private Health Insurance in India, Proceedings, 1999, New Delhi, India, p. 5.

Gesler, W., 'The Global Pharmaceutical Industry: Health, Development and Business' in David Phillips, and Yola Verhasielt (eds.), *Health and Development*, London: Routledge, 1992, pp. 97–108.

Guennif, S., *AIDS in India: Public Health Related Aspects of Intellectual Property Rights Policies in a Developing Country*, Occasional Paper No. 8, Centre de Sciences Humaines, 2004, p. 179.

Gupta, D.B. and A. Gumber, 'Decentralisation: Some Initiatives in Health Sector', *Economic and Political Weekly*, vol. 34, no. 6, February 1999.

ICRA, *The Indian Pharmaceutical Industry*, ICRA Industry Watch Series, 2002, p. 253.

Indian Drug Manufacturers Association (IDMA), *Annual Report 2004*, 2004.

Institute of Medical Sciences, Banaras Hindu University, *Pharmaceutical Study on Drug Policy: Uttar Pradesh*, Report in collaboration with World Bank, Institute of Medical Sciences, Varanasi, India, 2000, p. 54.

Kumar, A., 'The Indian Drug Industry Under the Raj, 1860–1920', in B. Pati and Harrison (eds.), *Health, Medicine and Empire: Perspectives on Colonial India*, Hyderabad: Orient Longman, pp. 356–85.

Lalitha, N., 'Drug Policy 2002: Prescription for Symptoms', *Economic and Political Weekly*, vol. 37, no. 30, July 2002.

———, 'Indian Pharmaceutical Industry in WTO: A SWOT Analysis', *Economic and Political Weekly*, vol. 37, no. 34, August 2002.

Lanjouw, J.O., *The Introduction of Pharmaceutical Product Patent in India: 'Heartless Exploitation of the Poor and Suffering'?*, Center Discussion Paper no. 775. Economic Growth Center, Yale University, 1997.

Lathwal, O.P. and A. Banerjee, 'Availability and Utilization of Major Equipment at District Hospital Gurgaon, Haryana', *Journal of the Academy of Hospital Administration*, vol. 13, no. 2, 2001, December, pp. 23–8.

Lopert, R., D.L. Lang et al., 'Differential Pricing of Drugs: A Role for Cost-effectiveness Analysis?' *The Lancet*, vol. 359, 2002, p. 2105.

Malik, V., *The Drugs and Cosmetics Act, 1940: With Rules & Orders*, New Delhi: Eastern Book Company, 1994, p. 480.

Mahal, Ajay (ed.), *Who Benefits from Public Health Spending in India?*, Report, National Council of Applied Economic Research (NCAER), 2000, p. 78.

Mahapatra, P., S. Srilatha and P. Sridhar, 'A Patient Satisfaction Survey in Public Hospitals', *Journal of the Academy of Hospital Administration*, vol. 13, no. 2, December 2001, pp. 11–15.

Malhotra, P. and H. Lofgren, 'India's Pharmaceutical Industry: Hype or High Tech Take-off?', *Australian Health Review*, vol. 28. no. 2, November 2004, pp. 182–93.

Mittal, D.K., *Drugs and Pharmaceuticals Industry*, New Delhi: Anmol Publications, 1993, p. 250.

Offner, J.M. and D. Pumain (eds.), *Réseaux et territoires. Significations croisées*, Groupement de recherche 'Réseaux', CNRS. Editions de l'Aube,1996, p. 283.

OPPI, *Annual Report 2000–1*, Mumbai: Organisation of Pharmaceutical Producers of India, 2001.

———, *Annual Report 2001–2*, Mumbai: Organisation of Pharmaceutical Producers of India, 2002.

———, *Annual Report 2003–4*. Mumbai: Organisation of Pharmaceutical Producers of India, 2004.

Pati, B. and M. Harrison (eds.), *Health, Medicine and Empire: Perspectives on Colonial India*, Hyderabad: Orient Longman, 2001, p. 408.

Phillips, D.R., and Y. Verhasselt, *Health and Development*, London: Routledge, 1992.

Purohit, B., 'Private Initiatives and Policy Options: Recent Health System Experience in India', *Health Policy and Planning*, vol. 16(1), 2001, pp. 87–97.

Qader, I., K. Sen and K.R. Nayar (eds.), *Public Health and the Poverty of Reforms: The South Asian Predicament*, New Delhi: Sage, 2001, p. 547.

Ramachandran, R., 'Unhealthy Policy', *Frontline*, vol. 19, no. 5, 2002.

Ranade, A. and R. Ahuja, 'Life Insurance in India: Emerging Issues', *Economic and Political Weekly*, vol. XXXIV, January 1999.

Rane, W., 'Essential Medicines and International Trade', *Economic and Political Weekly*, vol. XXXIV, no. 50, 1999, pp. 3490–1.

———, 'Prices of Prescription Drugs: Marginal Rise in Cardiovascular Products', *Economic and Political Weekly*, vol. 37, no. 33, August 2002.

Rao, M., *Disinvesting in Health: The World Bank's Prescriptions for Health*, New Delhi: Sage, 1999, p. 236.

Redwood, H., *New Horizons in India: The Consequences of Pharmaceutical Patent Protection*, Felixstowe: Oldwick Press, 1994.

Singh, S., *Multinational Corporations and Indian Drug Industry*, Delhi: Criterion Publications, 1985, p. 320.

Sen, E.S., *Opening Up to the World: India's Pharmaceutical Companies Prepare for 2005*, Asia/Pacific Research Center, Institute for International Studies, Stanford University, 2000, p. 45.

Shiva, M., 'Towards a Healthy Use of Pharmaceuticals: An Indian Perspective', *Development Dialogue: Another Development in Pharmaceuticals*, vol. 2, 1985, pp. 70–93.

Subramanian, A., 'Medicines, Patents and TRIPS', *Finance and Development*, vol. 41, 2004, pp. 22–5.

Swain, N.M., and C.S. Mishra et al., 'Indian Pharmaceutical Industry: An Analysis', *The ICFAIAN Journal of Management Research*, vol. 1, no. 6, 2002.

Thomas, J.W. and R. Penchansky, 'The Concept of Access: Definition and Relationship to Consumer Satisfaction', *Medical Care* 19(2), 1981, pp. 127–40.

Vaguet, A., 'Healthcare Systems Caught in the Twists and Turns of Globalization', in F. Landy and B. Chaudhuri (eds.), *Globalization and Local Development in India: Examining the Spatial Dimension*, Delhi: CSH-Manohar, 2004, pp. 46–62.

Watal, J., *Intellectual Property Rights in the WTO and Developing Countries*. Delhi: Oxford University Press, 2001.

WHO/DAP, *Comparative Analysis of National Drug Policies*, WHO/DAP/97.6 Report, WHO, 1997, p. 114.

WHO, 'Mieux utiliser les médicaments', *Médicaments essentiels: Le Point*, no. 23, 1997, p. 24.

WHO, *The World Medicines Situation*, WHO, 2004, p. 145.

Yesudian, C.A.K., 'Behaviour of the Private Sector in the Health Market in Bombay', *Health Policy and Planning*, vol. 9(1), 1994, pp. 72–80.

CHAPTER 7

International Legal System on Pharmaceutical Patents and its Impact on the South: Economic and Legal Analysis of India's Case

JULIEN CHAISSE AND SAMIRA GUENNIF

Introduction

The rationale behind the patenting of an invention can be traced to the community of interests between the society and the inventor. For the society, it means that an individual can be guaranteed access to new therapies that are safe and effective and obtain disclosures of an invention to promote innovation. The inventor, gets benefits in the form of a monopoly on the use of the patented product or process. Certainly, patents are an incentive for innovation in a sector where processes and products are the fruit of expensive R&D programmes, which often expose companies to problems of appropriation (Arrow, 1962 and Demsetz, 1967).[1] Thus, interests albeit not conflicting but nevertheless divergent in nature are brought into play. The society as a whole and more particularly the consumers would prefer that patents be issued for a limited period and monopoly granted in proportion to the benefit brought by the inventor. On the other hand, the inventors would prefer patents granting a wide-ranging and long-lasting monopoly that would provide them with a profit that far exceeds the investment in R&D (Scherer, 1998; Grabowsky, 2002; Sterckx, 2004).

This compromise between diverging interests was always at the heart of changes made in patent protection in the developed countries. Initially, these countries granted patents on processes alone in order to ensure the innovation's diffusion, a necessary condition for the growth of a competitive pharmaceutical industry. Later, from the 1950s onwards, they ratified product patents (Desterbecq and Remiche, 1996, and Mfuka, 2002).[2] Finally, bowing to constant pressure from the pharmaceutical industry, the term of a patent was extended to twenty years in developed countries. As of the same period, we witness in the history of patents a new phase of extending patenting on a global level, especially to the developing countries (Braga, 1989).

In fact, the round of negotiation launched in 1986 at Punta del Este sought to extend the GATT trade regime to new sectors such as trade in services and intellectual property. This round lasted eight years. It culminated in the establishment of the World Trade Organisation (WTO) and the ratification of the Agreement on Trade-Related Aspects of Intellectual Property Rights (TRIPS) at Marrakech in April 1994.[3] Beginning 1 January 1996, the developed countries were to amend their national legislation to comply with TRIPS. However, a moratorium was provided for the rest of the world: twenty years for the least advanced countries and ten years for developing countries and countries transiting towards a market economy.

Since then, there has been sharp questioning and criticism. While it has been constantly reminded that the agreement is not inconsistent with the legitimate aims of industrial development and public health, especially of the developing countries, there have been expressions of acute fear and sharp protests from Brazil, India and even the 'African group' within the WTO. The flexibility provided for in the agreement failed to reassure the developing countries. The main aim of this article is precisely to shed light on the ins and outs of the extension of IPR to the developing countries. We will especially deal with Indian fears: step by step (and with delay), India has amended the patent law to comply with TRIPS.

To understand better the stakes involved in the ratification of the TRIPS agreement in India, we will begin by establishing that opting for the intellectual property regime is not without consequences. It determines the extent of progress achieved in the industrial and health sectors both in the developed as well as developing countries (§1). Then, we shall see how the TRIPS agreement establishes a strong IPR system that aims to reconcile protection of innovation and public health promotion by providing for 'exceptions' at the global level (§2).[4] Finally, after having dealt in detail with Indian reticence and tardiness in making its legislation TRIPS compatible (§3), we will analyse the prospects available presently for India (§4).

Industrial Development and Betterment of Public Health: Importance of the IPR Regime

In one century, India has been witness to two IPR systems. The passage from one to the other has markedly changed its industrial path as regards domestic pharmaceutical production. From a strong IPR system (process and product patents) in which the local industry was only at the fledgling stage, the country changed course to a weak IPR system (process patents) that allowed the dynamic pharmaceutical industry to grow. This led to vast improvement in the country's self-sufficiency in health care.

First, a Strong IPR Regime

Historically the growth of Indian pharmaceutical industry started during the colonial period (Felker et al., 1997; and Smith, 2000) with the founding of the Bengal Chemical and Pharmaceutical Works in 1901, the King Institute of Preventive Medicine (tropical diseases research centre) in 1904 and the Pasteur Institute in 1907. It is only from the Second World War onwards that India started producing conventional medicines (serums and vaccines). The country also commenced manufacturing synthetic products meant for the fight against dysentery and leprosy. Later several government production units were established: Hindustan Antibiotics in 1954 with technical assistance from the WHO and UNICEF as well as Indian Drugs and Pharmaceuticals with technical support from the erstwhile USSR (Felker et al., 1997; Smith, 2000; Dubey, 2003). Despite these forays following India's Independence, the local pharmaceutical industry was still in its infancy and the country was heavily dependant on external supplies.

Faced with continuing dependence, experts found fault with the IPR regime inherited from the colonial days. In fact, India's patent policy dated back to 1856. The Indian Patent Act (IPA) amended in 1911 authorized issuing of both process and product patents. These patents were valid for a period of sixteen years and could be extended for another period of ten years if the patent holder believed that he had not been adequately defrayed for his innovation (Lalitha, 2002a). As of 1948–50, the Patent Enquiry Committee specified that 'the Indian patent system has failed in its main purpose, namely to stimulate inventions among Indians and to encourage the development and exploitation of new inventions for industrial purposes in the country so as to secure the benefits thereof to the largest section of the public' (Government of India, 1949, cited by Ramanna, 2002).

At the end of the 1960s, a second committee confirmed this finding: the IPR regime was only a tool in the hands of the multinational companies (MNCs) of the developed world to keep the Indian market exclusively for themselves. It was a fact that they held between 80 to 90 per cent of the patents. Having cornered monopolistic positions, they indulged in prohibitive prices, which were among the highest in the world (Mittal, 1993; Keayla, 1995; Watal, 2001; Ramanna, 2002). Based on the findings of an enquiry on the price of eighteen essential drugs, this committee pointed out that most often the same products were cheaper abroad. Therefore, it recommended amendments to the existing IPR regime and the, establishment of a new 'institutional arrangement' (Arrow, 1962) that was more flexible and permitted a 'fair-selling price'. All these institutional modifications were supposed to encourage the development of a high-performance domestic industry capable of making the country self-sufficient in health care and reduce the price of medicines.

FOLLOWED BY A RELAXATION OF THE IPR REGIME WITH POSITIVE EFFECTS

In 1970, the patent law was relaxed. The 1970 IPA stipulated that patents would be granted only for processes for a period of seven years as regards the pharmaceutical industry.[5] Furthermore, a company would only be able to enjoy one patent for one manufacturing process (Lalitha, 2002a). From then on medicines were exempted from the scope of patentability.[6]

Besides, only local production would validate the effective use of a patent. Contrary to the earlier practice, the import of pharmaceutical products no longer allowed the patent's effective use to be validated. As a result, the patent holder was given three years to exercise his right in the form of local production.

The IPA also provided for assignment of rights. If, at the end of the three-year period, a medicine was not available at all or not at a reasonable price, the Indian government could construe that the public need had not been met and could issue a compulsory license (CL). It could thus instruct a local company to manufacture the medicine and market it at a lower price. *A fortiori*, if two years after the issue of the CL, the medicine was still not available, the government could simply revoke the patent due to lack of satisfactory usage.

Along with industrial policy measures, the public authorities instituted price control the same year. The Drug Price Control Orders (DPCO) was established in 1970 in order to enhance people's access to drugs (Singh, 1985; Felker et al., 1997; Srinivasan, 2001; OPPI, 2001; Kunnapallil, 2003). In practice, the public authorities published a list of the most essential drugs with a large volume of sale. Henceforth, the retail price of these drugs was fixed at a reasonable level. This price was supposed to enable manufacturers cover the cost of raw materials, formulation, packaging and distribution while at the same time ensuring a reasonable profit margin. The price for most essential drugs was fixed in such a way as to ensure a margin of 75 per cent taking into account various production costs for the company. The margin for non-essential drugs was fixed at 150 per cent. Later, this price control system underwent recurrent changes (Gross, 1999; Govindaraj and Chellaraj, 2002; Lalitha, 2002a, 2002b).[7]

Thus, the 1970 IPA along with the DPCO, sought to reconcile the aims of diffusing innovation in the country and fulfilling the needs of people as regards quality drugs at affordable prices (Keayla, 1995). Since only processes could be patented, at that time it was possible for local companies to copy molecules developed by MNCs. Working on the basis of reverse engineering and learning by copying, these companies could market generic drugs or less expensive versions of drugs patented by MNCs elsewhere.

Coming into force in 1972, this new IPR regime had a substantial impact. First of all, it allowed the growth of the fragmented domestic pharmaceutical industry. In 1953, the sector consisted of 1,752 companies which grew to 5,126 in 1980. Today, there are 20,000 companies with 250 big timers and about 10 public sector enterprises (Mittal, 1993; OPPI, 2002).[8]

Moreover, the country was able to make good its backwardness as regards domestic production of raw material and formulations. Raw material production rose from Rs. 180 million in 1965 to Rs. 9 billion in the early 1990s and rose further to Rs. 45 billion in 2001. As for formulation, it recorded an even higher growth. At the end of the 1960s, the industry formulated drugs worth Rs. 1.5 billion. This turnover went up to Rs. 60 billion in 1993 and settled at above Rs. 183 billion in 2001 (Mittal, 1993; OPPI, 2002).

The pharmaceutical industry's exports to the rest of the world went up from the 1980s. Initially, these exports mainly concerned finished products: 76 per cent as against 24 per cent of raw material exports.

However, considerable growth in the export of both raw materials as well as finished products was observed at the end of the 1990s. Indeed, exports increased respectively more than 100 times and more than 300 times during this period. Finally, a more even distribution of exports in this sector was observed: 55 per cent of exports pertained to formulation as against 45 per cent for active substances in 2000 (Mittal, 1993; OPPI, 2002).[9] Besides, the dynamism of exports manifested in a trade surplus right from the end of the 1990s. Thus, the chronic deficits between the 1960s and 1980s began to decrease and disappear as of 1989. Today, the pharmaceutical sector trade surplus is nearly Rs. 51.3 billion (IDMA, 2001; Chaudhry, 2002).[10]

Since the 1970 IPA, Indian pharmaceutical industry's growth has meant enhanced self-sufficiency as far as the country's health care is concerned. The industry produces 70 per cent of raw materials and 80 per cent of finished products in the Indian market (Lanjouw, 1997). In addition, the grading of the top ten companies in the Indian market reveals the performance of the domestic industry. Four of these companies are from India and have almost 16 per cent share of the Indian market (OPPI, 2002).

Moreover, comparison between the drug price index and the price index of other goods between 1961 and 1989 evidences the positive effect of the DPCO. In the beginning of the 1960s, the drug price index was almost at par with the general price index: 2 per cent inflation for drugs as against 3 per cent for all other goods. Till 1966, a restrained price increase for drugs as compared to other goods could be noted; an effect that could be attributed to the first steps taken towards drug price control during the Sino-Indian War (Singh, 1985; Felker et al., 1997). Then, from the 1970s onwards, the gap between the drug price index and the price index of other goods began to widen. In general, between 1961 and 1989, the price index for all products increased by 676.60 per cent as against 386.60 per cent for drugs (Government of India, Indian Drug Statistics, cited by Prasad et al., 1993).

We should dwell a little further on this point. When we compare the relative prices of some of the essential drugs sixteen years after the DPCO came into force, we notice that the prices in India were among the lowest in 1986. Of eight essential drugs belonging to seven therapeutic classifications, Mittal (1993) maintained that the Indian prices were lower than the prices prevalent in countries like Pakistan or the United Kingdom. For example, the price of an antibiotic in India was 82.50 per cent of the price in Pakistan and 32.20 per cent of the price in

Britain. For the most expensive drug, a hypertensive drug, the Indian price was equivalent to approximately 69 per cent of the British price and 42 per cent of the Pakistani price. Similarly, according to a study conducted by Keayla (1995) on the costs of largest selling drugs during the years 1991 and 1992, India enjoyed attractive prices. For an antibiotic (Ciprofloxacin), the Indian price was 5.66 times lower than the Pakistani price. Even for an ulcer drug (Ranitidine), the American price was 25 times higher than the Indian price.

Recently, Indian pharmaceutical firms have been highly appreciated and have received wide coverage in the media for the supply of anti-retroviral drugs (ARVs) at competitive prices in the developing world.

GLOBAL EFFECT OF A RELAXED IPR REGIME: INDIAN COMPETITION AND PRICES OF ARV

ARV production began in India in 1991. At that time, Cipla wisely had a go at the manufacturing of the less costly ARV formulations, whose active substance content was low and whose manufacturing process was relatively less complex.[11] A decade later, there were five Indian companies (Cipla, Ranbaxy, Hetero, Aurobindo and Cadila) which had developed the wherewithal for this formulation and this allowed each one of them to market more than fifteen ARVs, especially in the form of double and triple therapies.

The entry of these generic drugs in the ARV market brought the cost of treatment crashing down. Médecins sans Frontières (MSF) (2003) clearly demonstrated that the sharp decline started with Cipla announcing in February 2001 that it would sell its triple therapy in the form of a cocktail at $350 per year per patient to NGOs.[12] At that time, a triple therapy cost $931 with brand-name medicines. From March 2001, the price of triple therapy with brand-name drugs fell to $727. Moreover, competition between Indian generic drug manufacturers triggered a new decline in prices. Two months after Cipla's announcement, Hetero joined the fray and declared its intention to sell its cocktail at $347 to NGOs. A few months later, Ranbaxy raised the stakes by fixing the price of its cocktail at $295 for NGOs. In its last report, MSF stated that prices were still decreasing. In 2003, Hetero was selling the tri-therapy at $152 to NGOs against $562 for brand-name drugs. Thus, between January 2001 and June 2005, the price of the triple therapy fell by more than 83 per cent thanks to the most effective means of lowering medicines price, i.e. generic competition (MSF, 2006).

On the whole, the beneficial effects of a relaxed IPR regime (patents on manufacturing processes alone) were confirmed as seen in the Indian experiment. By making its IPR regime more flexible, India had encouraged the growth of a pharmaceutical industry and improved accessibility to drugs. Further, this high-performance industry had recently succeeded in pushing ARV prices down and making the drugs affordable. As a WTO member, India had to amend its laws by 2005 to make them TRIPS compliant. What is the content of this agreement and what impact can it have on the Indian trajectory as regards pharmaceutical development and access to treatment? To answer these questions, it is imperative to spell out clearly the contents of the TRIPS agreement.

Strengthening of the IPR Regime at the International Level: Patentability under the Terms of the TRIPS Agreement

The TRIPS agreement attempts to reduce the differences in the manner in which IPR is protected around the world by fixing a minimum level of intellectual property protection that each of the WTO's member-states ought to guarantee. Thus, Articles 17 and 34 of this agreement lay down common minimum international regulations. These regulations specify what is patentable, what is not patentable and the extent to which the rights are protected under the patent (Gervais, 1999; Boulet and Velasquez, 1999).

GENERAL PROVISIONS

First of all, the agreement defines patent as 'any invention, whether products or processes, in all fields of technology, provided that they are new, and involve an inventive step, . . . , that they are capable of industrial application' or it be 'non-obvious and useful' (Article 27.1 and the linked footnote).

As regards the patent's term, it is fixed at a minimum of twenty years from the date of its application (Article 33). In this respect, the industrialized countries' standard has prevailed. Indeed, the lengthy administrative procedures to determine a product's safety and effectiveness before marketing approval (MA) tended to eat into the effective duration of the patent.[13] As *quid pro quo*, the American authorities, on one side and the European authorities on the other, granted an extension of the patent term to twenty years.

As regards patent validity, Article 27 lays down that 'patent rights shall be enjoyable without discrimination, whether products are imported or locally produced'. In other words, whereas the national laws of developing countries such as India and Thailand stipulated that local production alone could validate a patent, henceforth import would also validate the actual use of the patent. Thus, WTO member states no longer had any discriminatory tools to encourage access to technology and medicines.

PATENTABILITY CONDITIONS

The issue of patentability conditions, in other words the patentability criteria (positive and negative), is not merely technical. These criteria define what can be appropriated by private parties and what cannot be monopolized or withdrawn from free use. These criteria formalize the old social contract between the community and the inventor.

As per Article 27.1, the member states are beholden to offer protection granted by a patent for any invention whether it is a product (medicine) or a process (a method to produce chemical ingredients for a drug composition). Thus, whereas a number of developing countries had opted for patenting only the process, henceforth they are bound to grant patents both for the process and the product under certain conditions.

The first of these conditions is that, the process or product should establish its novelty. The agreement does not give any details on this point. However, it is generally considered that anything not previously included in a technique is new. Therefore, any previously unknown invention regardless of the place and time under consideration is accepted as new. Thus, any past disclosure, to be understood as any revelation, written or oral, express or implicit, including that which is known through usage, will limit the innovative character and exclude a product or a process from being patented. Similarly, prior art can encompass past patent applications not yet published and limit the eligibility of a patent application. Finally, knowledge of local communities, traditional practices can be included in prior art and on this basis become non-patentable.

Second condition, the innovation should be inventive, which corresponds to the 'non-obvious' criteria. It is a filter which makes it possible to refuse the grant of a monopoly for processes and products that are based neither on intelligence nor on any particular creative activity. The act of inventing is generally understood to have been achieved if, for a person skilled in the art, the invention does not obviously follow prior art.

Third condition, the invention is 'capable of industrial application' (Article 27.1). Here too, the agreement does not provide any details, thereby giving governments sufficient room for manoeuvre. This criterion is generally understood to be a means to ensure that the monopoly is granted solely to processes and products likely to result in material manufacture of a product and industrial production.

Last condition, supposing that the invention is new, inventive and capable of industrial application, 'Members shall require that an applicant shall disclose the invention in a manner sufficiently clear and complete for an invention to be carried out by a person skilled in the art and may require the applicant to indicate the best mode for carrying out the invention known to the inventor at the filing date' (Article 29).[14] Therefore, the product features shall be described in the patent application and made public. Disclosure is an indispensable factor in the contract drawn between the inventor and the society. In fact, in exchange for the grant of monopoly, the applicant shall make public the technical information that helps technology progress and guarantee that after the patent's expiry, the invention shall truly fall in the public domain. After the patent's expiry, based on the information disclosed by the applicant, it will become possible for professionals in that sector to easily copy the concerned process or product, without having to display any creativity on their part. In addition, a clear and complete disclosure helps in restraining the patent's scope. A clear and complete description limits excessive claims from the applicant, which, consequently, avoids the grant of a sweeping monopoly liable to stifle competition to a great degree.

LIMITATIONS TO PATENTABILITY

On the grounds of public order or morality. Article 27.2 provides that 'Members may exclude from patentability inventions, the prevention within their territory of the commercial exploitation of which is necessary to protect *ordre public* or morality, including to protect human, animal or plant life or health or to avoid serious prejudice to the environment, provided that such exclusion is not made merely because the exploitation is prohibited by their law'. The notion of public order is, however, not defined in the agreement. Room for manoeuvre is thus available to the member-states to meet their particular ends. Thus, it is possible to exclude certain drugs from patentability for reasons of public health. However, these exclusions can be contemplated only under exceptional circumstances, subject to the limitation laid down in the article that such restrictions can be applied only to inventions—'the prevention of the commercial exploitation of which is necessary'.[15] In any case, an object cannot be declared as non-patentable if its distribution or sale has been authorized in the national territory at the same time.

Medical methods. Article 27.3a authorizes the member-states to exclude from patentability 'diagnostic, therapeutic and surgical methods for the treatment of humans or animals'. Such exclusion is of great importance to developing countries inasmuch as the patenting of these methods may have repercussions on public health and reduce accessibility to health care.

Diagnostic, therapeutic and surgical methods or plants and animals and biological processes for the production of plants or animals. Under the terms of Article 27.3b, 'plants and animals and other micro-organisms, and essentially biological processes for the production of plants or animals other than non-biological and microbiological processes' can be excluded from patentability. In this matter, the latitude granted to the states is limited by the obligation to patent microorganisms. Now, inventions concerning microorganisms are common and useful in the pharmaceutical industry. For example, a surgical sequence or a new medical test can be excluded from patentability in that it is a diagnostic, therapeutic or surgical method. On the other hand, medicines can be patented as a microbiological process (antibiotic) or simply a chemical process used for therapeutic purposes. In all these scenarios, they are not considered as therapeutic methods (Luff, 2004).

On account of public health, nutrition and public interest. Article 8.1 allows certain pharmaceutical products to be excluded from patentability. This clause permits member-states to adapt their national policies based on public health concerns. It is thus possible to exclude from patentability certain pharmaceutical products, as a temporary measure, to deal with a national emergency as far as public health is concerned. However, the article sets limits to such measures by specifying that they must be indispensable and consistent with the agreement. These possibilities would thus be limited by nature and their use would require justification. These provisions complement Article 7 according to which IPR 'should contribute to the promotion of technological innovation and to the transfer and dissemination of technology, to the mutual advantage of producers and users of technological knowledge and in a manner conducive to social and economic welfare, and to a balance of rights and obligations'. On principle, protection of patent rights should, thus, be commensurate with the interest of the society and should establish 'social and economic welfare'. To do so, additional and necessary measures can be taken under the terms of Article 8.

LIMITS TO THE RIGHTS ENSUING FROM THE PATENT

In accordance to the principles laid down by the TRIPS agreement, a country can disregard the rights of the patent holder to promote public health objectives such as accessibility to medicines or for treatment in case of national emergencies such as an epidemic. Once the patent has been granted, WTO members are permitted to waive the protection conferred by the patent under circumstances that have been provided and enshrined in the agreement.

The general principle of exceptions to rights conferred. As per Article 30, the patent owner enjoys monopoly over the product or process with certain exclusive rights. Basically these rights pertain to the right to forbid a third party to manufacture and use the patented product or exploit the patented process, to sell or offer for sale patented products and products derived from the patented process and finally to import these products. Patent owners shall also have the right to assign, or transfer by succession, the patent and to conclude licensing contracts (Article 28).[16]

These rights are not without limits. In this regard, Article 30 leaves a certain latitude to the member-states to provide for 'exceptions' to patentee's rights, under the following three conditions: 'Members may provide limited exceptions to the exclusive rights conferred by a patent, provided that such exceptions do not unreasonably conflict with a normal exploitation of the patent and do not unreasonably prejudice the legitimate interests of the patent owner, taking account of the legitimate interests of third parties'. The aim of these exceptions is to create a competitive environment favourable to a decrease in drug prices and enhancement of people's access to medicines. However, the three conditions are cumulative, each being a separate and independent requirement that must be satisfied. 'Failure to comply with any one of the three conditions results in the Article 30 exception being disallowed', as underlined by the Panel in the Canada—Patent Protection of Pharmaceutical Products case.[17]

Exception for research and experiment and specific provision. Some countries allow manufacturers of generic drugs to use the patented invention to obtain marketing approval without the patent owner's permission and before the patent protection expires. The generic producers can then market their versions as soon as the patent expires. In addition, by allowing researchers to use a patented invention for experimental purposes, third parties are encouraged to work on or around the invention to understand it better and possibly surpass it. The declared purpose is to advance technological progress. This pharmaceutical sector specific provision, inherited from the American IPR regime, is called the 'Bolar' provision. It has been covered in Article 8 of the TRIPS agreement and confirmed by a WTO's panel report adopted by the Dispute Settlement Body (DSB).[18]

Extemporaneous preparation of medicines. This enables a pharma-ceutical board to authorize the preparation of a compounded mixture, in units, to meet the needs of a particular patient's medical prescription. Only this particular case is dealt with in this exception. Thus, it has a limited scope of application and is of lesser interest compared to the applications accepted in the Bolar provision.

Compulsory licensing.[19] In accordance with Articles 8 and 40 of the TRIPS agreement, governments can take steps to prevent patent owners from abusing their rights by 'unreasonably' restraining trade or hampering the international transfer of technology. In practice, public authorities can authorize a third party to manufacture a patented product or to use the patented process without the patent owner's consent. Most developed and developing countries provide for CL concession in their legislation.[20]

Recourse to CL is based on Article 31 of the TRIPS agreement devoted to 'other uses without authorization of the right holder'. The article aims to strike a balance between the concern to promote access to medicines and provide protection/incentive for R&D in the pharmaceutical field (Luff, 2004). The objective is to create a more competitive environment without, however, ignoring the rights of the patent owner, who ought to be adequately compensated whatever the circumstances.

It is possible to issue a CL under certain conditions to ensure that the legitimate interests of the patent owner have been protected.[21] In particular, an attempt should have been made to obtain a voluntary license (VL) from the right holder on reasonable commercial terms (Article 31.b).[22] However, this article provides for making the VL redundant in case of a national emergency, circumstances of extreme urgency, public non-commercial use (or government use) or anti-competitive practices. The CL is of particular importance for developing countries that are subject to epidemics such as HIV/AIDS. Their objective is to improve patients' access to drugs. Thus, certain countries see this as a means to stymie the negative effects of patents on prices and availability of medicines, in so far as it makes it possible to reduce prices of drugs protected by a patent in force and to obtain technology.

Nevertheless, certain difficulties continue to exist. First of all, the lack of a clear definition of these scenarios and the resultant legal insecurity has led developing countries to demand a specific statement on this matter. Further, a CL is normally granted mainly to replenish the local market. So what about developing countries reeling under a national emergency or victim of a monopolistic practice who do not have local manufacturing capacities?

Parallel import (*PI*). PI allows imports and resale in a country without the authorization of the patent owner of a product patented and marketed in another country by the patent owner himself or through a duly authorized agent. This measure also stems from the concern to strike a balance between adherence to the patentee's monopoly and the principle of free flow, in order to create as competitive as possible an environment. In practice, this has to do with drugs produced and marketed by the patent owner in one country that are subsequently exported to another country without his permission. Thus, if a drug X has been patented and manufactured in countries A and B and if the price of the drug is cheaper in country A, then country B would be tempted to import the drug from country A to benefit from a lower price. This practice is known as parallel import.[23]

Recourse to PI is governed by the principle of exhaustion of rights retained by the members. Exhaustion of rights can be at the national, regional or international level. According to the principle of exhaustion of rights at the national level, the patent owner's rights are considered to have fulfilled their objective once he has marketed the product anywhere in the national territory. This means that the patentee no longer holds any rights over his product's subsequent sale and resale, his rights having been 'exhausted', once it has been marketed. However, marketing of his product outside the national territory does not exhaust his rights. In other words, exporting the product to a third country is prohibited. This system is in force especially in the United States. At the regional level, there is exhaustion of rights the moment the product is put up for sale in the regional market. This mechanism also prevails in the European market, which for example allows a product marketed on Spanish soil to be subsequently exported to another European Union member country. Finally, at the international level, once the patent holder consents to market his product in one country, the international exhaustion of his rights takes place: the product can be exported to any other country without the consent of the patentee. As a result, if the principle of exhaustion of rights at the international level is retained, as soon as the patent holding company has sold its product in country A, its rights are exhausted as regards all other countries and therefore all other markets; country B can then proceed to imports from a more competitive source of supply.

On this point the TRIPS agreement lays down that 'nothing in this Agreement shall be used to address the issue of the exhaustion of intellectual property rights' (Article 6). By its refusal to arbitrate, the WTO thus gives wide latitude to members to legislate. As a result, if a country authorizes PIs based on modalities that infringe on the agreement, the matter cannot be brought before the WTO's DSB, unless the fundamental principles of non-discrimination are at issue under the terms of Article 6 of the agreement.

At the end of this overview, we can ascertain that the TRIPS agreement controls a certain number of factors. For example, product and process patents have a lifespan of minimum twenty years. Nevertheless, the agreement leaves other more or less important factors to the discretion of the members. In particular, a country must define what constitutes a national emergency or the choice of the principle of exhaustion rights to be retained. And finally, in the case of India, for instance, there are many differences between the IPR regime based on the TRIPS agreement and the IPR regime inherited from the 1970 IPA. These have been summarized in Table 7.1.

TABLE 7.1: 1970 INDIAN PATENT ACT AND TRIPS AGREEMENT

1970 Indian Patent Act	TRIPS agreement
• Patents only on processes in the pharmaceutical sector.	• Patents on processes and products.
• Fields in which patenting has been excluded: nuclear, agriculture.	• Fields in which patenting has been excluded: diagnostic, therapeutic and surgical methods for treating humans or animals.
• Patent duration: 7 years in the chemical and pharmacy sectors from filing of application and 14 years in other sectors.	• Patent duration: Minimum 20 years from filing for patent.
• Discrimination: Patent valid in case of local manufacture.	• Discrimination: Patent valid for both local manufacture and imports.
• Compulsory licensing; parallel imports and other assignment of rights.	• Statutory license; parallel imports not excluded.
According to the TRIPS agreement, the following falls under the States' discretion National emergency Exhaustion of right (at national, regional or international level)	

Ensuring the TRIPS-Conformity of Indian IPR Law

DETERMINATION OF NON-CONFORMITY BY THE DISPUTE SETTLEMENT BODY

The WTO system imposes stiff conditions regarding conformity to the international trade law. Any national law must conform to WTO requirements and this requirement is quite unique in international public law (Chaisse, 2005). All the WTO Members must then implement the TRIPS agreement. Indeed, Article 16.4 of the agreement lays down that 'each Member shall ensure the conformity of its laws, regulations and administrative procedures with its obligations as provided in the annexed agreements'. Also, WTO members must provide for civil and administrative procedures for the enforcement of intellectual property rights to holders. As had been pointed out earlier, the agreement provides for a moratorium for developing countries. For the least advanced countries, the agreement should be ratified before 1 January

2016. For other developing countries, the ratification must take place before 1 January 2005. Despite repeated protests, India was placed in the other developing countries' category. In fact, a low per capita income ($530) places it among low-income countries. However, it appears that India was done in by the demographic factor. Its high population was put forward as a reason for justifying its classification under the other developing countries' category. Therefore, it is obliged to amend its national laws pertaining to patenting in order to comply with the TRIPS agreement by 2005.

Apart from the discussions regarding the time frame granted to one or the other category for compliance with the TRIPS agreement, other difficulties too surfaced. They concern the violation and interpretation of certain provisions in the agreement. In this respect, the key element in the WTO is its DSB, which does exert a considerable influence on world trade and diplomacy (Chaisse, 2006). Its aim is to maintain the judicial rights and obligations of each of the WTO members. Moreover, unlike other judicial systems of this type, its mechanism is based on a large jurisprudence that clarifies and develops laws that stem from the Marrakech Agreement. On the whole, more than any other international organization, the WTO is truly capable of ensuring the effectiveness of all its regulations laid down in the agreement it administrates. The immediate consequence of such a system is that the developing countries take frequent recourse to this dispute settlement mechanism, bringing before it litigation against developed countries as well as other developing countries (Chaisse and Chakraborty, 2007). In fact, with the establishment of the WTO, dispute settlement under international trade laws has become judicial and much more efficient.[24] An important feature of the DSB system is that it has mandatory jurisdiction over all disputes arising out of the WTO agreement. The members cannot take recourse to any other process to settle disputes. In other words, litigation is centralized within a single body, which *de facto* results in the creation of a homogeneous jurisprudence. Finally, it must be underlined that once a report has been adopted, all the parties involved in the dispute must accept all its elements, which means that the 'loser' must make its legislation compatible with WTO laws as expressed and explained in the DSB report. This far-reaching change has surely made the DSB one of the most effective mechanisms in international law even if some improvements are still necessary (Chaisse and Chakraborty, 2006).

In the field of IPR and with regard to India in particular, we have already confirmed the important role played by the DSB. As examined earlier, with the amendment made to the IPA in 1970, India did not grant patent protection for pharmaceutical products when the TRIPS agreement came into force. But Article 70.8 states the obligation to create a system by which patent applications can be filed for such inventions. This provision is generally known as 'mail box application' and generated the 'India–Patent Protection for Pharmaceutical and Agricultural Chemical Products' case which is the first litigation on intellectual property settled within the WTO framework. Regarding the conformity with Article 70.8 of TRIPS, the DSB noted that 'the absence of judicial security in the functioning of the mail box system in India [was] such that the system did not [permit] Article 70.8 to be fulfilled appropriately and protect the legitimate expectations implied for the pharmaceutical products and agricultural related chemical products inventors'.[25] The DSB did not fail to support its argument by observing that 'foreseeability as regards the intellectual property regime is essential for citizens of WTO countries when they take decisions pertaining to trade and investment in their commercial transactions'.[26] Subsequently, this analysis was by and large confirmed. DSB added that members were not obliged to guarantee that patent applications deposited in the mail box would not be rejected or invalidated because they preceded the enforcement of any legislation.[27] It did not in any way challenge India's right, by virtue of the transitional provisions in paragraphs 1, 2 and 4 of Article 65, to defer the implementation of Article 27 pertaining to patents on pharmaceutical and agricultural chemical products until 1 January 2005.

1995–2005: INDIA'S SLUGGISH APPROACH ON PATENT LAW COMPLIANCE

After having signed the agreement, between 1994 and 1998, and despite the bilateral and multilateral trade pressures exerted by the United States and Europe, India did not amend its IPR regime. The sluggishness evidenced was due to the opposition of players who benefitted from the IPR regime inherited from the 1970 IPA. In particular, the generic drug manufacturer Cipla continues to plead in favour of a moratorium extending up to 2015. It is demanding that India be classified under the list of least advanced countries regardless of its large population. Another example of India's sluggishness pertains to a bill introduced in Parliament in March 1995 to amend the 1970 IPA. This bill was not approved by the Parliament and was sent back to a committee. It is only from 1998 onwards that there have been significant changes.

Around 1998 political parties changed their position under the delayed effect of the liberalization policy initiated in 1991 (Ramanna, 2002). The Congress party changed its stance in favour of amending the IPR regime. On its part, having come to power in 1998, the BJP went on record that it was for the establishment of a stronger IPR regime. At the same time, the lobbies also geared up. The Confederation of Indian Industry ensured that the IPR reform would help the country attract foreign direct investments (FDI) and gain access to new technologies, a factor necessary for a modern and professional management of the Indian industry, according to this body. The Federation of Indian Chambers of Commerce and Industry (FICCI) set up the International Institute of Intellectual Property Development in 1997. The latter has launched a campaign with the slogan 'patent or perish'. The public scientific bodies have taken a positive view of the possibility of patenting the knowledge they have developed. Following the lead given by the Council of Scientific and Industrial Research, these bodies have declared their support for strengthening the patent laws. Finally, in 1998, following a complaint brought to the DSB by the United States, India was asked ensure compliance of its legislation as of April 1999.

As the first sign of an effective modification of patent laws, India signed the Paris Convention on 8 December 1998 and ratified the Patent Cooperation Treaty (Kumar, 1998). In 1998, the BJP introduced a motion for amending the patent law. In 1999, the first amendment was adopted (Watal, 2001; Bhattacharya, 2002; Chaudhuri, 2002). It authorized product patenting in agro-chemical and pharmaceutical sectors. Patent applications could thus be deposited in a 'mailbox'. The applications were to be reviewed in 2004 and be possibly accepted in 2005. Since the TRIPS agreement came into force in 1995, only those molecules that were discovered and were the subject of patent applications in another WTO member after this date are patentable. Thus, the countries would have to ensure in 2005 that applications filed are indeed for drugs invented after 1995. In addition, as provided in the TRIPS agreement for the transition period, exclusive marketing rights could be granted for five years to companies that file their application under certain conditions.

In May 2001, India was placed under the 'Special 301 Priority Watch List', an instrument the United States employs to exert trade pressures on countries that adversely affect their economic interests either by adopting protectionist measures or by not bringing about a desirable change in their IPR regime. In 2002, a new amendment was adopted. Amongst other issues, it provides greater clarification about the definition of the term 'invention', non-patentable elements, patent owner's rights, CL and even PI (Bhattacharya, 2002; Keayla, 2003).

In short, making its legislation fall in line with the TRIPS agreement was not a smooth process for India and much still needs to be done. Based on the points presented above concerning the history of patent protection in India and its pharmaceutical industry, we can understand better the reticence shown in this matter by the public authorities. The implementation of the TRIPS agreement constitutes a renewed fortification of patent protection. Thus, the country fears that this renewed fortification would apply the brakes on the growth its industry had enjoyed till now and eat into the progress achieved towards self-sufficiency in health care and peoples' access to medicines. Furthermore, Thailand's experience, another country that had to bring about strengthening of patent protection earlier, has put the promises associated with TRIPS ratification in a different perspective.

Prospects of Reinforcement of Legal Pharmaceutical Patent System in Developing Countries

When the TRIPS agreement was being ratified, the developed countries had repeatedly stressed on the fact that the developing countries too would benefit by strengthening their IPR regime. First of all, it was stated that a strong IPR regime would promote FDI and technology transfer, which would at last help the developing countries stimulate their industrial growth and gain access to the latest therapeutic innovations (Correa, 2001a and 2002b). Then, it was stated that public health objectives would not be threatened by the TRIPS agreement in so far as exceptions had been built in to deal with medical emergencies or to remedy abusive trade practices such as market rationing or fixing of prohibitive prices. What has happened with these promises?

TWO DIFFERENT PATHS FOLLOWED BY DEVELOPING COUNTRIES: LESSONS LEARNT

First and foremost, let us recall that the analysis revealed that the Indian pharmaceutical industry's growth curve was largely due to the relaxation of its IPR regime. By switching from a stringent IPR regime to a more flexible one in 1970, the Indian authorities managed to ensure their pharmaceutical industry's growth and improve people's accessibility to medicines. Furthermore, the growth of the domestic Indian industry does present definite benefits for the rest of the world as suggested by the impact of the competition war unleashed between MNCs and Indian generic drug manufacturers in the ARV market (Guennif, 2004; Guennif and Mfuka, 2005). In this sense, this industry has helped to improve global welfare by offering treatment at more affordable prices to persons infected by HIV/AIDS.

Moreover, Thailand's experience in this matter is enlightening. The country took the opposite path compared to India's journey by strengthening its IPR regime as early as 1992 under US trade pressures and subsequently due to the ratification of the TRIPS agreement. To this date, if the benefits of this reinforcement remain hard to pinpoint as regards FDI and transfer of technology, the disadvantages in terms of patients' access to treatments are, on the contrary, clearly perceptible.

In fact, as regards FDI and transfer of technology, it seems that between 1984 and 1998, Thai companies remained mostly in the hands of Thai nationals (Supakankunti et al., 2001). Therefore, it appears that there has been very little FDI inflow in the local pharmaceutical industry since 1992. This is because MNCs have preferred to import rather than manufacture medicines locally as is evident from the growing share of imported medicines in Thailand since 1992. In real terms, following the amendment of patent laws, the imported products' share in the local drug market grew to 42.80 per cent in 1999 as against 23.50 per cent in 1984. In short, having obtained patents on drugs and not being bound to make actual use of their patents in the form of local manufacturing, the MNCs were tempted to simply take advantage of existing formulation capacity in the country (Guennif and Mfuka, 2003, 2005) and very rarely promoted technology transfers to the country.

As regards accessibility to treatment, between 1979 and 1992, a generic medicine usually became available in the market 1–2 years after the launch of the brand-name drug. However, following the strengthening of the IPR regime in 1992, a generic version could be made available only five years after filing of patent (Kwa, 2001). Thailand also experienced great difficulties in meeting public health objectives when for example the HIV/AIDS epidemic had to be dealt with and patients' access to treatment facilitated. The 'ddl affair' is a perfect example of the magnitude of these difficulties. Ddl is an ARV whose patent is held by the American company Bristol-Myers & Squibb (BMS).

Despite managing to develop a generic version of ddl, the public sector unit, GPO, under the aegis of the Thai Health Ministry, was forced to stop marketing it due to the modification in the Thai Patent Act and the introduction of patents on processes and products. For want of a generic version, ddl became an inaccessible drug for infected persons: it was offered for $0.50 a pill by BMS whereas GPO had sold it for $0.15 in 2001 (Guennif & Mfuka, 2003, 2005). Not willing to give up, in 1997, GPO filed a request for a CL in view of the national emergency created by the HIV/AIDS epidemic. BMS then exerted pressure on its government, which in its turn interceded with the Thai authorities. Under commercial pressure,[28] the Thai Government had to give in and refuse the grant of the CL. In 2001, an association of people living with HIV/AIDS sued BMS and asked for the revocation of its patent for lack of significant inventive steps or novelty. The patent was not invalidated but its scope reduced so that GPO could produce tablets larger than 100 mg dosage (Oxfam, 2004). The generic was marketed at half the price of the brand-name drug. At the end, under the pressure of the civil society, BMS gave up its patent.

After all, in response to the question whether a stringent IPR regime promotes transfer of technology and improves accessibility to medicines, the past Indian experience and the present Thai experience would raise serious doubts. Of much more concern is the recourse to exceptions provided for by the TRIPS agreement in theory, which remains problematic, especially when we take into account the developing countries' place in world trade and the import of trade pressures emanating from the developed world.

ROOM FOR MANOEUVRE FOR INDIA AND DEVELOPING COUNTRIES?

How can we ensure that patent protection does not impede access to medicines in poor countries, while at the same time preserving the patent's incentive role in the R&D field? A compromise seems difficult to reach. The developed countries are clearly at an advantage with respect to the developing countries (Ramappa, 2000). As a matter of fact, the industrialized nations, cradles of pharmaceutical firms that are patentees of most drugs, are the main exporters of both processes and products. It is natural that their interest lies in a stringent protective IPR regime in as many countries as possible. The TRIPS agreement affords them this protection and therefore further strengthens the

MNCs' predominant position and their income throughout the world.[29]

On the other hand, the developing countries are, for the most part, importers of both processes and products. They are likely to be subjected to a rise in prices for imported patented drugs. At the same time, the market launch of generic drugs, which provoke a significant drop in prices, would be delayed due to the extension of the protection period granted by a patent. Consequently, there is already a fear of foreign monopolies in the domestic market and the transfer of profits to industrialized nations, as well as loss of public control over drug prices, promotional campaigns and national drugs policy. It will then become very difficult for developing countries to protect their imperatives for public health—imperatives that had been put forward in the objectives and principles of the TRIPS agreement (Articles 7, 8.1 & 8.2) and reaffirmed at Doha (Article 4).

In fact, given the difficulties and pressures encountered by developing countries in making effective use of flexibilities provided for in the TRIPS agreement, the members at first reaffirmed at Doha their commitment to the principle of IPR protection as the driving force behind innovation: 'We recognize that intellectual property protection is important for the development of new medicines.' (Article 2 of the Declaration on the TRIPS Agreement and Public Health adopted on 14 November 2001 at Doha). Then, it was reiterated that the principle of IPR protection was subordinate to the principle of public health: 'We agree that the TRIPS Agreement does not and should not prevent members from taking measures to protect public health. . . . Accordingly, we affirm that the Agreement can and should be interpreted and implemented in a manner supportive of WTO members' right to protect public health and, in particular, to promote access to medicines for all' (Doha Declaration, paragraph 4). It was thus that the possibility available to the Members to take recourse to PI and CL in case of national emergencies, and the sole discretion to define what 'constitutes a national emergency' was reaffirmed (Paragraphs 5b and 5c). On the one hand, each state was left free to establish its own regime of exhaustion of IPR (Paragraph 5d), which will determine the practical possibility of recourse to PIs at the regional or global level. However, on the other hand, faced with the objections raised by African countries, which were unable to take recourse to CL due to insufficient manufacturing capacities in their territory, the ministerial WTO conference held at Doha instructed the members to find a solution before the end of 2002 (Paragraph 6). This proposal was rejected by, among others, the United States.[30]

Indeed, in August 2003, a few months before the Cancun Summit, an agreement was reached (WTO, Press Release dated 30 August 2003). It provided for an additional flexibility: the possibility for members to import medicines under CL. Thus, a country like Botswana could very well issue a CL and ask a company established in a third country (where the patents would possibly be recognized) to proceed with the manufacture of drugs and export them to its territory, enabling it to deal with a national emergency such as the HIV/AIDS epidemic. Further, the WTO General Council President's statement laid down a series of undertakings to avoid possible abuse and committing the country to use this mechanism in 'good faith'. The statement aimed at reassuring the United States about the unjustified use of the notion of national emergency as a cover for commercial interests. Similarly, the CL issued by exporting members would set out a series of strict conditions: a predetermined production volume, unequivocal identification of products, notification of these conditions and the country of consignment as well as adequate remuneration to the patent owner as provided for in Article 31h of the TRIPS agreement. All in all, since the Uruguay Round, though not reversed, a distinct change had taken place in the balance of power between developed countries and developing countries, as evidence by the Doha declaration adopted on 14 November 2001 and the agreement reached in August 2003.

Finally, in the matter of treatment accessibility, it must be added there is yet some more room for manoeuvre for developing countries in general, and India in particular. There is nothing in the TRIPS agreement that prohibits members from taking institutional price control measures once the principles of national treatment and the most-favoured nation treatment have been met. Indeed, in France, such price control processes do exist. On the one hand, drugs are classified either as reimbursable medicines or as non-reimbursable medicines. On the other hand, negotiations between the public authorities and pharmaceutical companies are arranged to fix the prices of the first category of drugs. Thus, unlike the United States, France has learnt to maintain a balance between compliance to patent laws and controlling public health care expenditure.

For all that, recourse to both the flexibilities contained in the TRIPS agreement and effective price control measures presupposes a very strong political will on the part of Indian authorities as well as adequate economic ability to withstand trade pressures from developed countries. Indeed, the last amendments to the patent law made in 2005 indicate that India is strongly committed to the protection of public health within its territory, and abroad. On the one side, the scope of patentability was restricted. As a consequence, new forms and new uses of a known drug are not patentable. Additionally, a pre-grant opposition is provided: people can oppose a patent application filed by a firm. Due to these two provisions, Novartis was denied market exclusivity rights for its Gleevec in 2005. The patent controllers state that Gleevec was not a new drug but a new use of a previously known drug. Presently, Novartis is challenging the decision. A number of NGOs opposed the patent application filed by the firm Gilead on Tenofovir (an anti-AIDS medicine) on the same ground. NGOs are willing so to ensure patients' access to this essential ARV. Since then, Gilead has announced its intention to grant voluntary licenses to Indian manufacturers for Tenofovir . . . after obtaining a patent in India. Earlier, an opposition was made to GlaxoSmithKline's exclusive market rights on Combivir, an anti-AIDS bi-therapy. On the other side, India has amended its patent law in order to allow exportation of drugs produced under compulsory licence. Thus, domestic firms can produce patented drugs and export low-cost generics to an African country, for instance, as soon as other regulatory conditions are met.

Conclusion

The IPR regime adopted by any country is essentially a tool that strives to ensure both the growth of the domestic pharmaceutical industry and people's access to medicines. But, contrary to the easily advanced theory, there is no paradox between the two. From this perspective, the Indian experience has shown that it is precisely the relaxation of its national IPR regime that promoted the growth of its domestic industry, thereby ensuring better patient access to medicines. However, the globalization process does not overlook any sector, which means that medicines too are submitted to the new legal framework established within the WTO.

Confronted with this new framework, which constitutes a reinforcement of the legal patent system the world over, India is witnessing a reappraisal of its industry and as a corollary, of patients' access to medicines. The problematic of self-sufficiency in health care has resurfaced with the danger of India once again becoming dependant on foreign products, which are themselves fortified by guarantees granted at the international level. It is the main stance taken by some developing countries, which would like the WTO to acknowledge the priority of patient care over drug manufacturers. In other words, these countries would appreciate it if the WHO logic is given more evident and effective weight, for it is a logic that recommends health care for all and the recognition of health as a global public good for this new millennium (Kaul et al., 1999; WHO, 2001; Correa, 2001a).

Admittedly, the Doha Declaration does highlight the right to health care and access to medicines, but the international rules as they exist today are still markedly in favour of manufacturing in developed countries to the detriment of poor countries. This is the entire point of the developing countries' and in particular India's position. These countries are currently engaged in fresh international negotiations in search of a better balance between the urgent necessity to guarantee the most underprivileged populations an as satisfying as possible access to medicines, especially to fight against epidemics, and the consideration of the drug industry's financial compulsions. In any event, this problem has transcended from the national level to the international level.

Yet, to conclude, we must add that for the past five years, far from the logic of 'multilateralism' recommended by the WTO, the US has been going on a tour of developing countries in Latin America, Africa and Asia, with a view to making them sign Free Trade Agreements (FTAs). Since 2000, bilateral or regional agreements have been signed with Jordan, Morocco, Chile and Central America. This tendency to develop trade diplomacy out of the WTO system will surely be reinforced since the WTO General Council formally suspended global trade talks on 27 July 2006, following the collapse of last-ditch efforts to overcome divisions on farm supports. To that extent, the growing number of these FTAs may be much more harmful in matters related to strengthening of IPR protection in the world and could very well make economic compulsions run counter to health care imperatives of developing countries. More precisely, many provisions may undermine the recourse to TRIPS flexibilities, prevent the supply of generic drugs and finally damage drugs accessibility in developing countries. Among others, efforts are being made to broaden the scope of patentability so that new forms and new therapeutic uses can be patented; data protection is ensured for five years, even ten years; and amend provisions governing CL and PI that are more restrictive compared to the ones in the TRIPS agreement. To sum up, these provisions could well strengthen in more than a reasonable manner the interests of the MNCs by ensuring the protection and the extension of monopolistic positions in developing countries (Cptech, 2004; Oxfam, 2004; Abbott, 2006; Guennif, 2006).

NOTES

1. In fact, companies experienced great difficulties in obtaining maximum benefit of their R&D activities and seemed unable to recover the considerable sum invested in the development of new treatment. They were under the constant threat of their competitors copying their products. So, it appears that in the absence of a suitable 'institutional arrangement' (Arrow, 1962) companies were evidently not inclined to allocate funds for their R&D, which resulted in the lowering of general welfare, as access to the latest innovations was being compromised.
2. To cite a few examples, the United Kingdom introduced a patent on medicines in 1949, France in 1959 and Switzerland in 1977.
3. The framework of international negotiations on IPR had thus shifted from the World Intellectual Property Organisation (WIPO), a specialized technical organization, to the WTO vested with a larger mandate, but literally and definitely driven by trade considerations.
4. The reinforcement of the IPR regime in the world is taking place at a time when the World Health Organisation (WHO), another international institution, has launched a programme promoting people's access to essential drugs, as these medicines go a long way in treating diseases that are the most prevalent in developing countries.
5. Seven years from the patent application date or five years from the date of obtaining the patent.
6. In the vital nuclear, agriculture and food supply sectors patenting has been totally banned. We should remember that by adopting short-term process patents, India was but following the example set by the developed countries, which belatedly opted for a more relaxed IPR to encourage the growth of national champions based on a sufficiently large reserved domestic market and to enhance health care self-sufficiency in their country (Mfuka, 2002).
7. At present, drugs with a sales volume higher than $1 million or which hold monopoly over the market come under the purview of the DPCO. Monopoly here means a medicine that has a turnover of more than $250,000 dollars and is supplied by a single manufacturer with at least 90 per cent of the market share. Medicines for which competitive pressure is deemed to be sufficient are exempt from this purview: at least five raw material

manufacturers and ten finished product manufacturers who have each less than 40 per cent of market share either for raw material or the finished product.

8. At present, the sector directly employs 250,000 persons and indirectly 750,000 individuals, especially in distribution (Felker et al., 1997).
9. This phenomenon can be explained by the very high taxation imposed by the Indian government on the import of finished products, which in turn induces domestic production of these products.
10. Indian industry exports a large chunk to the developed markets, especially to the United States. Generic drug manufacture has grown by leaps and bounds impelled by the public authorities seeking to bring health care expenditure under control.
11. In practice, generic drug manufacturers confess that they are not much inclined to market ARV whose production costs are very high, or whose active substance content is very high or whose manufacturing process is complex.
12. A cocktail is a treatment composed of three drugs that are present in a single pill to be taken 2 or 3 times a day. This innovative dosage brings down the number of pills to be taken everyday and improves patient compliance (WHO, 2002).
13. The time taken between the patent application as such and the obtaining of a MA can add up to several years, which brings down by as much the effective monopoly granted by the patent and eats into the pharmaceutical firms' profit meant to cover R&D expenditure.
14. The applicant can also be asked to give details of all the biological sources involved in the invention. Thus, by ensuring respect for the 1992 Biological Diversity Convention (BDC) clauses, biopiracy can be curbed. Further, by proclaiming the States' sovereignty over national resources, the agreement aims at preserving traditional knowledge and biological diversity. Therefore, the applicant has to be capable of proving that the materials' country of origin had given its prior informed consent as per the regulation in force in that country. This also helps in ensuring the creation of a just and equitable system of sharing benefits resulting from the use and marketing of this material. For problems of articulation between the TRIPS agreement and the 1992 convention, cf. Chapman (2002).
15. For the interpretation of the necessity criterion refer to Luff (2004).
16. The patent holder enjoys the rights of use of the product or the process (usus), the voluntary right of disposal of the said product or process (abusus) and the right to enjoy the benefits (fructus) (Mfuka, 2002).
17. Report of the Panel, *Canada: Patent Protection for Pharmaceutical Products*, WT/DS114/R, 17 March 2000, paragraph 7.20.
18. Ibid., paragraph 4.15.
19. For a critical legal review of the notion of CL, refer to Matsushita et al., (2003).
20. Besides, as can be seen from the anthrax episode, which pitted the American public authorities against Bayer that held the patent.

21. Article 31 of the agreement sets out to determine, as accurately as possible, a framework for the CL regime. The list of conditions for the use of CL consists particularly of the following points: authorization to use without the patent owner's consent should be reviewed based on the circumstances peculiar to this problem; a voluntary license should have been requested from the patent owner, at reasonable commercial conditions and within a reasonable period of time (except in times of national emergencies or other circumstances of extreme urgency or in cases of public non-commercial use purposes); the CL's scope and the duration should be limited to the purpose for which it was authorized; its use should be non-exclusive; the use is authorized mainly for replenishment of the domestic market of the member-state that granted this license; the right holder shall be paid adequate remuneration in the circumstances of each case, taking into account the economic value of the authorization and the remunerations are likely to be revised.
22. AVL means that the patent holder has given his consent to a local company to copy the concerned drug, against royalty payments, which shall be marketed only in the internal market.
23. Trade practice, which, in extreme cases, results in the reshipment of those drugs that MNCs sell at preferential tariffs in developing countries, to developed countries to be sold at a higher price by smugglers.
24. The GATT's effectiveness in settling disputes was limited, since the agreement (consensus) of all contracting parties was required for adopting a report (judgement) formulated to settle a case. The expected refusal from the losing party was sufficient to stop the adoption of the report. With WTO, the consensus rule has been reversed: henceforth a unanimous decision is necessary to reject a report (negative consensus). In other words, a report can only be rejected if the 'winning' State rejects a decision given in its favour by the DSB, a hypothesis that has never come true since 1995.
25. See Report of the Panel, *India: Protection Granted by a Patent for Pharmaceutical and Agricultural Chemical Products*, WT/DS79/R, 24 August 1998, paragraph 7.41.
26. Ibid., paragraph 7.30.
27. Ibid., WT/DS50/AB/R, 19 December 1997, paragraphs 57–71.
28. The United States used 'Special 301' against Thailand too.
29. Besides, the proposal came at a moment when companies were going through a serious crisis. Whereas the R&D programmes were becoming costlier by the day, the number of molecules being patented was decreasing substantially every year. To add to the woes, a large number of blockbusters were falling and would be falling in the public domain, eating into the profits of corporations holding patents that had expired or were about to expire (www.cptech.org, Pignarre, 2001).
30. For a presentation on the Indian position, refer to Sen, 2001.

REFERENCES

Agrawal, P. and P. Saibaba, 'TRIPS and India's Pharmaceuticals Industry', *Economic and Political Weekly*, 29 September 2001.

Arrow, K., 'Economic Welfare and the Allocation of Resources for Invention', in R. Nelson (ed.), *The Rate and Direction of Inventive Activity*, Princeton: Princeton University Press, 1962.

Bhattacharya S.K., *TRIPS, Indian Patent (Amendment) Act and India's Agendas in the Next Ministerial Meeting at Mexico*, Indian Institute of Public Administration, 2002.

Boulet, P. and G. Velasquez, *Mondialisation et accès aux médicaments: les implications des Accords ADPIC/OMC*, World Health Organisation, 1999.

Braga, C.A., 'The Economics of Intellectual Property Rights and the GATT: A View from the South', *Vanderbilt Journal of Transnational Law*, 1989, pp. 243–64.

Canal-Forgus, E. and T. Flory, *Recueil des contentieux GATT/OMC*, Bruylant, 2001.

Chaisse, J. and D. Chakraborty, 'Towards a Tumultuous China's Participation in WTO? Issues and Options', in Fanny Cheung, C.S. Tseng and Oliver Yau (eds.) *Harmony v Conflict: Euro-Asian Management in a Turbulent Era*, EAMSA Annual Conference 2004, City University of Hong Kong Press, 2004, pp. 383–94.

———, 'The Doha Development Agenda on Disputes Resolution: An Indian Perspective', *Amity Law Review*, September 2004.

Chaisse, J., 'Preserving the Rights and Obligations of WTO Members: The Indian Perspective in Dispute Settlement', in Alokesh Barua (ed.), *The WTO and India: Issues and Negotiating Strategies*, New Delhi: Sage, 2005.

———, 'Adopting the European Community Legal Structure to the International Trade', *European Business Law Review*, 2006, vol. 17, no. 6, pp. 1615–35.

Chandiramani, N.M., *World Trade Organisation and Globalisation: An Indian Overview*, Mumbai: Shroff Publishers, 1999.

Chapman, A.R., 'The Human Rights Implications of Intellectual Property Protection', *Journal of International Economic Law*, vol. 5, issue 4, December 2002, pp. 861–82.

Chaudhuri, S., 'TRIPS Agreement and Amendment of Patent Act in India', *Economic and Political Weekly*, vol. 37, no. 32, August 2002.

———, *Second Amendment of Patent Act: Scope for Improvement*, Kolkata: Indian Institue of Management, 2003.

Correa, C.M., 'Intellectual Property Rights and the Use of Compulsory Licenses: Options for Developing Countries', *Trade-related Agenda, Development and Equity*, Geneva: Working Papers, South Centre, 1999.

———, 'TRIPS, Development and Public Health', *The Journal of World Intellectual Property*, 3 April, 2001a.

———, 'Review the TRIPS Agreement: Fostering the Transfer Technology to Developing Countries', *Third World Network*, 2001b.

———, and A. Yusuf, *Intellectual Property and International Trade: The TRIPS Agreement*, Kluwer Law International, 1998.

Cptech (2004), www.cptech.org/ip/health/trade/fta-onebig.doc.

Demsetz, H., 'Toward a Theory of Property Right', *American Economic Review*, vol. 57, issue 2, pp. 347–59, May 1967.

Desterbecq, H. and B. Remiche, 'Les Brevets Pharmaceutiques dans les Accords du GATT : l'Enjeu ?', *Revue Internationale de Droit Economique*, t.X, 1, 1996.

Dörmer, S., 'Dispute Settlement and New Development Within the Framework of TRIPS: An Interim Overview', *IRIPCL*, vol. 31, no.1, February 2000, pp. 1–16.

Dubey, D.P., 'Globalisation and its Impact on the Indian Pharmaceutical Industry', *Revolutionary Democracy*, 2003, www.revolutionarydemocracy.org.

Felker, G., S. Chaudhuri, K. György and M. Goldman, 'The Pharmaceutical Industry in India and Hungary: Policies, Institutions and Technological Development', *World Bank Technical Paper*, no. 392, 1997, Work in Progress for Public Discussion, the World Bank.

Gervais, D.J., 'The TRIPs Agreement, Interpretation and Implementation', *European Intellectual Property Review*, no. 3, 1999, pp. 156–62.

Govindaraj, R. and G. Chellaraj, 'The Indian Pharmaceutical Sector: Issues and Options for Health Sector Reform', *World Bank Discussion Paper*, no. 437, 2002. The World Bank.

Grabowsky, H., 'Patents, Innovation and Access to New Pharmaceuticals', *Journal of International Economic Law*, vol. 5, issue 4, December 2002, pp. 849–60.

Gross, A. and S. Patel S., *Indian Pharmaceutical Industry: Market Regulatory, Import and Investment Regime*, Pacific Bridge Inc., 2002, www.pacificbridgemedical.com.

Guennif, S. and C. Mfuka, 'Impact of Intellectual Property Rights on AIDS Public Health Policy in Thailand', in Moatti et al. (ed), *Economics of AIDS and Access to HIV/AIDS Care: Issues and Challenges*, Edition de l'Agence Nationale de Recherche sur le Sida, 2003a.

———, *AIDS in India: Public Heath Related Aspects of Industrial Policy and Intellectual Property Rights in a Developing Country*, CSH Occasional Paper 8, Centre de Sciences Humaines, 2004.

———, 'Promesse et risque du renforcement du brevet au Sud. Transfert technologique, dévelopment pharmaceutique et accès aux traitement', *Cahiers de l'Association Tiers Monde*, 20, 2005, p. 184.

———, 'De la logique de sante publique a la logique industrielle: l'épidémie du Sida en Thaïlande', *Sciences Sociales et Sante*, 21(1), 2003, p. 45.

Kaul, I., I. Grunberg and M.A. Stern, *Global Public Goods: International Cooperation in the 21st century*, New York: UNDP, Oxford University Press, 1999.

Keayla, B.K., 'Patent Protection and the Pharmaceutical Industry', in K.R.G. Nair and A. Kumar (eds.), *Intellectual Property Rights*, New Delhi: Allied Publishers Limited, 1995.

———, 'Trips Patent System: Core and Important Issues of Concern', *National Working on Patent Law*, Government of India, 2003.

Kumar, N., 'India, Paris Convention and TRIPS', *Economic and Political Weekly*, 5 September 1998.

Kunnapallil, P., *Drudgery of Drug Price Controls: Who Benefits*, Center for Civil Society, 2003

Kwa, A., 'Dying for "Free Trade": U.S. or Us?', *Focus on Trade*, part 1, no. 65, August 2001.

Lalitha, N., 'Indian Pharmaceutical Industry in WTO Regime: A SWOT Analysis', *Economic and Political Weekly*, vol. 37, no. 17, August 2002a.

———, 'Drug policy 2002: Prescription for Symptoms', *Economic and Political Weekly*, vol. 37, no. 24, July 2002b.

Lanjouw, J.O., 'The Introduction of Pharmaceutical Product Patents in India: Heartless Exploitation of the Poor and Suffering', Center discussion paper no. 775, Economic Growth Center, Yale University, 1997.

Luff, D., *Le droit de l'Organisation Mondiale du Commerce: Analyse Critique*, Bruxelles: Bruylant, 2004.

Matsushita, M., P. Mavroidis and T.J. Schoenbaum, *The World Trade Organization: Law, Practice and Policy*, Oxford: Oxford University Press, 2003.

Médecins sans Frontières, *Untangling the Web of Price Reductions: A Pricing Guide for the Purchase of ARVs for Developing Countries*, 4th edn., 2003.

Mfuka, C., 'Accords ADPIC et Brevets pharmaceutiques—Le difficile accès des pays en développement aux médicaments antisida', *Revue d'Economie Industrielle*, no. 99, 2nd quarter, 2002.

Mittal, D.K., *Drugs and Pharmaceutical Industry*, New Delhi: Anmol Publications Pvt. Ltd., 1993.

Nair, K.R.G. and A. Kumar, *Intellectual Property Rights*, New Delhi: Allied Publishers Limited, 1995.

Organisation of Pharmaceutical Producers of India, *Drug Prices Control Order–95*, OPPI, 2001.

———, *Pharmaceutical Compendium*, OPPI, 2002.

Oxfam, 'Free Trade Agreement between USA and Thailand Threatens Access to HIV/AIDS Treatment', *Oxfam Briefing Note*, July 2004.

Prasad, A., Ashok Chandra and H. Shripad Bhat, 'Strenghtening India's Patent System. Implications for Pharmaceutical sector', *Economic and Political Weekly*, 22 May 1993.

Ramanna, A., 'Policy Implications of India's Patent Reforms: Patent Applications in the Post-1995 Era', *Economic and Political Weekly*, vol. 37, no. 21, 25 May 2002.

Ramappa, T., *Intellectual Property Rights Under WTO: Tasks Before India*, 1st edn. New Delhi: A.H. Wheeler & Co. Ltd., 2000.

Scherer, F.M. and J. Watal, *Post-TRIPS Options for Access to Patented Medicines in Developing Countries*, ICRIER, Working Paper no. 62, 2001.

Scherer, F.M., *The Patent System and Innovation in Pharmaceuticals*, Cambridge: Harvard University, December, 1998.

Sen, J. 'Negotiating the TRIPS Agreement: India's Experience and Some Domestic Policy Issues', research report, Jaipur: CUTS Centre for International Trade, Economics and Environment.

Singh, S., *Multinational Corporations and Indian Drug Industry*, New Delhi: Criterion Publications, 1985.

Smith, S.E., *Opening Up to the World: India's Pharmaceutical Companies Prepare for 2005*, Asia/Pacific Research Center, Institute for International Studies, Stanford University, 2000.

Srinivasan, S., 'Drug Price Control: Who is in Charge', *Economic and Political Weekly*, vol. 36, no. 12, 24 March 2001.

Sterckx, S., 'Patents and Access to Drugs in Developing Countries: An Ethical Analysis', *Developing World Bioethics*, vol. 4, no. 1, May 2004, pp. 58–75.

Supakankunti, S. et al., 'Impact of the World Trade Organization TRIPS Agreement on the Pharmaceutical Industry in Thailand', *Bulletin of the World Health Organization*, 79(5), 2001.

Watal, J., *Intellectual Property Rights in the WTO and Developing Countries*, New Delhi: Oxford University Press, 2001.

WHO, 'Macroeconomics and Health: Investing in Health for Economic Development', *Report of the Commission Macroeconomics and Health*, chaired by J.D. Sachs, Geneva: WHO, 2001.

WTO, *Agreement on Trade-related Aspects of Intellectual Property Rights*, Annexe 1C, 1994, www.wto.org

———, *Declaration on the TRIPS Agreement and Public Health*, Doha WTO Ministerial 2001, 14 November 2001, www.wto.org

———, *The Doha Declaration Explained*, 2001, www.wto.org

———, 'Implementation of Paragraph 6 of the Doha Declaration on the TRIPS Agreement and Public Health', Decision of the General Council, *WTO News*, 1 September, 2003a, www.wto.org

———, 'Decision removes Final Patent Obstacles to Cheap Drug Imports', *WTO News*, 30 August 2003b, www.wto.org

CHAPTER 8

Why Should We Produce More Doctors?: Socio-economic and Political Framework of a Doctor in India*

RAÏS AKHTAR

The unequal distribution of health care is a typical feature of developing countries including India. In these countries great majority of people suffer excess mortality and morbidity while in contrast the affluent enjoy a health status similar to that of most people in the developed world. Health services also show a lopsided pattern with expenditure primarily concentrated on sophisticated facilities in urban areas, leaving the rural majority practically unserved. The provision of a doctor is the most important component of health care facilities. However, rough estimates suggest that in India nearly 80 per cent of the doctor population work in urban areas which comprise about 25 per cent of the total population.

The amendment (1993) in the Consumer Protection Act, 1986[1] bringing private doctors also under the Act's purview has provoked loud protests from the doctor community. The focus of their protest is that there is a sacred tie between a doctor and a patient, and this relation will suffer with the implementation of this Act. Of course, there is a sacred tie between the two in many cases, but the large number of new generation doctors may not be practising such medical ethics. There is a need to elaborate this dimension of medical ethics and the framework of a doctor in the Indian context with relevant examples.

*I am grateful to the Institute of Development Studies, University of Sussex, for awarding me visiting fellowship and enabling me to carry out my work on Politics of Health Care in India. I am also thankful to Dr. Malcolm Segall for his valuable comments.

It is an open fact that majority of Indian medical graduates either wish to emigrate or practice in urban areas. Therefore, one find it very difficult to understand as to why we still continue to train over 13,170 doctors annually in 165 medical colleges, at a cost of more than Rs. 1 million each.[2] These doctors, according to Antia (1989),

> detest preventive and social medicine and the majority of whom wish to specialize in increasingly abstruse branches of curative medicine, more suited for those who migrate to the affluent countries or practice in affluent urban hospitals in the private sector . . . of the estimated three lakh allopathic doctors, over 70 per cent are at present working in the private sector and of these 80 per cent are in the urban areas, while 75 per cent of our population is rural. The reason for medicine being the students' first choice is not because of a sense of service to the people, especially the underprivileged, but because it ensures a lucrative practice with minimal risk and high social status. Hence the rush for admissions, payment of capitation fees, opening of private medical colleges for those (affluent group) who cannot get admission into the highly subsidized government ones.

This argument by Antia can be substantiated by Table 8.1, which reveals that the majority of Indian doctors who went abroad for specialization belong to surgery and only an insignificant number, i.e. 45 belong to public health, which is so vital from the point of view of the Third World. This is clear evidence that majority of the doctors don't want to serve their own country and wish to remain in Western countries—United States and United Kingdom, where surgery and general medicine are more in demand than public health, while TB and chest diseases and pathology are more relevant in Third World countries.

Antia has also stated (1989), that:

> Maximising of monetary gain and over-production of doctors has invariably led to corrupt practices like fee splitting, giving of unnecessary medicines and injections. The search for monetary gain has also led to the deliberate mystification of medicine. Patients are encouraged to seek the services of the doctors for every imagined illness and accept expensive and unnecessary investigations and therapies.

Banerji has rightly highlighted the crisis prevailing in the medical profession in India, which is, 'manifested in the form of a sharp decline in the ethical standards in the practice of medicine (Banerji, 1989). He quoted examples of the deaths due to use of contaminated intravenous fluids in the prestigious J.J. Hospital in Mumbai and allegation of irregularities in the award of a doctoral degree in medicine to the daughter of the former chief minister of Maharashtra state. The

TABLE 8.1: SUBJECT-WISE DISTRIBUTION OF INDIAN DOCTORS TRAINED ABROAD (1990–8)

Subject	Total Number	
	1990	1998
Surgery	1,601	1,678
General Medicine	1,187	1,216
Obstetrics/Gyanae	716	747
Paediatrics	414	443
Ophthalmology	297	306
Anaesthesiology	264	282
Pathology	89	100
Psychiatry	85	87
Radiology	75	78
Dentistry	65	66
TB-Chest Diseases	51	51
Medicine and Surgery	59	62
Public Health	45	45
Others	779	532
Total	5,813	6,084

Source: Health Information of India, Ministry of Health and Family Welfare, New Delhi, 1991, 1997 and 1998, p. 118.

Government of Maharashtra was forced to set up two inquiry commissions (headed by Justice Lentin). These two commissions have highlighted the malpractices committed in the two premier institutions in the country, namely J.J. Hospital attached to the Grant Medical College and the quality of postgraduate medical examinations being conducted by the University of Bombay.

Further examples of decline in medical ethics can be seen in the study conducted in Mumbai by R.S. Kumar, who uncovered some of the malpractices in the medical world. 'If you visit a doctor for treatment of common cold for instance, you may be pumped with antibiotics, analgesics, vitamins, tonics and decongestants, when all it needs is steam inhalation at home and a couple of words of caution' (Kumar, 1990).

Kumar quoted Pilgaonkar, a retired biochemist who had worked with the WHO, listing only 277 essential drugs and the country having no use for more than 1,000 formulations, even if multiple drug combinations for complicated diseases like tuberculosis are included. Yet the country has a floating market of 60,000 formulations, as drug stores stock many irrelevant medicines—a reflection of the patterns of demand created by the doctor–patient nexus. Kumar quoted one patient who revealed how he was lured into taking a blood test as well as an X-ray for a simple anaesthetic procedure. It is common knowledge that many practitioners are in collusion with agencies that own expensive equipments like computerized axial-tomography (CT) scans or laparoscopes who recommend patients to them for a commission from the organizations. The extent to which medicine is now viewed as a business is reflected in the rash of advertisements for diagnostic centres that have begun to sprout on the walls of the city and in trains and buses, as if the equipment were television sets or pressure cookers. Besides these, diagnostic centres in collusion with practitioners have been known to advise surgery, one more flourishing racket (Kumar, 1990).

Besides, the scheme of importing high technology medical equipments donated through the American Association of Physicians of Indian Origin (AAPIO) in association with the Medical Council of India may add fillip to the trend to acquire inappropriate and unnecessary technology. This will only push up the cost of medicine not only in private institutions, but in public hospitals as well (Kumar, 1988).

According to Tinaikar (1992), over the last decade, the growth of high-tech, five-star hospitals on the one hand, and medical colleges which thrive on astronomical capitation fees, on the other, have substantially contributed to the steep fall in medical ethics and the commercialization of medical profession in this country. Most of these hospitals enjoy the status of public charitable trusts, and as research centres enjoy further rebates and tax concessions. Tinaikar suggests that it is the responsibility of the management of these hospitals to establish internal mechanisms of independent committees to investigate substantiated complaints from patients of overcharging or clandestine charging of fees, excessive or improper drugging, failure to disclose the condition of the patient or the result of diagnosis or the line of treatment, or the absence and 'informed consent' and, above all, the use of patients for clinical research purposes (Tinaikar, 1992).

Such malpractices are not only confined to metropolitan cities, but are also increasing in smaller towns in India. One report suggests that private medical practitioners have never had it so good in Haryana, the state with the second highest per capita income in India. In Karnal, Hissar, Rohtak and elsewhere in Haryana, hysterectomy, cholecystectomy and appendesectomy clinics are seen everywhere (*Hindustan Times*, 1993). A report on the flourishing of medical 'shops' in rural areas of

Punjab reveals a grim story (*Hindustan Times*, 1995). The number of non-qualified and uneducated 'doctors' have increased the past few years in the border district of Amritsar due to non-availability of medical facilities. In the garb of treating patients these quacks befool the poor and innocent villagers and make a fast buck. With majority of government doctors absenting themselves from duty in the remote areas, the people are left with no choice but to get themselves treated from these 'doctors'. These 'doctors' include graduates and undergraduates in humanities and sciences who worked as helpers to senior doctors in the cities; Registered Medical Practitioners (RMP); Ayurvedic and Unani physicians who worked as allopathic doctors; and mobile doctors who just carried with them a few medicines (used for all kinds of diseases), injections and a stethoscope. It has also been noted that these so-called doctors have liaison with private nursing homes operating in cities.

Easy money has resulted in the mushrooming of nursing homes and diagnostic centres set up by not only doctors but quacks who are neither qualified nor hold any stake in the medical profession. The number of such centres has increased many folds with the introduction of computerized equipments which have become handy for the doctors to impress rural patients. In Delhi alone there are about 13,000 such nursing homes and diagnostic centres out of which only 1,000 are registered.

Doctor Dilemma

Table 8.2 shows the supply of doctors for the period 1950 to 1998. It is obvious that there has been more than a tenfold increase in the number of doctors. The latest figures reveal that India produces nearly 13,170 doctors a year. Contrary to this only about 9,000 nurses are trained, though even a rough estimate tells us that the actual need for nurses is over three times the number of doctors. As it is evident from the socio-political framework, the supply of doctors was deliberate. 'The demand for medical education which led to the rapid expansion of medical colleges in the 1960s and early 1970s was in part fuelled directly by parents who saw the chances of emigration for their children' (Jaffery, 1988).

In 1986 alone 238 doctors left for abroad, more than 50 per cent to Arab countries, through Government of India's Foreign Assignment Section. However, large numbers of doctors who join foreign jobs are not covered under Government's Foreign Assignment Section.

TABLE 8.2: NUMBER OF DOCTORS, MEDICAL COLLEGES AND ANNUAL OUTPUT OF DOCTORS

	Doctor	Medical Colleges	Annual Output of Doctor
1950	65,000	30	959
1990	365,000	128	12,292
1998	503,900	165	13,170

Sources: Ministry of Health and Family Welfare, New Delhi, and R. Jaffery (1988) *The Politics of Health in India.*

Doctor Shortage and Unemployment

On the one hand there is acute shortage of doctors particularly in rural and remote hilly areas; on the other hand, large numbers of doctors are unemployed and their number is on the increase. Table 8.3 shows the number of medical graduates and postgraduates on the live register of employment exchanges in different states and union territories. It is significant to note that the number of unemployed doctors is the highest in states with four metropolises namely, Delhi, Mumbai, Chennai and Kolkata. From the figure of nearly 25,612 unemployed doctors in 1986, the numbers rose to 31,360 in 1996 (Table 8.3).

In this context the suggestion put forward by Gish needs serious consideration. According to him, 'it may very well be that if the alternative of emigration is closed to these graduates many may then find their way into smaller and smaller population clusters' (Gish, 1971). Thus there is urgent need to implement the parallel stream of medical practitioners to improve the health care system in rural areas (Mudur, 2007).

Doctors in India: Working Conditions

Gish quoted one foreign returned doctor who wrote an article 'Brain-drain in Medicine', published in the *Times of India* in November 1969, as saying,

> Today politicians and leader-writers never tire of repeating that there is a great need for doctors in rural areas; that while there may be one doctor for a thousand persons in the towns, there is often less than one doctor to a hundred thousand population in villages in the remote parts of the country. This is true and the

TABLE 8.3: NUMBER OF MEDICAL GRADUATES AND POSTGRADUATES (1986–96)

States/Union Territories	1986	1996
Andhra Pradesh	1,894	5,067
Assam	138	105
Bihar	1,514	1,289
Gujarat	785	285
Haryana	405	607
Himachal Pradesh	113	507
Jammu & Kashmir	10	40
Karnataka	1,078	1,138
Kerala	1,492	3,764
Madhya Pradesh	1,133	858
Maharashtra	3,844	3,745
Manipur	45	132
Meghalaya	5	1
Orissa	528	1,825
Punjab	732	395
Rajasthan	673	2,382
Tamil Nadu	2,419	1,960
Tripura	17	85
Uttar Pradesh	1,814	1,110
West Bengal	2,145	1,221
Chandigarh	606	720
Delhi	3,873	3,561
Goa, Daman, Diu	113	146
Lakshadweep	7	6
Mizoram	4	17
Pondicherry	228	348
Total	25,612	31,360

Source: Health Information of India, Ministry of Health and Family Welfare, New Delhi, 1987 and 1997–8,

need for medical facilities in the rural areas cannot be denied, but can one seriously expect a highly trained specialist or surgeon to go and settle down in a rural hospital? He has been trained, often at great expense to himself and the country, to perform a specialised task and his talents and skills would be completely wasted in a rural dispensary. Of the rural hospitals, the less said the better. The equipment is Victorian and often does not work. These hospitals lack laboratories

> and investigative facilities. The only way to get highly trained medical men to settle down in a rural area is to establish a University atmosphere of the kind which is found at the Christian Medical College in Vellore. (Gish, 1971 also see Kalantri, 2007)

Another Indian physician, quoted by the *New York Times* (24 March 1974) put it as, 'there is not even a hut in many villages to work from, there is no medicine, equipment is zero. . . '. In my opinion there is some exaggeration in the statement. However with such a lucrative framework in mind, it looks impossible to persuade urban doctors to settle down in rural areas. To quote Maru, 'even in China where the government assigns jobs to every college graduate, and where dissenting leaders of the medical profession and the party were purged during the Cultural Revolution, it has not been possible radically to alter the distribution of high-level medical manpower in favour of the countryside' (Maru, 1977: 535).

It is obvious from the observations of doctors that the majority of them would not accept working in rural areas, and the available resources in the country cannot create Vellore-type atmosphere in our rural areas. It is worth noting that the vast majority of rural and urban population does not require specialized treatment though urban areas in India as in most developing countries are experiencing fast epidemiological transition similar to Western world. We in fact need a basic doctor who could treat the general communicable and water-borne diseases. Moreover, the present situation related to the non-acceptance of rural jobs is against the accepted policy of the Government of India in respect of undergraduate medical education in the country. This policy clearly states 'That the ultimate goal of medical education should be to enable its products to deal, in the most effective measures, with the health problems of the society.' In view of this Bajaj has laid greater emphasis on the teaching of infectious diseases like amoebiasis. Nevertheless the real significance of such economic losses lies in the fact that money spent on the education of these emigrant physicians or urban-based doctors would have been better spent on other forms of health personnel and healthcare (Bajaj, 1988: 34).

Election Promises

Notwithstanding the fact that the existing medical colleges in the country have not benefitted the majority of the population, especially in the rural areas, politicians are not tired of promising the opening up of new medical colleges during elections, obviously for gaining political support. The example of the State of Gujarat can be cited in this context (*Hindustan Times,* 1989).

It is significant to note that Gujarat in 1989 had 613 unemployed doctors and certainly there was no need for an additional medical college to produce more doctors. Contrary to this the state minister of health had announced in October 1989 that the Gujarat government has decided to open four new medical colleges with 50-seat capacity one each in Bhawnagar, Rajkot, Palanpur, and Surendranagar. According to the Gujarat government the decision was taken in view of the shortage of doctors in the State. It is also evident from Table 8.3 that both Andhra Pradesh and Karnataka had a large number of unemployed doctors. Yet, both the state governments had attempted to establish more fee-paying medical institutes. This had also contributd to the downfall of the two governments in late 1992. In the context of Gujarat the decision to establish more medical colleges was taken by the state government, almost one month before the General Election in November 1989. In 1994 the minister of education in Gujarat had resigned due to the shifting of the location of one proposed medical college from his home constituency. This is a clear indication that the location of a medical college determines the influence of a politician.

Government Efforts

In 1990 the State Government of Uttar Pradesh (the most populous state of the country), finalized a new policy for transfer of doctors. According to it doctors will have to serve at a rural place for a period of three years. They could remain in a district for five years; specialized doctors could be posted for six years. In a division, comprising of 4–5 districts, a doctor could stay for no more than 12 years. However, lady doctors were exempt from these rules. A doctor who did not render services in rural or hilly areas for at least two years would not be entitled for promotion (*Times of India,* 1990). The policy has some rural focus and can benefit the people if implemented strictly. Nevertheless, in addition to promotion, some financial benefits to doctors serving in the rural areas would certainly go a long way in the successful implementation of this policy.[3]

In 1990, the Ministry of Health and Family Welfare, Government of India, proposed that it should be incumbent on all doctors to serve in rural areas before being awarded degrees. According to the then health minister, the situation in rural areas is truly dismal as of a total of 4.5 lakh doctors in the country, only 21,000 are working in villages, while the rural areas contain about 75 per cent of the total population. It has been pointed out that such proposal had been under discussion for quite some time, but has failed to take off because of stiff resistance from the medical fraternity.

Private Practice by Government Doctors

Doctors working in India remained seriously concerned with both private practice and urban preference. A large number of doctors in the state of West Bengal Health Service, agitated against enacting a legislation in 1990 making all teaching posts in medical institutions as non-practising ones. They argued that the legislation would not stop private practice as teachers were the supporters of the left Front Government and would continue their private practice. According to this report, some senior officers such as a vice-chancellor and some deans of medical faculties are engaged in private practice though officially debarred from doing so. In this context it is interesting to note that a study carried out in 1991 decried private practice by doctors in medical colleges in India as it is the major reason for poor quality of their research output. The study conducted by the *National Medical Journal of India* (NMJI), aimed at assessing research done in India's 128 medical colleges over a nine year period (*Hindustan Times*, 1991). The study noted that among the six institutions with highest publications, private practice is not permitted in five institutions.

Capitation Fee

Another serious problem is the establishment of private medical colleges. The criterion for admission in these medical colleges is mainly the paying of the capitation fee. Many such colleges have cropped up in Bihar and in the southern states. As a result, a large number of foreign students mainly from the Middle East and some from Africa, who cannot get admission in their own countries, and children of affluent parents (NRI) find their way into these medical colleges. These medical colleges not only run on the money they collect but have become a source of income leading to commercialization of medical education. According to Sinha 'more and more medical colleges are being started every year and there is no way in which Medical Council of India can stop private medical colleges. Not only students with poor merit get entry into these private medical colleges but even the atmosphere is not conducive to medical education' (Sinha, 1986). Interestingly, it was reported that the Indian Medical Association decided to start medical colleges in various parts of the country with an objective to provide quality education and eradicate several 'unethical systems' prevailing in the medical education, including charging of capitation fee (*Times of India*, 2005). Recent intervention by the Supreme Court in the allotment of seats and fee structure in private medical colleges in Maharashtra will go a long way in streamlining the fee structure in medical colleges.

It is interesting to note that in 1990 a self-financing private medical college had started functioning at Vadakkankulam in south Tamil Nadu without the approval of the MGR Medical University, Medical Council of India or the state government. Similar self-financing dental colleges seemed to be suddenly mushrooming' in the state. The Tamil Nadu Medical Students Association started an agitation against the establishment of these private medical colleges in the early 1990s. The association's argument was that the doctor-population ratio was actually in excess of the norms recommended by the Mudaliar Committee and that the students passing out of private medical colleges were not being properly trained due to the inadequate infrastructure. According to the association the evil of capitation fee will vitiate all aspects of education and reduce medical and dental colleges into commercial establishments (Ramachandran, 1990).

The question is why India has failed to check the deterioration in medical education. The answer lies in the commercialization of medicine because of political patronage as discussed earlier.

To quote Madan

> many of the newly opened medical colleges are, in the words of the President of the Medical Council of India, 'monuments to political influence'. The over production of doctors leads to unemployment since they are unwilling to serve rural areas despite the fact that large number of health centres in rural areas need doctors. Political support to the over production of doctors is evident from the fact that in India, as in Pakistan and Bangladesh, there are more doctors than nurses. Since the training of nurses has no material advantage, no private training centres are being established. Even the government is not keen in the establishment of new nurses training centres though there is acute shortage of paramedical staff in the country. (Madan, 1980: 26)

MEDICAL EDUCATION ABROAD

Since the 1990s and immediately after the breakup of the Soviet Union, there has been a heavy rush of Indian students who seek admissions in medical colleges in Russia, Ukraine, Turkmenistan, Kazakhstan. Thousands of students are being trained in these countries as well as in China, Romania, Bangladesh and Nepal. In several cases, even students of humanities and ineligible science students have been admitted in medical courses abroad (*Hindustan Times*, 2008).

Medical Council of India, has taken a serious view of this, and in 2001 modified the Act, pertaining to medical education in foreign universities. The amended Act states that a person shall not be entitled to be enrolled on any medical register maintained by a State Medical Council or to have his/her name entered in the Indian Medical Register unless he/she qualifies the screening test in India prescribed for such a purpose. It is only after the successful qualification of the list that the foreign medical qualification is deemed to be a recognized medical qualification.

The Act further states that to be eligible to get admission and obtain medical qualification granted by any medical institution in any foreign country the candidate should obtain an eligibility certificate issued by the Council. Otherwise he shall not be eligible to appear in the screening test referred to in sub-section (Part III Section 4).

In the light of the above socio-economic and political framework of doctors, the policy makers need to look into the system of present medical education in India. Establishment of medical colleges should be banned and all capitation fee colleges be closed down. Medical education should be available purely on merit. It may not be out of context to mention that majority of the doctors who completely ignore medical ethics might be coming from capitation fee based medical colleges. However, we need to research on this aspect before arriving at a definite relationship. Nevertheless, poor patients are being exploited. As regards private clinics and diagnostic clinics, it is suggested that all the private clinics be registered only when run by qualified persons. A policy should be evolved under which the distribution pattern of private practitioners is governed, whereby all the residential areas are benefited with the availability of private medical services. Thus it was a timely decision by the government to bring the private medical practice under the Consumer Protection Act.

NOTES

1. Consumer Protection Act, 1986 (Amendment 1993) passed by the government in 1993 is aimed at examining complaints against private doctors for negligence if any.
2. Current exchange rate Rs. 39.69 is equal to USD 1.
3. The proposal of the Indian Health Ministry panel to create a parallel stream of a 3-year course of community health workers to improve the delivery of health care in rural areas, which generally suffer from basic communicable, nutritional and environment-based diseases is a welcome suggestion (Mudur, 2007). Similar proposal was suggested by the author 23 years ago in his joint paper (with Nilofar Izhar), 'Inequalities in the Distribution of Health Care in India', in R. Akhtar and A.T.A. Learmonth (eds), *Geographical Aspects of Health and Disease in India*, New Delhi: Concept, 1985, pp. 437–60.

   Also see, R. Akhtar and N. Izhar (1986), 'The Spatial Distribution of Health Resources Within Countries and Communities: Examples from India and Zambia', *Social Science & Medicine*, 22, pp. 1115–29.

REFERENCES

Antia, N.H., 'Poor Health: Who is to Blame?', *Economic and Political Weekly*, vol. 14, no. 39, pp. 2214.

Bajaj, J.S. , 'Issues in Medical Education', *Indian Journal of Medical Education*, vol. 17, no. 1, 1988.

Benerji, D., 'Crisis in the Medical Profession in India', *Economic and Political Weekly*, vol. 14, no. 20, 1989, p. 1091.

Gish, O., *Doctor Migration and World Health*, Occasional Papers on Social Administration, no. 43, London: G. Bell and Sons, 1971, p. 74.

HT, 1989, 'Four New Medical Colleges in Gujarat', *The Hindustan Times*, New Delhi, 22 October 1989.

———, 1991, 'Doctors' Private Practice Hampering Research', *The Hindustan Times*, New Delhi, 29 July 1991.

———, 1993, 'Doctors Thrive, People Suffer', *The Hindustan Times*, New Delhi, 1 September 1993.

———, 1995, 'Medical Shops Flourishing in Amritsar Villages', *The Hindustan Times*, 10 January 1995.

———, 2008, 'Aspiring Doctors Set Sight on Nepal, and Operation MBBS', *The Hindustan Times*, New Delhi, 8 June 2008.

Jaffery, R., *The Politics of Health in India*, Berkeley: University of California Press, 1988, p. 247.

Kumar, R.S., 'Health: Market for Outdated Technology?', *'Economic and Political Weekly'*, vol. XXIII, no. 35, 1988. p. 773.

———, 'The Great Medical Scam', *The Times of India*, 7 January 1990.

Kalantri, S.P. (Editorial), 'Getting Doctors to the Village: Will Compulsion Works?, *Indian Journal of Medical Education*, no. 4, 2007.

Madan, T.N., *Doctor and Society*, New Delhi: Vikas Publishing House, 1980.

Maru, R.M., 'Health Manpower Strategies for Rural Health Services in India and China, 1949–75', *Social Science and Medicine*, vol. 10, no. 11, 1977.

Mudur, G. 'Doctors Criticise Proposal for Community Practitioners in Rural India, *British Medical Journal*, 334: 12 (6 January), 2007.

Ramachandran, T., 'Row Over Private Medical Colleges', *Indian Express*, New Delhi, 24 March 1990.

Sinha, A.K.N, 'Procedure and Policy of Medical Admission', *The Indian Journal of Medical Education*, vol. 15, no. 1, 1986, pp. 65–8.

TOI, 1990, 'Rural Stint Before Degree', *The Times of India*, New Delhi, 16 September 1990.

———, 2005, 'IMA to Start Medical Colleges', *The Times of India*, New Delhi, 9 May 2005.

Tinaikar, S.S., 'Ethics in Medical Profession: Need for Prescription of Conduct', *The Times of India*, New Delhi, 26 October 1992, p. 10.

PART II

LOW SPEED HEALTH LANDSCAPES

A. Pending Globalization Landscapes

CHAPTER 9

Delhi NGOs Take Charge of the HIV/AIDS Epidemic: An Obligation for Proximity

MATHILDE CLERC

From the 1980s onwards, health has been a global priority. Defined by the WHO as 'a state of complete physical, mental and social well-being', it forms part of the established indicators of a society's level of development, with the process of development being defined by the World Bank as 'the satisfactory incorporation of human societies within their ecosystems'.

The 'HIV/AIDS tornado', which swept all the regions of the world, destroyed, in a few years, what the developing countries had accomplished in terms of 'development' in several dozens of years in the form of an increase in life expectancy, the dynamism of economies or enhanced schooling of children. In the process, it reaffirmed health as a 'privileged field for the fight against social inequalities and the redistribution of wealth, a lever of collective as much as social development' (Massé, 2001), which, therefore, naturally became an integral part of international policies for aid to the countries of the South.

Indeed, from 1986 onwards, WHO's executive board decided to develop the organization's activities against AIDS. The organization had to act as a coordination agency for multilateral and bilateral assistance. But with the rapid propagation of the epidemic in all the countries of the world, the essentially medical orientation of WHO was no longer sufficient to fight HIV in an effective and complete manner. In 1996, in order to respond to the demand of a better coordination of activities, the United Nations' organizations were grouped within a new structure, UNAIDS, so that the epidemic could be tackled in all its dimensions, medical, but also, economic, political, cultural and social.

In the absence of vaccinations and effective and accessible treatment, a check on the HIV epidemic could only be envisaged in the developing countries as the result of solid public health policies aimed at preventing risks of new infections. Public health, whose maxim 'prevention is better than cure' trivially sums up its philosophy, is based on the prescription of positive norms and recommendations, whereby 'behaviours needed to be changed'. According to Raymond Massé (2001), however, it should not appear as 'normativeness that is being imposed, leading to the citizen's alienation, but with an emphasis on its complimentary aspect, it should take the form of a strategy that allows control over one's destiny, social participation, involvement in a collective cause, in other words, a healthy society'.

In this perspective, NGOs have become privileged partners in the fight against HIV/AIDS. By working in the field, NGOs enable direct contacts with people and indeed, have become a symbol and tool of proximity. Carol Lancaster, USAID administrator in the 1980s, had highlighted this growing need for proximity in development programmes: 'Not only do NGOs help in realising our programmes, but they also strengthen civil society by working with local groups' (CETRI, 1998).

In the course of this article, we shall attempt to define the role played by NGOs in the current fight against the HIV/AIDS epidemic in Delhi, India. In the first part, it would be appropriate to first define what NGOs, and to place them in their historical context in order to understand the reasons why their activities have grown in the health sector in India. The second part would describe the content of the Indian HIV/AIDS policy according to the different levels at which the programmes have been implemented, with special attention paid to the state of Delhi. Then we shall try, in the third part, to define the spatial logic that leads NGOs to mark out 'their territory of action' within the city of Delhi. A fourth part will finally question their role and the advantage they offer to the different actors in the fight against HIV/AIDS. Does their proximity to the local population make them genuine 'local alternatives'?

This work was enabled by a field study carried out between January and July 2002 in Delhi. A survey was held in the capital of India within the framework of a Master's dissertation (Clerc, 2003). It studied eighty Delhi-based NGOs, their donors (multilateral and bilateral cooperation institutions, international NGOs and private philanthropic organizations, government agencies) as well as a sample of their users. The results presented and the conclusions drawn in this article are the outcome of this work carried out almost five years ago. It is therefore apt to underline the outdated nature of the statistics given here. While 2002 does not seem so far away, five years constitute a long period in the scale of the recent history of the fight against the epidemic in India. The programmes and institutions responsible for the fight against HIV are actually quite 'young'. However, there has been a rapid development in their activities since 1999.

THE NGO-HEALTH LINK

NGOs?

NGOs vary enormously in their size, their approach and their orientation, their physical, financial and technical resources, the scale of their intervention, the degree of support that they receive from the government, and the socio-political context in which their actions are carried out. This diversity is explained by the fact that the term NGO by itself does not clearly define the type of organization in question. Their name is in fact purely negative—these are organizations that are not included in government structures. So, there might be organizations designated as NGOs, which sometimes have nothing in common, apart from the fact of having been created within a framework other than that of State organizations. For the Louvain-la-Neuve Tricontinental Centre, NGOs are 'autonomous *vis-à-vis* governments and have their roots in what one today terms civil society. . . . They form a body of socially diversified players, acting in the field of development, outside of State organisations, but in close contact with the State' (CETRI, 1998).

However, they can be distinguished from each other by the nature of the activities that they undertake:

- Humanitarian type of activities responding to the immediate needs of material survival, in fields such as health, housing, food, clothing.
- Activities in support of local development take the form of interventions of an economic, social and cultural nature, at the micro level and in favour of local, rural or urban communities, or of specific social groups.

- Activities in support of social struggle, in the economic, social and political fields and those of defence of rights and the protection of peace, are carried out through financial support, organizational support, political pressure, research and analysis, or through the international representation of marginalized groups, with the aim of achieving the transformation of the social structures in place.

NGOs exercising humanitarian type of activities or those of local development can be designated as reformist: they devote themselves to correcting the effects of social inequalities without modifying the structures. When they are engaged in social struggle activities, NGOs are often described as radical. The causes of inequalities, not their consequences, are the focus of attention of such NGOs.

Certain characteristics are, nevertheless, common to all NGOs: the flexibility of their organization and of their decision-making mechanisms, which turns them into structures that are capable of rapidly adapting to the local conditions in which they operate. From the financial point of view, they all have a 'non-profit making' goal, i.e. they do not make any profits. Their funding comes from public subsidies or from private donations, but in no case from capital accumulation.

THE GENESIS AND DEVELOPMENT OF INDIAN NGOs

In India, NGOs are generally known as voluntary action groups or community-based organizations. Theoretically, NGOs were created to educate, create awareness, mobilize or provide for the needs of marginalized groups, the poor and the oppressed. Much before Independence, many enterprises or princes had set up schools, colleges, hospitals, and residences (dharamshalas) for handicapped and disadvantaged people. Health and education continued to be priority sectors for non-governmental activities after Independence, in the 1950s and 1960s. But NGOs only started to visibly emerge in the 1970s, and experienced a real 'explosion', in terms of numbers but also in terms of recognition, in the 1980s.

If the number of NGOs grew considerably in the 1970s, it was because national policy, since Independence, had created a favourable ground for their birth. According to K.L. Sharma (1998), 'After Independence, until the start of the 1970s, the political arena remained one of the main vehicles for social transformation, an autonomous process of change and challenge. . . . Trust in the democratic process encouraged a large acceptance of values and norms proposed for the construction of a new India.' For Nehru, the architect of the new Indian State, the priority was prosperity. It would create appropriate conditions for equality and peace. This position took the form of what Sangeeta Kamat (2002) calls 'State managed capitalism', where the power of decision-making and the administration of the economy in its totality were entrusted to the State, and particularly to the national bourgeoisie.

The dominant objective until the 1980s was therefore that of a strong and powerful State capable of regulating and engaging measures of massive industrialization, of economic production for the global market, and of capital accumulation. But from the beginning of the 1970s, the contradiction between economic growth and egalitarianism was experienced. In the rural zones, where more than 75 per cent of the Indian population was concentrated, the 'flaws' in the development policy affected first the petty peasants and the landless. The miracles of technology, supposed to increase food production, and demanding high financial investment, benefited only the rich farmers. Moreover, water and energy resources being primarily intended for industrial production, drinking water and adequate irrigation resources became inaccessible for the poorest farmers.

The magic of rural development, which took the form of the 1965 Green Revolution, actually benefited only peasants who were proprietors, whose financial means enabled them to adopt methods of intensive agriculture, and to thereby benefit from different types of credit and investments meant to increase production. At the same time, the Indian Communist Party, representing the rights of the poor, particularly of the lower castes and of the landless peasants, was becoming eroded. Its dismemberment gave rise to more or less radical factions, such as the Maoist Party or the Marxist-Leninist Party, and to reformist parties, such as the Communist Party of India (CPI), or the Communist Party of India-Marxist (CPI-M).

The erosion of the belief in a communist revolution, coupled with growing inequalities among the rural populations, created a favourable playing field for the formation and the multiplying of non-governmental and non-political organizations. For K.L. Sharma (1998),

> enormous power was concentrated in the Central Government, and yet, it suffered from powerlessness due to the weakness of systematic links between the political centre and the social peripheries. . . . The State became an agent of the dominant class and of its interests. Greater centralisation of power made it less

autonomous. Confidence in the State's positive role and in its legitimacy was also eroded.

The 1970s likewise marked the decline of official Development Assistance at the global level: the amount of Official Development Assistance (ODA) reduced from 0.44 per cent of the donor countries' GNP in 1960 to 0.33 per cent in 1970 (Sharma, 1998).[1] The reduction in the ODA intended for the developing countries in this case foreshadowed the austerity measures that would mark the 1980s, during which Structural Adjustment Programmes would be set up in the poor countries. Intended to integrate the developing countries into the market economy, and orchestrated by the International Monetary Fund, 'thanks' to austerity measures such as debt service payments, privatizations, reduction of State expenditure, these programmes had disastrous social consequences. International organizations such as the World Bank, specialized institutions of the UNO, and bilateral partners then agreed to create 'safety nets'. In order to avoid a real and dramatic increase in poverty, private organizations capable of substituting for the state in the social sectors had to be subsidized.

The spread of neo-liberal ideology for some, the necessity for better distribution of money to population groups for others, the State renouncing part of its social functions, be that as it may, favoured the expansion and the proliferation of NGOs in the education and health sectors. Indeed, overseas funds were massively poured into NGOs towards the end of the 1980s, and provoked a spectacular increase in their numbers in India. In 1988, the Home Ministry listed 12,000 NGOs receiving overseas funds.

Today, the concept of sustainable development that includes gender relations, environment protection, public health, community participation, applied in the context of economic liberalization, enables Indian NGOs to cover a great diversity of sectors in public life and in society.

THE ADVENT OF COMMUNITY HEALTH: FAVOURABLE AREA FOR NON-GOVERNMENTAL ACTION

'Community participation' is contemporaneous of 'Health for All' and the arrival of 'primary health care'. In September 1978, 130 countries participated in the International Conference at Alma-Ata, organized by WHO and UNICEF, unanimously adopting a declaration emphasizing that primary health care, being as much a part of national health as of general economic and social development, was the means of instituting acceptable health standards for everyone. In May 1979, the World Health Assembly endorsed the declaration and adopted the strategy 'Health for All' as the WHO's dominant priority.

'Health for All' is based on five principles defined in Alma-Ata: equality as far as the availability and the distribution of treatment was concerned; people's active participation in health development; health promotion and prevention of disease should occupy the same place as curative treatment; technology should have a solid scientific base while being socially acceptable and should be available at a cost that the community and the country are able to meet, all sectors of human activity should be taken into account, depending on their direct or indirect effects on health.

The strategy objective applied to all people, whatever be their level of social and economic development. However, 'social justice' requires that special attention be paid to the disadvantaged, in order to enable them to escape from the trap in which poverty has enclosed them. Primary health treatment responds to this expectation. It is based on the following eight points: education concerning different health problems, as well as prevention methods and efforts undertaken to fight them; the promotion of proper food and nutritional conditions; an adequate provision of clean water and basic sanitation measures; maternal and child care, including family planning; vaccination against major infectious diseases; prevention and control of local endemic diseases; treatment of common diseases and lesions; and provision of essential medicines.

Yves Beigbeider perceives in this strategy 'a radical evolution—indeed, a social revolution in the conception and policy of public health, which should reorient government priorities and the activities of the professional health milieus, act on health structures and systems as well as modify the behaviour of population groups by encouraging community participation in preventive action, health education and curative treatment' (Beigbeider, 1997). For Bernard Hours (1998), however 'Health for All' is the continuation of missionary activities of colonial times. The historical context, from 1970 to 1985, in which the number of NGOs working in the health sector went up considerably marks the pinnacle of Third Worldism. According to the anthropologist, 'Western belief in that era imagined development as a cumulative pedagogical process with political, social and health emancipation as its objective, which would define development as a contemporary humanistic project of decolonisation supported by "progressive" Christians or Marxists'.

Indeed, NGOs inspired by Christianity dominate the health sector. In Delhi, for example, out of all the NGOs and donors surveyed, a majority of organizations claiming religious affiliation are Christian. Christian Medical Association of India, Emmanuel Hospital Association, Navjeevan Sewa Mandal, Catholic Relief Services, Church of North India, are just so many organizations claiming Christian affiliation and working in the field of HIV/AIDS, in conformity with ecclesiastical principles. Promoting condoms is not included in the programmes that they subsidize or set up. Only the 'Bapu Nature Cure and Yogashram' organization, which runs educational campaigns on HIV, adopts disease treatment practices based on naturopathy, yoga, massages and acupuncture, since it believes in a holistic conception of well-being and of health. While the NGO relies on the use of traditional Hindu methods, it does not claim any religious affiliation.[2] There certainly exist Hindu, Muslim and Buddhist religious organizations engaged against the spread of epidemics in India, but these are few or do not claim themselves as such, in contrast with Christian organizations. For Bernard Hours (1998),

> this is due to the influence and the experience of missionary activities, with military medicine and missions dispensing most of the treatment intended for the natives. The way of life of the missions on the field explains the familiarity and true proximity to the local population, despite the surrounding paternalism. It is probably here that one should look for the origin of community health, which heralded the 'auto-centric', self-managed and local nature of primary health treatment as it would be later defined by the WHO in Altma Ata in 1978.

Just like community health was the natural approach for NGOs in the 1970s, which they inherited from the missionary 'welfare' practices, primary health treatment was a necessary reference, in line with Third World aspirations for the liberation of men and societies. The strong states set an example by turning health into a public priority. In the weaker states, local communities, with the support and guidance of NGOs, were supposed to contribute to constructing operational and equitable national health systems.

STRUCTURAL ADJUSTMENT AND THE CREATION OF 'SECURITY NETS'

From 1985 onwards, the WHO noted that the economic crisis that raged in many countries was a serious obstacle to realizing the new strategy. Poor countries, which were subjected to an austere policy of reducing public expenditure for balancing their balance of payments, were unable to undertake all the primary health care programmes.

The 1980s' Structural Adjustment Programme and the World Bank's 1993 World Development Report encouraged the governments of poor countries to select public health programmes on the basis of cost-effectiveness.

For Imrana Qadeer (2001), 'While "Health For All" in many countries could be attained by a comprehensive or integrated approach to primary health care, that is to say, by taking into consideration the political, economic and social dimensions, it was rapidly reduced to a selective approach of the latter.' The World Bank World Development Report 1993, entitled 'Investing in Health', prescribed five recommendations for India: cuts in public expenditure on health services, particularly medical services at the tertiary level; the transfer of curative treatment to the private sector; the introduction of a cost recovery system in public hospitals; defining public health 'packages' and those of 'essential' clinical services; elimination of poverty thanks to structural adjustment policies, education and women empowerment.

To compensate for cuts in public health expenditure, the government was encouraged to develop a partnership with 'communities', NGOs, teaching establishments and other community organizations, in order to put their creativity and their commitment at the service of the 'Health for All' strategy. The 'communities', which initially were to serve as the driving force in formulating an operational and just national health system, thus found themselves, from the mid-1980s onwards, entrusted with the mission of almost completely planning and managing their health care.

Today, in the context of the fight against HIV/AIDS, it seems that they play a fundamental role, in view of the inaccessibility of existing treatment, which implies the predominance of preventive action. HIV is a sexually transmissible virus. To prevent its transmission necessitates tackling the question of sexuality, and therefore, of exceeding the boundaries of privacy. Sexuality concerns the personal life of families, couples and individuals. Therefore, the prevention of transmission risks is bound to apply to private space, and consequently, entails the need for cultural and social proximity among the interlocutors. What could symbolize this proximity better than 'communities'? In 1997, UNAIDS claimed that 'action at the community level . . . had always played a major role in the overall response to AIDS'. As for the International HIV/AIDS Alliance, it sets for itself the goal 'of supporting community activities against HIV/AIDS in developing countries, by organising local associations'. These associations are described as community-based associations, since they work at the community level, are well-acquainted with it, and speak on its behalf. As for people suffering from the disease, it seems taken for granted that 'the community' has to ensure that they are well-looked after. For the Voluntary Health Association of India (2001), 'Without the community's substantial participation, HIV prevention and treatment projects are nothing but a bank without money.'

NGOs: INCARNATIONS OF A COMMUNITY FANTASY?

Soizick Crochet (2000) examined the definition and history of the concept of community:

> In the social sciences, the basis of what con-stitutes a 'community' has been the subject of debate since at least a century. After more than forty years of research, a list of 94 definitions was published in 1955 by George Hullery, but the only common denominator that he could find in them was that communities have to do with people. So the 1960s sociologists ended up abandoning the concept. However, administrators and technicians of humanitarian aid readily speak about it as about a physical person: the community mobilises itself, the community shows its willingness to participate and so on. It was demonstrated on several occasions that the notion of community was often defined and applied from the outside, by intervening parties or observers who do not identify themselves as members of the group thus designated. Most often, therefore, 'the community, it's others'.

In India, the phenomenon of community participation in development activities is also known by the name of community development. It seems that the term 'community', in India, is reserved for the poor or for socially marginalized people. Thus, people often speak of a 'community-based approach' when they seek to involve the inhabitants of a slum or a village in a HIV prevention project. When the projects are directed at students, or at the general population, the term 'community' is not used and the project beneficiaries are simply designated by their names.

For Sangeeta Kamat (2002),

> the leadership of community development organization is usually from upper caste men who may be followers of the Mahatma Gandhi, or former military men, or senior professionals who are imbued with a strong sense of civic duty and responsibility, that also meshes well with the Hindu notion of dharma

(duty). Thus, the model visualized in community development is that of the more fortunate, more learned citizen dedicating himself to the improvement of the community as a whole. Accordingly, the strategy for change is their self-identification as role models for the community, especially the poor, who, they anticipate, will emulate them and change accordingly.

Sangeeta Kamat's explanation thus confirms the idea of 'the community, it's others', and more specifically the poor, for whom the rich are responsible.

These views corroborate those of Soizick Crochet, who worked in the field of HIV/AIDS in Cambodia, and one of whose interpretations of community corresponds to a certain type of space or habitat. It designates the inhabitants of a village, in rural areas and the inhabitants of slums, in the urban milieu. In both cases, the space identified as community emerges as a unit of sharing. According to the ethnologist, this vision of the Third World as a place where men, fine and gregarious, know a way of life characterized by consensus and solidarity, can therefore materialize only by the construction of the object 'community'.

Were NGOs created to give concrete shape to the bucolic fantasies of donors, who were concerned about a development adaptable to 'local' conditions? Are they instruments of a 'low-cost policy of solidarity', or are they genuinely endogenous organizations, capable of representing the identities, the aspirations, and the claims of population groups as far as health is concerned?

The Indian HIV/AIDS Policy: A Multi-scale Strategy

Programmes set up at different echelons

The National Aids Control Programme (NACP) includes several components entrusted to different players, at different levels: strengthening of institutional capacities, monitoring of blood and blood products; epidemiological surveillance, HIV prevention, treatment and support for seropositive people. Keeping decentralization in mind, these different missions are sometimes entrusted to National AIDS Control Organization (NACO) or others through it at the national level, sometimes to states through the State Aids Control Societies and sometimes to NGOs.

It is up to the central government to provide strategic and technical assistance to states and to distribute the budget amongst them, to plan monitoring of blood and blood products by funding the purchase of equipment and the modernization of blood banks and laboratories. The responsibility for epidemiological surveillance too lies with it. The central government has also been entrusted the task of funding 'low-cost' treatment of HIV and opportunistic infections in all public health care infrastructures in India, as well as the treatment dispensed by NGOs in low and moderate prevalent states.

Different states and territories, through their States Aids Control Societies, are entrusted with ensuring the planning and funding of prevention measures, and in high prevalent states, of HIV treatment dispensed by NGOs.

The responsibility for 'field' work lies with NGOs: preventive actions, most of the 'care and support' programmes for people living with HIV, and the pre- and post-HIV test counselling sessions in public hospitals. NGOs, who work in the area of HIV/AIDS, can also operate outside the state's framework. Thus, funding might come from other sources but the programmes carried out remain essentially the same.

THE PROBLEM OF LISTING NGOs IN DELHI

According to estimates, some 37,000 people were living with HIV/AIDS in the state of Delhi in 2003,[3] and 925 cases of AIDS were declared between 1986 and 2004.[4] In contrast with the most populated Indian city, Mumbai, the Indian capital does not belong to the category of 'high prevalent cities'. The territory of Delhi is considered as belonging to the category of 'moderate prevalent states', where the epidemic is said to be 'concentrated' since it has exceeded 5 per cent of the population having high-risk behaviour, but has not, however, reached 1 per cent of pregnant women.

When the epidemic is concentrated in 'high-risk group', the priority set by NACO and its partners consists of preventing the virus from percolating from the high-risk groups to the general population. It is then that the NGOs are called to undertake prevention operations.

The listing of NGOs in Delhi posed a problem in 2002. Indeed, the absence of centralized information, along with a very high fluctuation in the number of NGOs that have been developing projects centred on HIV over the years, necessitated cross-referencing between different sources for an exhaustive vision of a 'non-governmental coverage' of the concerned area.

More than 200 Delhi-based NGOs must be working or must have worked in the sphere of AIDS in Delhi. Nonetheless, it would be appropriate to draw up a typological classification, and to extract from it NGOs that are conducting significant and sustainable action in the field. Indeed, a NGO whose 'HIV-component' represents only one or two days of work per year, when it is a matter of participating in an annual information campaign, or a NGO working in the education sector which devotes one session to sexual education for children and adolescents during a school year, cannot be considered on par with NGOs whose mission consists of preventing and treating the infection regularly and frequently, with specific tools and personnel.

In addition, there are many NGOs, which are engaged in the sphere of health or education and which received funding for a short period for regular information operations. However, their subsidies were taken away at the end of the project, thereby causing the disappearance of HIV-centred programmes.

Finally, from the second half of the 1990s onwards, an increase in the number of subsidies intended for non-governmental HIV/AIDS control projects, motivated, without a doubt, the birth of a small number of 'phantom NGOs', which were created to channel funds without really establishing significant activities on the ground. Thus, some NGOs exist 'on paper', without for all that, conducting concrete activities in the city. A chronological study of the number of Delhi-based NGOs working in HIV/AIDS projects shows marked 'growth' between 1994 and 1998, with an acme during this last year: 75 per cent of the 80 NGOs surveyed in Delhi had established HIV/AIDS-related activities between 1994 and 1998. And 18 per cent amongst them had engaged in these between 1998 and 2002. Thus, only 7 per cent of the NGOs worked at fighting HIV before 1994. The figures observed in 2002 in Delhi correspond to the figures reported by Frédéric Bourdier (2001) at the time of a study completed in 1988, in the three cities of Tamil Nadu—Chennai, Coimbatore and Madurai. With reference to these figures, the anthropologist wondered about the rapid increase in the number of NGOs during this period. For the author (Bourdier, 2001),

> a liberalisation policy goes together with an increase in the volume of NGO operations. These experienced an expansion, which was proportional to the foreign funds that poured into the country. Thus, along with older NGOs that had integrated for the most part AIDS prevention in their activities and those that had definitely changed their focus to the fight against the epidemic, there were now new ones that specialised in the field of prevention and information dissemination. . . . Indeed, a whirlwind of funds coming from international organisations caused new candidates with a (sudden?) desire to fight the epidemic to spurt every day.

Consequently, if we remove NGOs that intervene only in an occasional, rare or 'bogus' manner from our list, the number of NGOs operating in Delhi in the area of HIV/AIDS reduces by half. In 2002, 'only' about a hundred NGOs worked in regular HIV/AIDS control programmes.

IN DELHI, 'PREVENTION IS BETTER THAN CURE'

Non-governmental activities in the field of HIV are grouped around four poles: prevention, HIV test, care and support, and fighting against discrimination.

Prevention incorporates different types of interventions, such as, 'Information-Education-Communication' (IEC),[5] the promotion and distribution of condoms, as well as detection-related incentives and counselling. IEC is one of the most widespread activities. It consists of spreading information related to HIV, either through material means such as posters, books, brochures, or through means of the media such as television or radio, or through direct contact with people. So conversations, discussions, theatrical representations and group work serve as means of information.

Detection itself is not undertaken by NGO members, but two of its essential components are: pre- and post-test counselling sessions. In the course of the former, people are prepared for a possibly positive result, and go through an individual IEC session. The post-test counselling session repeats the 'lesson' if the result is negative, and, if the result is positive, marks the transition from detection to treatment. It is actually in the course of this session that the patient is informed about his or her serology result. This is followed by an information session on 'life with the virus': the methods by which others can be protected, dietary practices to be followed, the necessary medical follow up, the development of the disease, existing treatments. In short, the patient is guided towards different support and treatment structures available in the Indian capital, depending on his or her financial means and habits. The post-detection counselling session therefore opens the door to treatment.

The terms care and support encompasses all those activities which enable people living with HIV/AIDS to be attended to from the medical and psycho-logical points of view: delivery of medicines, hospitalization of patients, discussion, counselling, end-of-life support, follow up and financial support for children's education and so on.

Finally, fighting discrimination incorporates activities such as legal support to the seropositive person. If he or she was a victim of discrimination in his or her place of work, hospital or clinic, the NGOs working in this area see to it that his or her rights are protected. As far as the family is concerned, NGOs also work for children of infected people, who would have found themselves expelled from school because of the serological status of their parents, or couples who might be refused marriage for the same reason. Beyond legal support, NGOs acting at this level are also involved with what is commonly called 'rehabilitation'. They are responsible for ensuring the mainstreaming, or, at the very least, fighting against the expulsion of a person living with HIV, from his family, friends or professional circle.

The classification of NGOs according to the type of activity underscores the priority given to prevention activities in the Indian capital (Figure 9.1).

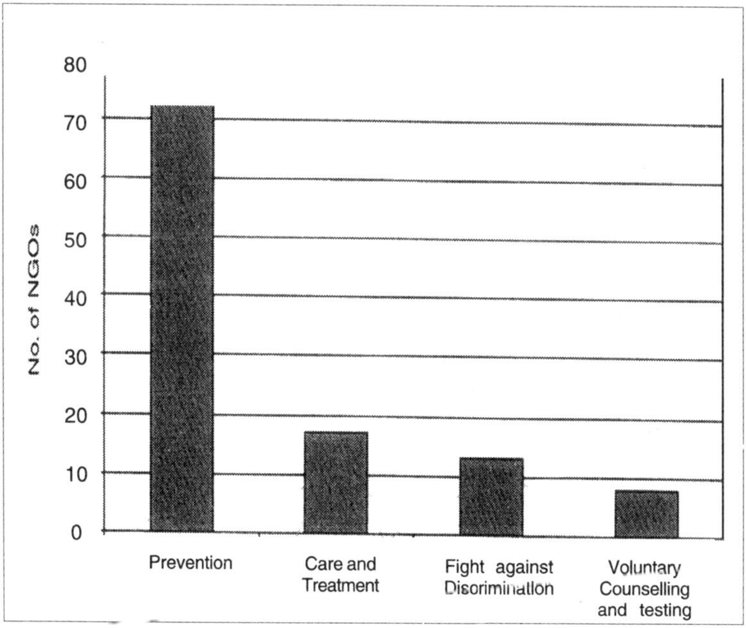

Source: Personal surveys, 2002.

FIGURE 9.1: ACTIVITIES OF 80 NGOs SURVEYED IN DELHI IN 2002

So, from the quantitative point of view, it is clear that preventive measures are given preference. Out of the 80 NGOs that receive funds for fighting against HIV/AIDS in Delhi, 73 are involved in prevention activities, of which 13 carry out both prevention and care and support operations. Sixty are only engaged in prevention activities. And among the 17 NGOs working in the care and support sector, four do not provide medical treatment. They are Positive Life, Delhi Network of Positive People, Navjeevan Sewa Mandal, and Lawyers Collective. These NGOs work on psychological support and on the social rehabilitation of people living with HIV/AIDS, like Navjeevan Sewa Mandal which helps in children's education and morally supports the diseased parents. Besides providing psychological support to seropositive persons, these NGOs defend their rights from the legal perspective as in the case of the Lawyers Collective Association, or, as the other two cases, and constitute a place of exchange of resources and information for persons infected or affected by HIV. They are also engaged in advocacy activities, for access to antiretroviral treatment.

There are very few donors involved in the sphere of care and support in Delhi. International NGOs such as HIV/AIDS Alliance, Catholic Relief Services, and Family Health International, by themselves alone fund the programmes of 11 NGOs. The European Commission supports two NGOs, Sharan and Lawyers Collective, just like the Indian State, whose share in the funding of non-governmental treatment in the capital is only several million rupees, corresponding to 20-bed operations in two care homes until the end of 2002, and those of 30 beds since 2003.

In Delhi, as in most Indian states, emphasis is therefore laid on prevention. Since the state is placed at the infection's intermediary phase, the priority for the Delhi State AIDS Control Society is to prevent the virus from percolating from the 'groups at risk' to the general population.

Actually, until the beginning of the year 2004, HIV/AIDS care was envisaged in India only in the form of treatment of opportunist infections in NGOs or public hospitals. NACO calls this 'low cost AIDS care'. However, it was rare for dispensaries and hospitals to be able to dispense free and regular treatment and care. Indeed, patients suffering from HIV are regularly confronted with refusals of hospitalization under the pretext of lack of place, of means, etc. Even if the situation has developed favourably in public health infrastructures, there is still discrimination towards persons living with HIV/AIDS. And there are also scarcely any initiatives by donors, Indian or foreign, to promote the development of public health infrastructures' capacity for admitting HIV-infected patients. 'Community-based care', also called 'home-based care' or 'community-care' is actually like having the wind in your sails. The term 'community' signifies all that happens outside the hospital, while 'home-based', or 'community-based' clearly spells out that treatment is carried out in the patient's residence or in the midst of his 'community'.

However, due note must be taken of an essential event that occurred during the year 2004: the introduction of anti-retroviral treatments in the national HIV/AIDS control programme and their free distribution in the public hospitals of seven pilot states, including Delhi. The state of health of people living with HIV will therefore improve considerably in the years to come, and one can only be delighted at this policy orientation, though late and selective, since only seven states and certain population groups, based on their resources and age, will have access to this for the time being.

NGO Territory

A Very Heterogeneous Spatial Distribution

Besides the unequal distribution of funds assigned for prevention and treatment, the spatial distribution of NGOs and their activities indicate major heterogeneity in the response to the spread of HIV within the territory of Delhi. As the map in Figure 9.2, non-governmental interventions are concentrated in Delhi's urban areas. And even in the heart of the city, the supply of prevention measures and treatment is very heterogeneous. While there is a relative 'blank' over the entire area occupied by New Delhi, as well as in the Cantonment, south-west and north-west areas of Delhi, you can see 'concentration hubs' in Central Delhi, in the census towns of Jahangirpuri and Narela in the North Delhi district, and Nizamuddin and Govindpuri in South Delhi. In the rest of the city, particularly in the urban neighbourhoods of the west, south, north-east and south-east districts, where the population density is high, you can see relatively homogeneous and significant coverage of prevention measures. Why such a distribution?

While population density allows us to form several hypotheses concerning the location of non-governmental activities, another factor is essential to understand the unequal spatial distribution of NGOs in Delhi. It concerns the location of marginalized population groups. For if NGOs are concentrated in specific areas, it is because they are concentrating on population groups termed 'at risk'. NGO activities are not located according to a particular area to be occupied or covered, but according to the population to be targeted. Therefore, to find NGOs, 'the risk must be located'.

GEOGRAPHICAL LOCATION OF NGOs, GEOGRAPHICAL LOCATION OF POVERTY

Which are the population groups 'at risk'?

NGO 'users' are not people chosen randomly among Delhi's population. Genuine 'social networks' exist within NGOs' 'user population'. In the case of HIV, 90 per cent of the associations work with the socially disadvantaged or marginalized classes[6]: sex workers, whose numerous unprotected sexual relations would place them 'in the front ranks' of HIV infection; injecting drug users who, by sharing injecting devices, would be exposed to high contamination through the medium of blood; and men who have sex with men, whose sexual practices would make them more vulnerable to the infection than heterosexual practices. Street children, because they are vulnerable to drug addiction, easily integrated into prostitution networks, undergo sexual violence, or are precociously sexual, while not having information related to 'sexual health', for want of going to school or growing up in a family, are also part of population groups that are considered very vulnerable to the infection by the virus. Truck drivers and migrant workers living in the slums, on account of their mobility, and consequently, the distance from their spouses, are more likely to frequent sex workers than the population termed general.

While it has been statistically proved that sex workers and intravenous drug users are more contaminated than the general population in India, there are no official figures concerning the virus prevalence rate amongst street children or slum dwellers. Associating 'poor, dirty, pathogenic', to use Alain Vaguet's expression (Vaguet, Rihouey and Eliot, 1995), with the representation of health, in India as elsewhere, could partly explain the attention that is cast on these population groups as regards the fight against HIV.

Figure 9.2 represents the number of non-governmental interventions in Delhi in 2002, in terms of the targeted population group. Almost 59 per cent of the interventions conducted by NGOs concerned 'migrants' or 'slum dwellers'. Programmes directed at street children

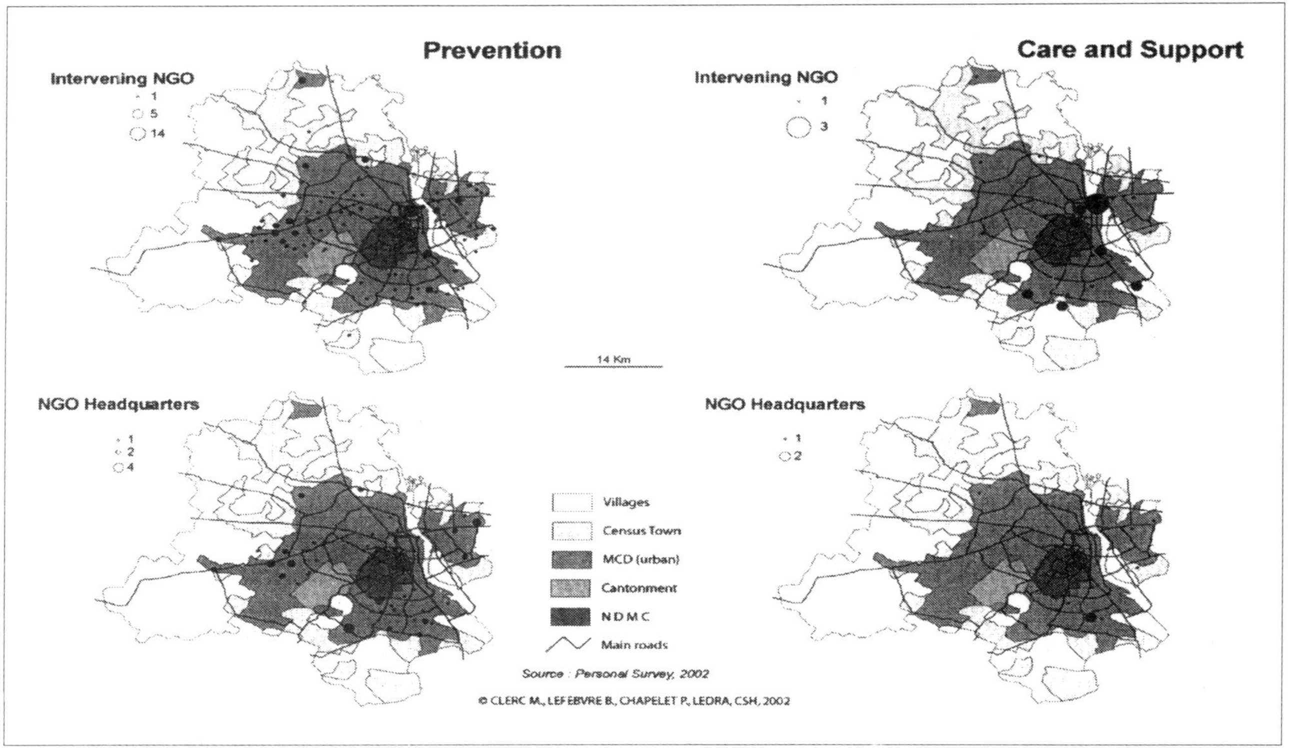

FIGURE 9.2: LOCALIZATION OF NGOs AND THEIR AREAS OF ACTION

constituted 27 per cent of the interventions. Truck drivers and drug users, were priorities for 9 per cent of the projects. Sex workers constituted the next 'target group': more than 3 per cent of the activities were devoted to them. Men who have sex with men formed a very tiny target group for NGOs in the Indian capital, along with the general population (population whose members do not present any special characteristics). Indeed, together they represented only 1 per cent of the interventions.

The location of the first three population groups in Delhi therefore explains to a great extent the location of NGOs. Figure 9.3 represents the areas most frequented by street children, drug users, as well as the spatial distribution of slums. It allows us to observe the geographical relationship between 'slums and drug-addiction zones'. While the opposite is not valid, it nevertheless seems that where there is drug addiction, there are slums. The correlation is however less visible in Central Delhi.

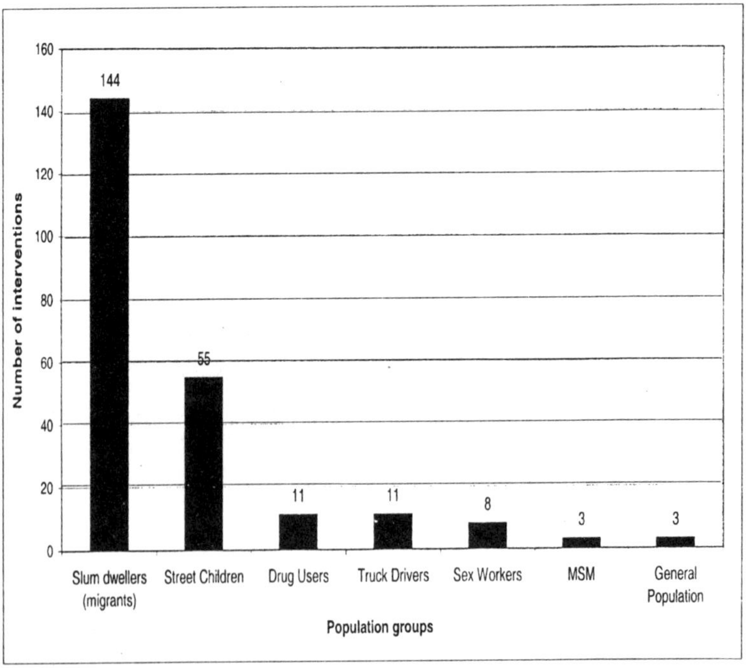

FIGURE 9.3: THE TARGETED POPULATIONS BY THE NGOs IN DELHI (2002)

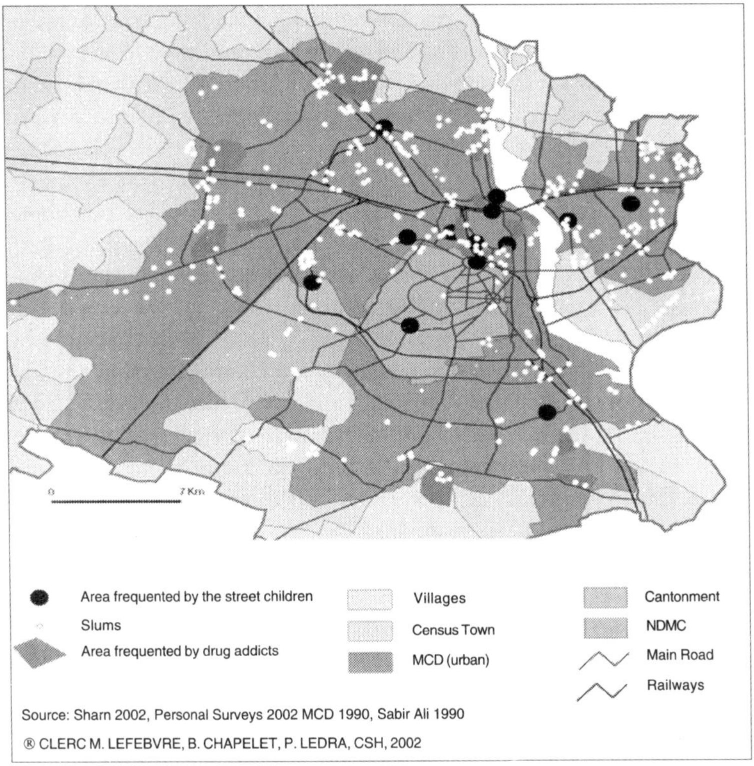

FIGURE 9.4: THE AREAS OF SOCIAL EXCLUSION IN DELHI

DISPERSAL OF SLUMS, DISPERSAL OF NGOs

If the city of Delhi, especially the neighbourhoods in the west, south, south-east and north-east districts benefit from a relatively important and uniformly distributed 'preventive' coverage. This is because slums in these areas are distributed in the same manner. The geographical dispersal of slums in the city of Delhi corresponds with that of NGOs. This dispersal of slums in Delhi is explained by the different sources of jobs that exist within the city, and by the location of 'land left vacant'. For Frédéric Landy (2002), 'They (the slums) have a tendency to follow, or even, to precede the direction taken by the growth of urban areas, because the best opportunities for survival are found in these dynamic areas.' In West Delhi, the neighbourhoods of Uttam Nagar, Mohan

Garden, Vikas Puri, and Hastsal, recently integrated into the Municipal Corporation of Delhi correspond to the 'urbanization fronts', which Frédéric Landy speaks about. Here, slums saw the light of day at the same time as the integration of these neighbourhoods into the city. The presence of large non-built-up areas and construction sites enabled the setting up of temporary housing and the employment of migrant workers at the same time. The same is true for the peripheral neighbourhoods of South Delhi, and the colony of Rohini, in the city's north-west. These areas have been the subject of a lot of non-governmental attention as regards HIV/AIDS prevention. In two districts east of the Yamuna, there are many slums, and many NGOs. This area too has recently seen a lot of growth. It has many small industrial zones, notably textile, and many construction sites. In North Delhi, the Census Town of Jahangirpuri, encircled in the west by railway tracks, in the east by swamps and in the north by a canal, is actually a large industrial zone. Here, four NGOs carry out preventive activities targeted at the inhabitants of temporary housing in this vast area, while two NGOs work specifically with injected drug users.

But it is in Central Delhi, more precisely in Old Delhi, and in Nizamuddin that the largest number of NGOs is to be found. Old Delhi and its peripheral neighbourhoods are actually the places where there is a concentration of non-governmental activities unequalled in the rest of the city. Indeed, the adjoining areas of Kashmere Gate, Chandni Chowk, Yamuna Pushta, Delhi Gate, Paharganj, Motia Khan and Jhandewalan, in Central Delhi host nearly forty NGOs.

CENTRAL DELHI: THE AREA OF CONCENTRATION OF 'RISKS'

Apart from the interventions intended for sex workers, located in a single street called G.B. Road, street children and migrant workers receive the maximum amount of non-governmental attention in Central Delhi. The trading area of Chandni Chowk is a never-ending source of formal or informal employment. Most of the children and migrant workers here are employed in many restaurants and *dhabas*, shops or small manufacturing units. Others work for themselves. They pick up and sort out scrap, beg (mainly around Jama Masjid).[7] Children and adults who have temporary jobs in Chandni Chowk live in the neighbouring slums, or are homeless, and sleep on the neighbourhood's pavements. In fact, it is in this neighbourhood of Delhi that you find the highest number of homeless people (see Dupont, 1997).[8]

Many children and migrant workers are also frequent visitors to the areas of Turkman Gate and Motia Khan, in the south of the walled city. They find jobs with the numerous manufacturers and mechanical repair businesses that operate here. In the north of Chandni Chowk, six NGOs operate in Kashmere Gate. All the activities here are meant for street children. This locality is very popular among marginalized children because Delhi's largest train station is located here. The children are 'self-employed' and work as porters, boot-polishers, or 'guides' for lost tourists. Others work as vendors in the small food stalls and tea shops that proliferate around the station.

South of the walled city, the neighbourhood of Paharganj has seven NGOs, of which six are involved in prevention measures for children. The New Delhi Railway Station located here is a 'street children's paradise'. Fifteen to twenty children arrive here everyday, after having left their families to escape poverty or domestic violence. For these children who are not familiar with the city and 'whose pockets are empty', the station is an ideal place. Here, they easily find work, shelter for the night, and groups of children, of which they can be a part and in which they feel protected. More than 700 children are listed in Paharganj, within and around the station. Children questioned at Paharganj said they preferred the New Delhi station and it surroundings, to the Chandni Chowk bazaar: 'At the New Delhi Station, they are their own bosses, work flexible hours, are able to earn money quickly, and the station provides them sanitation facilities and drinking water.'[9]

While the city centre seems to be a favourite spot for vulnerable population groups and for numerous NGOs, the single street of G.B. Road alone receives the attention of eight NGOs. It is Delhi's 'red light' area; the most important market as far as 'trade in women' is concerned. Women are sold here by the hundreds everyday. While the non-governmental HIV/AIDS-related activities' map shows an incredible concentration of activities at G.B. Road in Central Delhi, it does not mean, for all that, that all the sex workers are concentrated in the same place. Apart from the women in the brothels of G.B. Road, there are prostitutes scattered all over the city. It is therefore very difficult to locate them. A fixed and well-demarcated place such as a 'brothel' allows NGOs to identify and 'reach out to' a large number of prostitutes in the same area. It is technically more difficult to meet sex workers scattered away from each other, and away from the city centre. While the concentration of sex workers facilitates the work of NGOs among prostitutes, their dispersion forms an obstacle. To surmount this difficulty, NGOs target prostitutes' clients, who have been identified as such: truck drivers or migrant workers. That is why the prevention activities' map also shows several interventions located along or near important routes, and at the outskirts of the city. In the context of their work, they rarely enter the city's centre. Thus, NGOs work with them in places of their arrival or departure.

The concentration of truck drivers when they are stationary enables NGOs to get around the obstacle presented by the dispersion and the distance of the prostitutes from the city centre. However, truck drivers are not the only clients and 'inaccessible' prostitutes do not only work along highways. Thus, NGOs get down to preventing HIV/AIDS among the second group reckoned as 'clients of prostitutes' and therefore at risk—'the migrant workers'. And so they foist themselves on the most dynamic and the most attractive labour market, in Old Delhi.

'Central Delhi' thus appears as a hub of NGOs, as they are able to find all sorts of their 'preferred' population groups in this not so large area: sex workers, street children, and migrant workers, who account for more than 86 per cent of the beneficiaries of NGO prevention activities surveyed in 2002 in Delhi.[10]

NIZAMUDDIN: PREVENTION MEASURES TARGETED AT A MUSLIM AREA

The second centre of attraction for NGOs is located in South Delhi, in Nizamuddin, where there is a cluster of seven NGOs, four of which work with children. This neighbourhood is divided into two areas: Nizamuddin East and Nizamuddin West. In the eastern part, well-to-do Indians and expatriates enjoy luxurious housing. In the west, the structures suddenly transform into close-set and dilapidated housing. This is one of the city's Muslim neighbourhoods.

Most of Nizamuddin's children are neither orphans nor migrants. Just like slum children, they live amidst their families whose incomes are insufficient to feed and educate them. In contrast with children in Central Delhi and Connaught Place, who work to ensure their own survival and are homeless, the children of Nizamuddin, by working, contribute towards the family income. Here, small girls make and sell baskets or are employed as servants in the eastern part of the neighbourhood. Most of the small boys gather and sort scrap. Some come to beg in the mosque in the evenings. The Nizamuddin Station enables some to be self-employed as porters, shoe-polishers or vendors in tea shops and *dhabas.* The poor neighbourhood of Nizamuddin West, with a predominant Muslim population, therefore appears as an area apt for an assiduous prevention of HIV/AIDS, notably for NGOs that work with children.

There is also a NGO working among injected drug users. Poverty stricken areas seem to form the most fertile breeding ground for drug users. Indeed, drug use is an overlapping problem of socially excluded population groups that draw NGOs to Central Delhi or Nizamuddin. The correlation between poverty and drug addiction can be confirmed by the results of surveys[11] conducted amongst drug users by the Sharan Association: out of a total of 465 people surveyed, nearly 37 per cent of the respondents earned less than Rs. 100 per day; more than 40 per cent of the people interviewed earned between Rs. 100 and 200 per day; 10 per cent had a daily income between Rs. 201 and 400 while only 6 per cent earned more than Rs 400 per day. More than 45 per cent of drug users' income came from the informal sector: unskilled jobs in areas such as construction or mechanics, jobs of motor or cycle rickshaw drivers. Nearly 14 per cent of the people surveyed picked up and sorted scrap, and 58 per cent were employed in the private sector, in shops or in studios. Jobs 'outside the ambit of the law' such as theft, begging or prostitution represented nearly 17 per cent of the jobs held by psychotropic substance consumers surveyed by Sharan.

Thus, the majority of persons using opiate drugs live in precarious conditions. According to Sharan surveys, 48 per cent of them are illiterate, and 40 per cent homeless. Drug use contributes to fuelling the 'spiral of marginalization', since it creates a new social or spatial segregation. Indeed, people using drugs are de-socialized, live amongst each other in a world 'removed from the law'. Drug addiction is concentrated in less frequented public areas, such as abandoned parks or buildings, public toilets, the banks of the Yamuna, and prisons, including of course, prostitution areas. These are well-demarcated areas, more exposed to risks than any other. Drug consumption, besides the known risks of overdose, weakens the body, and leads to a certain number of illnesses peculiar to or 'facilitated' by drug addiction: venous problems, abscesses, lung diseases, poisoning, etc. Apart from diseases linked to inhalation or injection of substances, the spread of infectious diseases through the blood constitutes one of the major risks. In Delhi as elsewhere, drug-addicted population groups are the most affected by Hepatitis C and HIV/AIDS.

Therefore, socially excluded population groups seem to naturally draw NGOs. Thus, the keyword of these organizations—'proximity'—has a definite spatial connotation: the geographical location of NGOs working in the sphere of HIV/AIDS prevention in Delhi corresponds to the geographical location of risks.

SPATIAL PROXIMITY ENABLED BY EXTENSIVE MOBILITY

HIV/AIDS prevention can be divided into two types of programmes: 'Information-Education-Communication', and 'Primary Healthcare', which includes the detection and treatment of superficial Sexually Transmitted Diseases (STDs).

Two methods are used to carry out the IEC programmes. The first consists of visiting places selected by the NGO, and of spreading information from 'door-to-door'. Thus, members of the targeted population group see social workers streaming into their neighbourhood, knocking on doors to request individual or family interviews. This method implies 'pendular' mobility of NGO workers, who need to regularly visit the selected sites in order to spread information, replenish condom stocks, and evaluate the effectiveness of their interventions through surveys. This involves a regular but intermittent presence. The second method consists of establishing permanent 'Drop-in Centres' in the neighbourhoods. These are sort of small outpatient or social centres that enable the targeted population to obtain oral or written information, counselling, psychological support, or condoms that they need. Drop-in Centres are meeting and interaction places, and in the case of some NGOs working among street children, night accommodation or educational places. Associations such as 'Project Concern International', 'Torch', 'Salaam Balak Trust' or 'Prayas' have all set up Drop-in Centres, which provide not just daycare facilities to street children, but also night accommodation, literacy classes and in certain cases, even meals.

In Delhi, the first stage of HIV/AIDS prevention, which is that of IEC, is carried out mostly in an intermittent and pendular manner, and is therefore a 'one-way street'. Only NGOs move towards population groups, when this is included in their planning. Drop-in Centres, which population groups, especially children visit, once they have been targeted by 'intermittent canvassers', are concentrated in the Indian capital's 'high-risk areas', i.e. Central Delhi and Nizamuddin.

The spatial distribution of primary health care is less imbalanced. NGOs that are involved in this activity are partly mobile, partly sedentary.

Fixed facilities, such as dispensaries or 'STD clinics', are concentrated in Central Delhi, Nizamuddin, and in the outskirts of the city, along the main highways. In the latter case, the STD clinics have been set up for truck drivers. 'Mobile care' is dispensed in small trucks that regularly pass through the targeted neighbourhoods, on an average of once or twice per week.

Consequently, HIV prevention, which requires significant spatial proximity to population groups at risk, is enabled only by a large degree of mobility by NGOs. But does reducing the distance between NGOs and excluded population groups truly reduce the gap between poverty and health?

In the case of IEC programmes, in which most NGOs are mobile, the population groups are not active. Requests for information or health care do not come from them. Can one then consider them as users? Can NGOs in this case be considered as a resort?

Population groups that 'draw' NGOs do not do so intentionally. When NGOs move towards a place and towards the people who live there, it is not in response to a need for treatment or information, but because the NGOs had previously defined this place as a pathogenic area. Moreover, NGOs involved in HIV/AIDS prevention are not open to everyone. The information that they spread, the condoms that they distribute, or the medicines that they use, are intended for a previously determined number of people, according to the financial means assigned to the organization to carry out the programme. The NGOs' sphere of activities is limited, and non-governmental medical services are consequently restricted.

Indeed, every donor provides a NGO with a certain amount of money for a specific time, a particular area (neighbourhood, village, city, etc.), a specific type of population, and a certain number of people. The objectives are quantified before the project is even set up, which compels the NGOs to perform the tasks for which they are subsidized without being able to enlarge their programme for a larger number of people, when this is necessary. Some NGOs surveyed in Delhi in 2002 communicated their frustration as regards the impossibility of extending their programme to the neighbouring slum when they had received funds only for one slum. Others, subsidized for preventing HIV among street children, confessed to being unable to integrate projects linked to homosexuality, prostitution, or drug addiction because their budgets did not allow it.

To that may be added the intermittent nature of their services. Only structures set up permanently, Drop-in centres, STD clinics, or dispensaries could be considered as being an integral part of the health care system, as they are able to respond to the health requirements of Delhi's population unless, of course, these structures are suddenly wiped off the map when funding ends. This was the case for example, with the STD clinic set up by 'Casp-Plan' for three years in Govindpuri; it closed down because the 'project ended'. Can we then speak of the provision of and recourse to information and treatment? Can we speak of the accessibility of health services, when access to these services, determined by the material capacity of population groups, is reduced to nothing?

However, fixed facilities, such as Drop-in Centres, are essentially outpatient and information centres placed at the disposal of different population groups who consequently become their users. Thus, they can be considered as facilities 'offering' information.

The 'Drop-in Centre-Dispensary' set up by Sharan at Yamuna Pushta responds to an ever-increasing demand on the part of drug users. This small structure receives between 140 and 160 people per day. Established on the right bank of the Yamuna, a few dozens of metres from two parks that stretch out under the Yamuna Pushta bridge and that shelter nearly 40 per cent of drug users recorded in Delhi, the infrastructure offers basic medical treatment, counselling, condoms, oral replacement therapies and a syringe exchange programme. Initially expected to receive 500 people the first three years, since it opened in 1998, the Drop-in Centre has already received more than 3,500 persons. Indeed, health care services offered by Sharan respond very precisely to the specific needs of drug-addicted population groups. Above all, it is a place for treatment and counselling, where the idea of 'increase in demand' is taken into account. The first stage consists of limiting the risks associated with drug use, without compelling the users to 'give up'. Hygiene, distribution of condoms and sterile syringes as well as basic health care are essential elements of the first stage. In the second stage, replacement therapies are offered. If they fail, users can restart when they feel the need. Finally, the last stage consists of offering 'a cure' to the users in Sharan's de-addiction centre, located in the Neb Sarai village. The permanence of its programmes in Yamuna Bazar has enabled Sharan's Drop-in Centre to be included among health care infrastructures available in Delhi. Indeed, the ever-increasing number of people that visit it regularly testifies to the fact that it is a genuine facility which meets the specific requirements of drug users.

So, spatial proximity to population groups takes the form of two types of mobility: an alternating mobility, largely prevalent in the IEC programmes, which intermittently provides prevention measures focusing on targeted populations rather than users. The second form of mobility, resulting in the decentralization of NGO programmes, works according to an inverse process. By establishing themselves in a lasting manner near population groups, NGOs appear as a genuine resort. The population groups throng towards these to meet their need for information or treatment.

However, mobility is not the exclusive right prerogative of prevention. Indeed, most HIV/AIDS treatment is carried out in a 'pendular' manner.

LIMITED, HETEROGENEOUS AND UNEVEN AVAILABILITY OF HIV/AIDS TREATMENT

In Delhi, twenty-one home care services and five Care Homes sum up the facilities available for persons living with HIV/AIDS Figure 9.5.[12]

Home care, developed under pressure from international organizations, is much more widespread than 'institutionalized' care, or Care Homes, which are more expensive, but enable true care of people suffering from AIDS and serious opportunistic diseases, thanks to the full-time presence of competent medical personnel and an infrastructure that allows hospitalization of patients. Table 9.1 presents the characteristics of six Care Homes in Delhi.

Only four among these can be considered as care centres that are 'open to all'. These are Sahara, Naz Foundation, Chelsea Care Centres, and, since 2003, Ashraya Holistic Care Centre, established respectively in Neb Sarai and Saket in South Delhi, Shahadra in East Delhi, and near the international airport in West Delhi. Two Care Homes are meant for a specific type of population. At Neb Sarai, the Care Home run by the NGO Sharan is open to only drug addicts. And in Rohini in the north-west, the Navjeevan Sewa Mandal Association Care Home is open to only HIV-infected or affected children.

These Care Homes offer very limited capacity, for if you only consider facilities open to everyone, there are in all 64 beds available in Delhi's NGOs. These facilities, despite the fact that they do not have all the necessary equipment to provide complete care to persons suffering from AIDS and serious opportunistic infections, are currently the only places, which provide relatively complete management of the

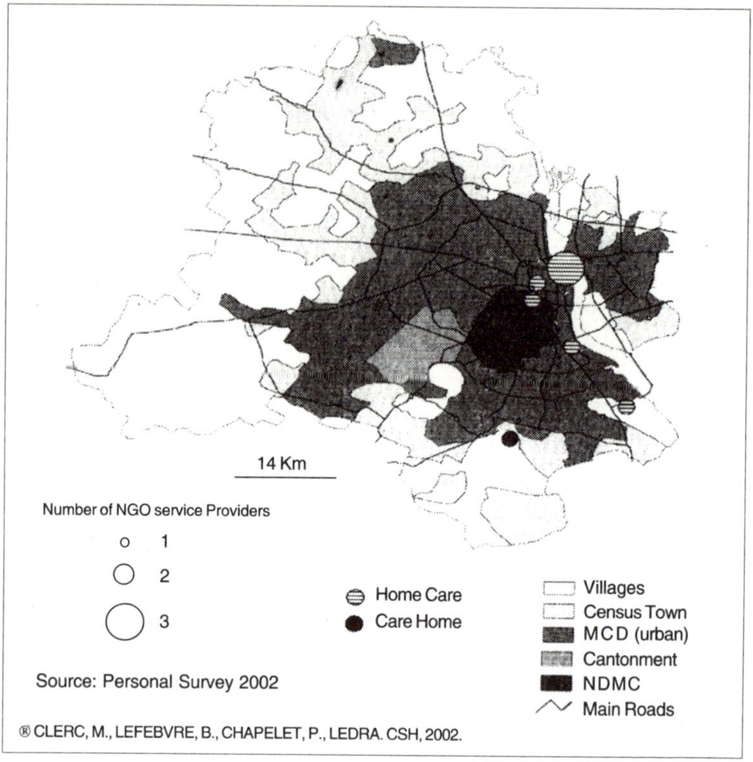

FIGURE 9.5: MEDICAL CARE FOR PERSONS LIVING WITH HIV/AIDS IN DELHI: LIMITED NON-GOVERNMENTAL ACTIVITIES

disease. Home Care is by definition very limited, since it consists of delegating part of the medical management of patients, whose state of health often necessitates 'specialized' treatment, to non-professionals. Thus, patients, their families, and their neighbours have to learn to treat diarrhoea, skin problems, fever and other symptoms of opportunistic diseases. Moreover, the unequal capacities of NGOs in treating diseases render non-governmental availability of treatment heterogeneous and disparate.

The financial means and professional competence vary from one NGO to another. All NGOs are not in a position to treat serious opportunist infections, which necessitate specific treatment and special medical follow-up. Basic vitamins and medicines (paracetamol, ointments, and treatments for ordinary lesions) are distributed by all

TABLE 9.1: CARE HOMES AND THEIR CHARACTERISTICS

Characteristic	Non-Governmental Organizations					
	Sahara Michael's Care Home	Naz Foundation	Chelsea	Sharan	Navjeevan Sewa Mandal	Ashraya Holistic Care Centre
Type of population	All	All	All	Drug users	Children infected/ affected	All
Number of beds	26	18	10	16	12	10

NGOs. Treatment for more serious opportunistic infections, such as tuberculosis, on the other hand, is less widespread. It is provided by only seven NGOs, within the framework of twelve health care programmes, five of which are carried out inside Care Homes, which means that only seven Home Care programmes include treatment for serious opportunistic infections.[13] Thus, the availability of non-governmental medical treatment for people living with HIV/AIDS is very restricted and very unevenly distributed in the Indian capital. If HIV/AIDS necessitated only medical care, then you could say that in Delhi, people living with HIV/AIDS have only a very limited access to treatment.

There are, however, other structures and other programmes, that enable people suffering from retrovirus to be looked after, from the legal and psychological point of view, and to be integrated from a social point of view. You do not die of AIDS. You die of a disease that thrives in a weakened body. Diet, moral well-being, the possibility of being integrated in the midst of a society, are the many factors that slow down this weakening. According to WHO, 'Health is not the absence of disease. It is a state of physical, mental and social well-being.' Although access to antiretroviral treatment is indispensable for the survival of millions of people in the world, the fact remains that people living with HIV/AIDS need psychological, emotional and social support, in order to slow down the virus' progression in their body. While medical treatment provided by NGOs in Delhi is not very widespread and shows a high degree of heterogeneity in terms of quality and quantity, patient management cannot be reduced to mere medical treatment. It includes moral and social dimensions.

Psychological support is a vast area. It incorporates counselling sessions, putting patients in touch with other seropositive people, and fighting discrimination. The latter is not systematically addressed at infected or affected people, but is intended to facilitate or maintain their integration into their family, their friends, and society in general. The fight against discrimination includes information activities among 'civil society', hospital personnel or prison personnel, support to families for providing care to patients, and incorporating people with HIV/AIDS into programmes and projects that concern them. Psychological support can be offered by NGOs that do not offer medical treatment. This is the case of associations such as Delhi Network of Positive People and Positive Life. These two NGOs are essentially reception and resource centres for people living with HIV/AIDS. Besides fighting discrimination, they also serve as intermediaries. They admit and organize meetings among seropositive people, offer documentation and works on the disease, the means of protecting oneself from it, advice related to diet and opportunistic infections, and guide people towards different medical, social or legal infrastructures that they might require.

Legal support, provided by Lawyers Collective, is divided into several stages. The first is that of increasing awareness in legal and political circles about problems encountered by people with HIV/AIDS: dismissals, expulsion from hospitals, from schools for children, ban on marriages, forced abortions, lack of access to medicines, and so on. The second consists of informing people of their rights: the right to confidentiality, a say in the use and dissemination of information contained in medical files, the right to refuse a detection test, the right to medical treatment, the right to work, to pregnancy, to marriage, to education. The third stage consists of lobbying for the adoption of laws specific to HIV/AIDS, access to antiretroviral treatment, the protection of sexual minors, sex workers and women. Lawyers Collective has also initiated proceedings on behalf of victims of contaminated blood, and is campaigning for systematic and effective monitoring of blood distributed in hospitals.

Further, the last three NGOs have a political vocation. Apart from their activities among people living with HIV, they work for the defence of human rights, with activities in an area much larger than that demarcated by the boundaries of the territory of Delhi. Campaigning for universal access to antiretroviral treatment, they work at representing patients at an urban but also national and global scale.

NGOs: Vehicles of Social Transformation or Alibis of an Unequal System?

The End of the State?

While NGOs might appear as a stop-gap measure, used as a substitute to the Indian public health sector by international and foreign agencies, it is, however, important to consider the role of the State that, despite outward appearances, is very much present.

Indeed, from the legislative point of view, two elements allow the State to keep a hold on non-governmental activities. First of all, the Indian State lets in international and foreign NGOs in very small doses in its territory. They are allowed access as potential donors and providers of technical assistance, but cannot work directly with the people. Only in cases of extreme emergencies, such as natural disasters, famines, or wars, is this authorized.

The second legal instrument that the central government has at its disposal for monitoring non-governmental activities is called FCRA: Foreign Currency Regulation Act. It binds every NGO that receives funds from abroad to obtain a certificate from the Home Ministry that allows it to perform tasks that it is supposed to detail in advance. This is to keep the central government informed of activities that it does not administer directly. The Act's history, brought to light by Sangeeta Kamat (2002), shows the dominant role that it plays in the State's control over foreign investments and the Indian civil society's movements. In the 1970s, following development failures in rural areas and an increase in inequality in urban zones was observed, which resulted in the spectacular rise in the number of slums, the resurgence or the formation of more or less extremist movements, such as the Naxalites in West Bengal, or the Communist-Maoist Party in several parts of India. The Narmada Bachao Andolan, an organization formed by landless peasants, low-caste farmers and tribals, who focused their claims on an equitable redistribution of land and resources for the benefit of the poor, succeeded in attracting the sympathy and support of international environmentalists as well as those of the progressive Indian middle class. The agitation led by small farmers and the landless, combined with the discontent of the socially disadvantaged classes and young urban activists, led to a legitimacy crisis for the Congress party. Indira Gandhi, the then prime minister, declared a state of Emergency in 1975, which enabled her to legitimize a certain number of repressive actions (imprisonment of political dissidents, forced sterilization of working class men and minorities, especially Muslims). To that was added the famous FCRA, justified by the need to control separatist movements. Thus, henceforth, the distribution of funds intended for non-governmental organizations required the Home Ministry's approval.

Consequently, today, two legal instruments allow the State to exercise its power of review over NGOs and their foreign partners: a ban on foreign organizations to establish themselves locally, and the FCRA.

However, the State's presence in the non-governmental domain of health does not stop at these two laws. For Frédéric Bourdier (2001), 'Whereas in other sectors of activity, NGOs continue to be pressure groups and are straightaway able to establish a presence in the political and social spheres, rarely any NGO, which has devoted itself to AIDS, manages to preserve a broader range of perspectives and maintain genuine ideological independence'. In reality, NGOs that work in the area of HIV/AIDS are pursuing activities that are nothing but an extension of governmental programmes, and cannot oppose them in any case. As far as prevention is concerned, NGOs help in reaching out to population groups to which state institutions do not have access, on account of these groups' marginalization. NACO and its State AIDS Control Societies fund more than 600 NGOs to conduct preventive interventions targeted and recommended in the national programme.

NGOs, involved in HIV/AIDS control activities, and particularly those working on prevention measures, can, therefore, be neither anti-State, nor provide an alternative to the State, simply because the State has inducted them into its own policy and into its own programme of action. Thus, NGO activities in the sphere of health do not suggest the State's absence nor a weakening of the State, since NGOs further the latter's activities.

NGOs: ALTERNATIVE OR STOP-GAP MEASURE?

Though NGOs have been integrated into the national HIV control programme, there are nevertheless sectors where NGO activities substitute for those of the government. Without calling into question national policy, certain NGOs create programmes for making up for governmental lacunae.

This is notably the case with HIV/AIDS treatment and prevention among certain types of population, such as homosexuals and drug users. Here, it is not a question of an alternative strategy, but of a palliative strategy. Because the State shows its weaknesses in these areas, and because 'hunger cannot wait for a revolution',[14] it is for the NGOs to take over.

In the sphere of prevention among homosexual populations, it was the State's attitude of denial that motivated the creation of non-governmental palliative structures. It was because no Indian public funding could be envisaged that NGOs working with homosexuals resorted to financial assistance from foreign organizations such as Ford Foundation, MacArthur Foundation, or Swedish International Development Agency (SIDA).

In the case of drug addiction, Indian policy is not really marked by an attitude of denial, but rather by a refusal to take into consideration the specific needs of people using drugs. Indeed, State-funded non-governmental organizations as well as public health services that have been made available to drug addicts work only on programmes based on abstinence, supplemented in certain cases with yoga sessions, manual labour, sports sessions, and, sometimes, with medicinal support of the homeopathic, ayurvedic or naturopathic type.

The distribution of sterile injection material is considered by government policy as incitement to consumption, and the oral administration of Buprenorphine, an allopathic replacement therapy treatment, is conceived as the replacement of one addiction by another. In such cases, NGOs are both a stop-gap measure and an alternative. They are a stop-gap measure when they distribute sterile injection material, deemed indispensable by AUSAID and the European Commission for an effective prevention of HIV among intravenous drug users, and an alternative when they propose another 'de-addiction programme' in place of the Indian strategy, based on abstinence, backed in certain cases by 'traditional' medicinal treatment. NGOs that distribute Buprenorphine prefer a method based on allopathic replacement therapy, widely prevalent in Western countries, and meant to reduce physical suffering related to withdrawal.

It is in the area of HIV treatment that the stop-gap nature of NGOs is more visible. For, if it was justified in the 1980s and in early 1990s to consider the HIV control policy in developing countries as only a risk prevention policy. Today, it is intolerable that antiretroviral treatments not be included in the fight against AIDS. Now, the States whose bilateral cooperation organizations fund low-cost care through NGOs are the same who opposed the spread of antiretroviral treatment in all countries of the world. 'Large-scale pillage goes well, for the time being, with small-scale salvage that gives the West a clean conscience', wrote Bernard Hours in 1998. His reflection is still relevant.

Thus, funding of non-governmental activities by developed countries can appear as a means for lessening imbalances—an outcome of unequal political and economic regulations—deliberately brought about by these same countries. Humanitarianism in this case is not aimed at fighting injustices or inequalities. It is used to conceal them. Rony Brauman, former president of Médecins Sans Frontières, himself described this phenomenon (2002): 'To the question "What is Man?", humanitarian philosophy simply responds that he is not made for suffering. Humanitarian principles forbid thinking of suffering by the yardstick of history and politics.' NGOs have since then appeared as instruments meant to mitigate the devastating effects of unequal liberal policies, all the while presenting a 'local' character, which gives them their so very respectable democratic dimension.

Conclusion

The spread of HIV/AIDS within the Indian Union necessitated, as in other countries in the world, an effective risk prevention policy intended to modify behaviour and sexual practices.

The population groups approached by NGOs working in HIV/AIDS prevention are those that are socially excluded. Their access to social services, especially educational and health services, is limited. From a material perspective, which includes financial and temporal aspects, these population groups do not have the necessary means to move about and take care of themselves. Thus, it falls upon NGOs to 'disseminate health' in these areas of exclusion. Being 'vehicles of health', NGOs have to be mobile. However, this mobility has taken the form of alternating migration. This means that in terms of time or area, information or primary health care provided is limited or selective. You may then wonder 'who has access to what?' Is it the NGOs that have access to the poor, or the poor who have access to the NGOs?

The 'community' and intermittent nature of AIDS care also raises the question of its 'authenticity'. Does this not give the impression of a stop-gap measure? Because public health services do not have sufficient means to meet the demands of patients suffering from AIDS, so patients, their family and friends circle, and organizations that sometimes have no medical specialization, are encouraged to provide proper care themselves. Indeed, the priority granted to prevention and Home Care programmes gives the impression that there has been a dismantling of the Indian public health system, in keeping with a neo-liberal ideology already contained in the 1980s Structural Adjustment Programmes.

However, rather than a series of clashes between NGOs and the State, or between the State and the Market, the advent of NGOs also marked the advent of a shared belief in a 'risk managing' and consequently profitable public health model. Indeed, NGOs appear as either extensions, or stop-gap measures of governmental activities. But whatever be their position, they do not ideologically oppose the State, which itself does not oppose the international HIV control policy. According to Bernard Hours (1998), we are experiencing today

> global co-management between, on the one hand, donors that hold most of the power to post a single public health model and NGOs, on the other, which implement the model, test its main aspects, make the connection with the field where the model has to be established, with the agreement of the State authorities, which does not have its own resources for proposing another policy.

NGOs therefore serve as ideological intermediaries for a development model that has come from elsewhere, for which health has become both the indicator and the objective.

> The social right to health has progressively generated a health obligation, a duty to follow recommendations that are capable of averting the onset of diseases that prove costly for the community. But health obligation is not just the response to a need for cost control. It is also a social and cultural process of impregnating values of perfect health, a conception of life and happiness. (Hours, 2001)

While we can justify such considerations regarding public health policies dictated by 'Western morals' in developing countries, the fact remains that today, 40 million people live with HIV/AIDS in the world, and for the most part, they do not have the necessary time to reflect on and criticize the measures that are intended for them. For Rony Brauman (2002),

> From a purely moral point of view, it is simply impossible to quantify the suffering inflicted and the suffering spared. Despite all the contradictions that go with it, the fact of trying to save people, alleviating their distress, remains fundamental. This cannot be shrugged off as small change in the broader perspective of political calculations.

Although NGOs are used by international and state organizations as 'tokens of democracy' or 'consensus builders', they work to minimize suffering. In the HIV/AIDS field, they try to apply a policy, which has undoubtedly been orchestrated by political and economic interests of the most powerful, but which all the same, aims at reducing rates of mortality, morbidity, and the suffering of thousands of patients, for whom HIV/AIDS, before being an economic or ideological instrument of subservience, is a fatal disease.

NOTES

1. *Source*: Comité d'Aide au Développement, *Annual Report*, OECD, 1998.
2. See the article 'Bapu Nature Cure and Yogashram of Naturopathy, a Gandhian Way of Healthy Living': http://www.organiser.org, 24 July 2004.
3. This figure was taken from the site 'http://www.indiastat.org'. The source of this figure indicated on the site is the following: 'Rajya Sabha Unstarred Question No. 571, 8 December 2003'. Nevertheless, this figure is to be used with caution, as the method of calculation is not mentioned on the site. NACO noted, for Delhi, in 2003, a prevalence equal to 0.13 per cent among pregnant women, and equal to 7.20 per cent among patients suffering from sexually transmissable diseases.
4. Source: National Aids Control Organisation, August 2004.
5. Activity currently termed IEC, both in English and French, in all official documents.
6. Personal surveys, 2002.
7. More than 100 children were listed as beggars in Jama Masjid by the Deepalaya Association.
8. Cf. Véronique Dupont, 'Les "rurbains" de Delhi', *Espaces, Populations, Sociétés*, nos. 2–3, 1997.
9. Results of surveys carried out by the Deepalaya Association, unpublished.
10. Personal surveys, 2002.
11. See Sharan, 'Rapid Situation Assessment of Drug Use in Delhi', unpublished New Delhi, 2002.
12. Personal surveys, 2002.
13. Ibid.
14. Brazilian theologist Leonardo Boff's sentence, used in relation to the need for humanitarian aid.

REFERENCES

Beigbeider, Yves, '*L'organisation mondiale de la santé*', Que sais-je? no. 3234, Presses Universitaires de France, 1997.

Bourdier, Frédéric, 'Ideo-logiques des prises de décision : le cas des ONG face au gouvernement indien à propos du Sida', in Bernard Hours, '*Systèmes et politiques de santé*', Karthala, 2001.

———, '*Sexualité et Sociabilité en Inde du Sud. Familles en péril au temps du Sida*', Karthala, 2001.

Brauman, Rony, *Humanitaire le dilemme ; Entretien avec Philippe Petit*, Paris: Literal, 2002.

Centre Tricontinental de Louvain La Neuve (CETRI—Louvain La Neuve Tricontinental Centre), *Les ONG, instruments du néolibéralisme ou alternatives populaires* ?', L'Harmattan, 1998.

Clerc, Mathilde (under the guidance of Alain Vaguet), 'Les ONG face au VIH / sida: entre institutions internationales, Etat, et Société Civile', Master's thesis in Geography, University of Rouen, 2003.

Crochet, Soizick, 'Cet obscur objet du désir : la participation communautaire', in Rony Brauman, *Utopies Sanitaires*, Paris: Le Pommier Fayard, 2000.

Dupont, Véronique, *Les rurbains de Delhi*, Espaces, Populations, Sociétés, no. 2–3, 1997.

Eliot, Emmanuel, 'Les lieux du VIH dans l'espace indien', Doctorate in Geography, University of Rouen, 1999.

Hours, Bernard, *Systèmes et politiques de santé*, Paris: Karthala, 2001.

———, 'Pour une anthropologie de la santé en sociétés', in B. Hours (ed.), *Systèmes et Politiques de Santé*, Paris: Karthala, 2001.

———, *L'idéologie humanitaire ou le spectacle de l'altérité perdue*, Paris: L'Harmattan, 1998.

Jain, Kalpana, *Positive Lives*, New Delhi: Penguin Books, 2002.

Kamat, Sangeeta, *Development Hegemony: NGOs and the State in India*, New Delhi: Oxford University Press, 2002.

Landy, Frédéric, *L'Union Indienne*, Nantes: Editions du Temps, 2002.

Massé, Raymond, 'La santé publique comme projet politique et projet individuel', in B. Hours (ed.), *Systèmes et Politiques de Santé*, Paris: Karthala, 2001.

NACO, 'Estimation of HIV/AIDS in India', www.naco.nic.org, 2003.

———, *Combating HIV/AIDS in India 2000–1*, Ministry of Health and Family Welfare, Government of India, 2001.

———, *Combating HIV/AIDS in India 1999–2000*, Ministry of Health and Family Welfare, Government of India, 2000.

Qadeer, Imrana, *Public Health and the Poverty of Reforms*, New Delhi: Sage Publications, 2001.

Rao, Mohan, *Disinvesting in Health: The World Bank's Prescription for Health*, New Delhi: Sage Publications, 1999.

Sharan, 'Rapid Situation Assessment of Drug Use in Delhi', unpublished, 2002.

Sharma K.L., 'L'Etat indien et les ONG: quelques réflexions', in CETRI, *Les ONG, instruments du néo-libéralisme ou alternatives populaires?*, Paris: L'Harmattan, 1998.

Steffen, Monica, *Les états face au Sida en Europe*, Presses universitaires de Grenoble, 2001.

Vaguet, Alain, Florence Rihouey and Emmanuel Eliot, 'Santé et culture en contexte urbain indien', *Espace, Populations, Sociétés*, no. 1995-1, Lille, 1995.

Voluntary Health Association of India (VHAI), *Community Action on HIV for Indian NGOs*, VHAI Press, 2001.

World Bank, *World Development Report 1993: Investing in Health*, 1993.

CHAPTER 10

From Global Policy to Local Politics: The Eradication of Leprosy in India

FABIENNE MARTIN

INTRODUCTION

International agencies such as the World Bank and the International Monetary Fund turned up in India in the early 1990s. No one has forgotten their involvement in the funding of the highly controversial Narmada Dam construction project. However, other collaborations that were not as extensively covered by the media also occurred, especially in the field of health. Thus, it was in collaboration with the World Bank that the Indian government launched the first phase of the National Leprosy Eradication Programme (NLEP) in 1993.

A National Leprosy Control Programme (NLCP) had been started in 1955. Its characteristic was the early detection of the disease and regular treatment of the patients with Dapsone monotherapy. The strategy was to control the disease through reduction in the quantum of infection in the population and thereby breaking the chain of disease transmission. With the availability of new treatments the programme was rebaptized National Leprosy Eradication Programme in 1983 with the aim of a complete eradication of leprosy. In 1991, the World Health Assembly resolved to eliminate leprosy as a public health problem by the end of the century, i.e. with a prevalence rate (number of cases per 10,000 inhabitants) of less than one. This goal has been taken up by the NLEP which received funding worth Rs. 6 billion from the World Bank in 1993–4. The first phase of World Bank funding was completed in September 2000. The project was then further extended for a period of five years. In addition, in 1999, the Global Alliance for Elimination of Leprosy (GAEL) was initiated with the aim of: 'carrying out a concerted and coordinated effort to eliminate leprosy in all countries by 2005'. The GAEL included representatives (ministers of health and/or directors of health services) from twelve main endemic countries, the Nippon Foundation/Sasakawa Memorial Health Foundation, the Novartis Sustainable Development Foundation, International Federation of Anti-Leprosy Associations (ILEP), Danish International Development Assistance (DANIDA), World Bank, members of the WHO Technical Advisory Group and the WHO Headquarters and regions. In 2000, the first chairmanship of the Alliance went to the Indian government.

Both at the global and national levels, leprosy management comes within the competence of public health policies like other diseases such as AIDS, cancer, malaria and TB. The way the policies are conceived and then applied call for a plurality of organizations (national and international, state and private) and a diversity of actors (administrators, scientists, doctors, social workers) to work together with a common goal: the eradication of leprosy. On the one hand, there are national and international issues involved concerning the definition of a common policy *vis-à-vis* leprosy. On the other hand, there is an importance of actors at the local level in the form of specialized and/or sectorial NGOs who are in charge of the implementation of measures. Thus, this diversity of partners and issues questions the articulation of the micro and macro level.

Depending on the different states of India and the availability of existing structures, the implementation of the NLEP was entrusted either to public health institutions (hospitals, dispensaries or health centres) or to private associations and NGOs.

In the state of Rajasthan, the implementation of this programme was entrusted to the Indian NGO Sarthak Manav Kushtashram (SMK), the name literally meaning 'leprosy community with a humanitarian purpose'. SMK had already been working in the leprosy field in India for about fifteen years by managing leper groups. It was precisely this experience that contributed to a decision in its favour for registration within the NLEP. Today, SMK stands as a model in the treatment and rehabilitation of leprosy patients.

As underlined above, the NLEP brings together a number of actors and institutions with the aim of controlling and in time eradicating leprosy. In this article we will examine how NLEP is structured around its different partners and the relations that govern them, covering both the decision-making authorities responsible for its framing as well as the structures entrusted with its implementation at the local level. We will focus on the political aspect of this type of programme at every level. We will show how the measures and guidelines that are adopted in the initial stages become the focus of political choices and strategies which cannot be implemented and applied unless they are incorporated within the game of local politics. To do so, we shall begin with a few remarks concerning the ideological presuppositions and the modes of action that are the salient features of the NLEP. Subsequently, we will present an analysis of the Indian NGO SMK's relations with the environment in which it works as well as its mode of functioning, which will make it possible to highlight how political mechanisms present at the global level are reappropriated and incorporated at the local level. We shall conclude by underlining that the NLEP and more generally public health policies manage and control not just diseases but also individuals. In other words, it embodies biopolitics in Michel Foucault's sense of the word.

National Leprosy Eradication Programme: Ideologies and Modes of Action

LEPROSY A PUBLIC HEALTH ISSUE

From a strictly medical point of view, leprosy is described as a non-hereditary disease, barely contagious, against which a high percentage of individuals are naturally immunized. By nature, it is neither an epidemic nor fatal, at least not directly. Given all this data, the existence of global leprosy eradication policies raises the following questions: Why is there such a great preoccupation with leprosy at the policy level? In which way is leprosy a public health problem? How is it a challenge that calls for the mobilization and implementation of specific measures? The responses to these questions stem not just from the nature of international administrative policies, but also from the matter at stake: leprosy. Let us begin by examining some characteristics of these policies and of the disease.

The formulation of international administrative policies as well as their implementation at the local level requires a relatively complex maze of power games, actions and interactions between actors: exerting of influence, authority and power as well as pressure by financial interests. In relation to disease management in particular, other factors too emerge in this interplay. The description of diseases and the designation of patients is one of these factors, which is a major challenge in itself. For instance, the fact of describing a disease as epidemic, pandemic or endemic in turn determines the priorities of action and modalities of intervention. The definition of a disease as 'contagious' or 'communicable' does not produce the same social perceptions. The designation of the patients too has its own implications: to speak of 'victims of Hansen's disease' and not of 'lepers' says a lot about strategic and socio-political choices. Beyond these questions and positions, the singular history of the disease, its past and the perceptions associated with it are also important. In this sense, leprosy has a heavy millstone around its neck. It is considered a disease of the poor, associated with an unhealthy body and environment, and is perceived as a scourge of the past. The presence still nowadays of leprosy does not coincide with the idea of modernity and social progress as defended by different partners.

Thus, the presence of leprosy triggers a whole series of interpretations which say a lot about the health and economic situation of certain regions of the world. The reason why leprosy is considered such a problem that it becomes the subject of international and national administrative policies is partly linked to the images it calls to the mind. But it is also associated with the side-effects of the disease which are both physical ('incapacities' according to the terms used by major international agencies) and social (ostracism or radical exclusion) and which are often the lot of the affected individuals. We shall see later that rehabilitation issues which have been increasingly at the heart of discussions, forums and new projects include the existence of physical disabilities and social stigma.

CIRCULATION BETWEEN PARTNERS

In the formulation of these observations we did not make any distinction between actors involved in the NLEP. In fact, it seems that in the view of the Programme's partners—at least at the general level of representations—intentions and objectives are homogeneous in nature. This points towards what seems to be a characteristic feature in NLEP's implemen-tation: the circulation of ideas, words, products, figures and people between different partners and at different levels of intervention.

To begin with, all the actors involved in the NLEP use the medical perspective while describing and defining leprosy: a disease caused by a germ, barely contagious, non-hereditary, with only 20 per cent of cases that are infectious and, above all, a disease that can be cured.

Further, they all reject the idea that leprosy could be fatal, a curse of god, the outcome of reprehensible or immoral behaviour perpetrated in the past. All share similar values—those of modernity, social progress, health and work. Thus, poverty, the lack of education and the occurrence of handicaps are implicit in the fight against leprosy.

These points of view and perceptions have been spreading. They are taken up by actors at every level of action. Such a circulation of ideas usually happens through meetings, forums, regroupings of associations into federations, circulation lists and bulletins, publications as well as through the definition of instructions and requirements. To fight leprosy, the strategy is defined upstream at the international level and is subsequently adopted at the national and then at the local levels. It is based on three fundamental principles:

- Early detection much before irreversible effects begin to occur.
- Immediate administration of a Multi Drug Therapy (MDT) which is a combination of three antibiotics.
- Education of patients, their families and the community at large about leprosy and its curability.

This is how medical knowledge and drugs flow through a chain from the WHO down to local actors, thereby establishing scientific expertise and rationality as a standard.

Basically, this is a circulation that percolates downwards from the members of the decision-making bodies who set up the measures to be followed by the various agents whose task is to implement them. Decision-making bodies and donors assess these agents' actions and their results at the local level, either on the basis of activity reports or by directly visiting the site. Thus, members of the WHO, World Bank or international associations such as Raoul Follereau send expert or appraisal committees to the field. While protagonists might present themselves as partners of the same programme and might be fully involved in a common project to eradicate leprosy, they do not act on an equal ground: this 'unidirectional' flow is the result of the hierarchization of the different actors involved.

The flow thus generates and consolidates a sharing of definitions (medical perspective), of values (health, work, integrity of the body), standards and objectives. These broad outlines provide a bracket within which perpetual readjustments are made on the basis of medical research and developments in drugs, as well as the human and financial means available. The possibility of such perpetual adjustments can itself be considered as the sign of a smoothly functioning operation and of an operational circulation of ideas and information, reports, aims and achievements.

TEMPORARY AND EFFICIENT: ACTION IDEOLOGY

While adjustments might be directed at efficiency, they are also a testimony to certain failures. We can take for example the re-evaluation of both the NLEP's objectives and due dates: 'Eradicate leprosy by 2000' became 'Eeliminate leprosy as a public health problem by 2005'. India achieved elemination as planned in December 2005—A Disability Prevention and Medical Rehabilitation—DPMR—plan is actually under consideration for implementation during the Eleventh Five Year Plan (2007–12). Not only the due date which could not be met with was redefined, but even the terminology was changed: the emphasis is no longer on 'eradication' but 'elimination'. It is no longer leprosy itself but leprosy 'as a public health problem'. The aim now is towards the disappearance of leprosy by itself, which would be a logical consequence of the disease's evolution once a certain prevalence rate has been achieved—less than 1 case per 10,000 inhabitants—according to various studies and appraisals. Today, the aim consists of achieving this prevalence rate, in other words, of decreasing the infection pool.

Beyond these redefinitions, as far as orientations and strategies to be adopted are concerned, the temporal dimension is an essential part of the ideology of these policies, as revealed by the importance of due dates and beyond that the notion of the 'programme' itself.

Different stages, durations and due dates are assessed upstream by the major decision-making agencies according to projections induced by principles of efficiency. A timeframe is set for each level: treatment, medical follow-up, resource management and realization of aims.

One of the consequences of this perspective is that the reduction of time becomes a major challenge. This challenge leads the government to rely on the different structures available, from local public structures to private associations and NGOs, thereby orchestrating an array of actors. It drives the government to make choices as far as the costs/means/results ratios are concerned.

For instance, time can be invested in medical research in order to reduce the treatment duration. Reducing the treatment duration would amount to savings in quantities of drugs and therefore, cost reductions (it would evidently be less costly to dispense a treatment for eighteen months than for two years). Reducing the treatment duration would also make it possible to reduce the time for medical follow-ups (the SMK teams visit the patients every month to distribute a fresh dose of drugs and ensure that those of the previous month have been taken). Furthermore, the chances of success increase. Indeed, one of the major obstacles to the treatment is its duration: the longer the treatment, the lesser the chance of patients continuing with it. Finally, a reduction in treatment time would make it possible to decrease much faster the number of registered cases (one case corresponds to one person detected and undergoing treatment) and therefore, allow for a faster diminution of prevalence rate (registered cases 'are removed' more quickly from the records).

Thus, the pace of the Programme is based on a certain liberal ideology of action, the notions of cost and yield depending on the aims to be achieved in a period always calculated as tightly as possible.

If you do not keep a schedule it is not only a sign of failure but also of poor management. This can then lead to the loss of allocated funds and of the free supply of medicines from the WHO and Nippon Foundation. It is a threat that the World Bank is exerting on the states of Bihar and Jharkhand.

Thus, aims are defined in terms of figures, prevalence rates to be achieved and due dates to abide by. The different partners have to assess the needs, plan stages and determine priorities. They make choices in accordance with emergency or health and safety criteria, but also by deferring to the pressures that weigh on them, along with funding sources and opportunities. It is this set of orientations and strategies that has led the policy towards the elimination of leprosy itself (achieving a certain level of prevalence) and not the development of research which would target the production of a vaccine.

Based on these remarks, we can say that on the face of it, global policies are not really directed towards individuals or communities as much as they are towards a specific object: the disease itself. Indeed, from the perspective of these policies it is leprosy that is the object of national and international challenges and it is leprosy that must be monitored, controlled, overcome, contained and in time made to disappear. Disease management has somewhat taken precedence over patient management. In fact, it seems that in general the patient as a subject rarely makes an appearance, whether at the global level of the Programme or at the local level as we shall see now through different activities of SMK, the Indian NGO in charge of NLEP implementation in the state of Rajasthan.

NLEP Conditions at the Local Level

SMK's Activities: An Integrated Whole

SMK is a voluntary organization which was officially registered in Rajasthan in 1984. The organization's existence and its work in the field of leprosy thus predates the launch of NLEP's first phase which began in 1993. The organization was already managing three lepers' communities (*ashram*) by providing them with medical care and food. Further, as part of NLEP, the NGO's activities developed and were systematized.

To fight against leprosy under the NLEP, Survey, Education and Treatment (SET) centres have been created to cover endemic pockets and to support the general health care infrastructure. SMK works with the same SET technique for the elimination of leprosy in Rajasthan. The medical teams of the organization conduct major case-finding campaigns in the form of a systematic census going from house to house in rural and urban areas where people live below the poverty line. They try to detect hidden leprosy cases. They then provide treatment free of cost to identified leprosy patients. The drugs are provided free by the Nippon Foundation and pharmaceutical firms such as Novartis and then are routed by the WHO through the central government and subsequently through the government of the state of Rajasthan. The NGO ensures a medical follow-up during the treatment and after its completion. Social workers also conduct education and awareness campaigns in order to change ideas associated with leprosy.

In addition, apart from activities that fall strictly within the competence of the programme, SMK carries out rehabilitation projects in collaboration with European NGOs. They make training centres operational as a way to re-integrate cured leprosy patients through work.

Our hypothesis is that, at least at the local level, actions that directly concern the NLEP and those that are peripheral form a whole that cannot be separated. A feature of the activities that runs parallel to the programme actions is their media dimension. Indeed, rehabilitation projects and activities are extensively covered by media, in particular by the written press and by television news to a lesser extent. Projects and activities give rise to opening ceremonies (a new training centre) and inaugurations (new premises, new housing) to which journalists are invited. Memorial days such as 30 January, Gandhi's death anniversary, are occasions for public events or ceremonies, which too are extensively covered. For instance, on 30 January 2002, the governor of Rajasthan visited the Galta lepers' community. After observing two minutes of silence in the memory of the Mahatma, he proceeded to distribute blankets to the community's inhabitants. He was accompanied by several Congress party representatives and by a few Rajasthan ministers, including the finance minister. The latter had also been present at the opening ceremony of the Ramghar centre, a vocational training centre set up by SMK and its European partners for cured leprosy patients. He was then accompanied by the chief minister of Rajasthan.

It must be pointed out here that the media coverage is not so much for the event as such but for the quality of personalities present. The re-integration centres and lepers' communities provide a space for the presentation and representation of political and industrial personalities at the local level. SMK, which is not a state organization, enjoys nonetheless close links with local political personalities (district collector, chief minister, maharaja) and influential industrialists. In fact, the association's president is himself a former high official of the transport ministry. In this capacity, he had built upon a large network of acquaintances comprising influential personalities whom he does not fail to mobilize in the course of his social activities for lepers. The presence of local personalities gives the programme credit in both senses of the term (credibility and funds) and all the stakeholders derive undeniable social and spiritual consideration. At the local level we can say that relationships of authority and prestige, possibilities of funding and the notion of *seva* (service) are closely intertwined.

In other words, the prerequisite to conducting social activities resides in the capacity to provide to local political personalities a stage where they can express themselves and be seen.

NETWORKING, PARTNERSHIP AND FUNDINGS

Beyond its local 'anchoring' SMK has also woven relationships with NGOs, international associations and foundations such as Raoul Follereau. These organizations are mainly Western and all concerned with leprosy. Whenever SMK diversifies its activities and initiates new projects, it is this network of partners that is mobilized afresh. For instance, the organization sets up re-integration centres and sales handcrafted articles by lepers in Europe through its partners.

It is essentially funding that the Indian association derives from these partners. According to SMK, it is this funding which keeps it going. In fact, the NGO receives no financial support from the government (and drugs are provided free of cost as we have already seen above).

Information about the flow of funds and their use remains rather vague; it is not easily accessible. All that we can state is that the possibility of getting land, access to water or electricity which are fundamental elements for any project requires constant support and substantial help from a network in India. The flow of funds between administrations, politicians and industrialists during elections is quite well known. Reference can be made here to an extremely realistic novel by Akhil Sharma, *An Obedient Father*, which provides a good description of the system of corruption and co-option in the Indian political scenario of the 1990s. The author describes well the collection, funds flow and allegiances through the story of a civil servant, Ram Karan. While we cannot develop further this aspect of the flow and use of funds, we can however note that the money mobilized within the framework of NLEP is significant and a part of it is evidently being integrated in these parallel circuits which also guarantees the programme's actions.

COMMON VALUES

While we have underlined the importance of media coverage and opportunities for the expression of local authorities, it must be specified that activities of the NGO and its partners do not merely give rise to gatherings that provide them with visibility. If partners are working on common projects, it is also because they echo each other's values and ideologies.

The different actions that have been mentioned above modulate and give expression to an entire system of values related to the health-rehabilitation duo through work and employment, education, integrity and the productive force of the body. We have already seen how these ideologies, values and representations of the body, the disease and the individuals flow through a vertical axis which connects agencies such as the WHO with various local entities via national governments. They also flow via a horizontal axis which corresponds to the European NGOs partners of SMK.

Thus, the Ramghar re-integration centre project stemmed from a common desire among members of SMK and three European NGOs to give back bodies their ability to work—a condition for their independence and re-integration into society. The project is the fruit of reflection about the first leper community run by SMK at Galta (near Jaipur). As explained in this brochure of a French NGO working with SMK on this project:

> Lepers live with each other in Galta and have very little desire to leave the centre because they are not ready to tread the path of re-integration alone and with no advantages or preferences over their peers in finding work. It is in this spirit that SMK and certain European NGOs felt that action needed to be taken in training and teaching lepers a craft or profession, but one that will not make them stay for ever in the centre that would be set up.[1]

It seems that it is only through the aspect of rehabilitation which erases the disease, that the individual could emerge. However, if the individual does make a reappearance it is only from the perspective that it too, like the disease, can be managed, shaped, submitted to planification and programmes if not productivity.

Michel Foucault has shown how capitalism is characterized by the application of power techniques which he described as 'disciplinary'—focusing on the 'man-body'—and 'bio-politics'—focusing on the 'man-species'. Concerning the latter, he wrote:

> In bio-political mechanisms, forecasts, statistical estimations, global-level measures would certainly be at the forefront. The emphasis would not be on modifying such and such phenomenon in particular, not even so much an individual insofar as he is an individual, but essentially, the need of the hour would be to intervene at the level of the very determination of these phenomena in all that is global within them. . . . Above all, regulatory mechanisms would have to be put in place, which would fix an average, establish a sort of homeostasis, and ensure compensations in this global population with its sphere of unpredi-ctability. In short, set up security mechanisms around this unpredictability itself, inherent in a population of living beings, in the way it optimises a state of life, if you wish.[2] (Foucault, 1997: 219)

NLEP measures and accompanying mechanisms recall some of the features of both disciplinary measures, focusing on the individual as a body that needs to be worked on and broken-in, and bio-political mechanisms that address the population as a mass that must be regulated. We now tackle these aspects that can be found in detection and awareness campaigns which play a vital role in the implementation of NLEP at the local level.

Indeed, the affected individuals are not considered individuals in their own right but viewed through the prism of the disease. The disease becomes somewhat their attribute, their unique identity, a nominal identity that reappears with the designation *leprosy patients*. Thus, the focus above all is on leprosy. It is leprosy that is the subject of the production of a whole series of figures, reports and statistics. It is, therefore, leprosy, which is been tracked through population surveys and case detection.

SCREENING

During leprosy elimination campaigns SMK tries as much as possible to diminish the social consequences of the identification of a leper. In a quasi-systematic manner the name of the disease is not revealed to the affected individual. Medical teams keep silent about the name of the disease and do not speak of leprosy but of a 'skin disease' while administering anti-leprosy drugs.

This perspective is implicit in SMK's anti-leprosy work, as it identifies and essentially ensures that the patients remain where they are. Indeed, they would otherwise leave if their disease were to become known as leprosy.

Case-finding campaigns are carried out systematically within a locality or a village, house by house. The houses are marked with references painted on the walls to signify that they have been checked. However, these campaigns do not concern the entire population. They aim categories deemed to be at risk: poor populations, inhabitants in unhealthy localities, slums (*kacchi basti*), or low caste communities.

The poverty-leprosy association introduces a form of paternalism and downgrading of individuals—individuals that need to be educated. Further, awareness campaigns are associated with case-finding campaigns whose aim is to change behaviours (awareness about hygiene for instance) as well as change the image of leprosy and get rid of reactions of rejection with regard to lepers.

AWARENESS CAMPAIGNS

For instance, SMK teams visit certain localities or villages, equipped with instructional material such as posters, banners, photo-boards or cartoons. Films too are sometimes shown. The aim is not just counteracting ideas and perceptions associated with leprosy—a contagious disease, fatal, the fruit of the errors committed in the past—but also inculcating behaviour to follow in the event of one being afflicted with leprosy.

As the fashion of a number of socio-health-related campaigns in India (alcoholism, illiteracy, etc.), children are the main target. Plays are enacted in schools with leprosy and hygiene awareness for backdrop. In fact, a team of actors that is on the SMK payroll has been entrusted with the task of inventing different scenarios depending on the location, audience and themes being tackled.

Recently, the Indian health ministry launched the distribution of informative material related to leprosy in schools, with small cards bearing a sketch of the body, inviting children to examine their family for any mark whatsoever and report them on the control sketches before returning them to their teachers.

Thus, it is bio-politics that is at play here, which invites people to check for marks on themselves—along with teachings of self-detection with the help of a needle to test the sensitivity of the marked skin—and others. It also calls for the observance of certain conduct related to private body functions, those that concern hygiene for instance.

These campaigns, on the lines of NLEP as far as its strict implementation is concerned, give barely any space to the patient as a subject—the author of his/her own treatment, capable of making choices. They do establish certain practices concerning the way you treat your body. In other words, they do establish a body's use policy. To reiterate what Anne Golse had said, we can say that regarding leprosy a sort of health medicine is emerging. The author describes how health 'is losing its logical and temporal otherness from the disease and redefining itself in the interplay of another otherness, that of a dialectical game between the individual and the milieu—or environment—within a bio-psycho-social holism' and whose place 'seems to redefine a new standard, that of adaptation' (Golse, 2001: 275-6).[3] In this regard, measures aim at developing a productive individual, as shown by SMK activities increasingly turning towards rehabilitation.

Conclusion

To end this article we would like to make a few general observations concerning the configuration of partners around a public health policy as was evident within the framework of NLEP.

The encroachment of these policies on national sovereignty has sometimes been put forward. This leads to strong opposition between on the one hand, international institutions and non-governmental organizations, and the governments on the other. A programme such as the NLEP shows that such a dichotomy is not operative. While at times there might be divergence of opinions and real pressure on states, the NLEP is based above all on understandings and conventions that orchestrate action and divide actors on the basis of perfect complementarity. As we have seen, the rank of actors is quite evident at all decision-making levels, just as the expression of influences, authorities and powers was present at all these levels. In concrete and practical terms, partners share monitoring and information means. It must be said that India had been in good hands as far as the British colonial administration was concerned. Partners here shared not just the means of assessment and expression but also the content (sharing of common values).

The complementarity of actors does not, however, do away with hierarchical dependencies which often turn NGOs into 'the left hand of the Empire' to quote Michel Agier, i.e. essential collaborators in a global control society. As noted by the author, the humanitarian has become 'an indispensable element for the social and moral edification of the "Empire", the unified world as a single 'control society' at the global level (Hardt and Negri, 2000)' (2003: 68). The indispensability is based on three principles: 'care, cure and control' which attributes the humanitarian its place and role in global control movements.

Thus, far from creating any opposition, the distribution of roles between NLEP partners is in line with the liberal ethics of responsibility and aptitude, from patients to actors who have to prove their actual ability at all levels. These ethics are coupled with humanitarian values and demands that are moral and rational with justificatory virtues. They should not be sought exclusively among civil or humanitarian society actors. For it is all the actors who draw from it the meaning of their acts. As noted by Paul Rabinow in a recent article, ethics, rights or the truth are forces that are not external to capitalism or domination, exploitation or subjugation. On the contrary, they are deployed in their midst through different collaborating actors and institutions (Rabinow, 2005: 48–50).

The issue at stake is undoubtedly the general orientation of NLEP protagonists, whose effects reflect in radical and interventionist domination and paternalistic subordination, which marginalize the ailing while they focus on the disease. And while public health policies may indirectly introduce the idea of a right to health and thus pave the way for claims, the fact remains that the demands made by patients for truth and morality are well and truly absent.

NOTES

1. The Original French runs as follows: «Les lépreux vivent entre eux à Galta et éprouvent peu d'aspiration à quitter le centre car ils ne sont pas prêts à faire le chemin de la réinsertion seuls et sans aucun avantage par rapport à leurs pairs pour trouver du travail. C'est dans cet esprit que SMK et certaines ONG européennes ont considéré qu'une action ultérieure devrait essentiellement porter sur la formation et l'apprentissage d'un métier pour les lépreux, mais sans que ceux-ci s'installent définitivement sur le centre qui sera créé.»
2. The Original French runs as follows: « Dans les mécanismes mis en place par la bio-politique, il va s'agir d'abord, bien sûr, de prévisions, d'estimations statistiques, de mesures globales ; il va s'agir, également, non pas de modifier tel phénomène en particulier, non pas tellement tel individu en tant qu'il est individu, mais, essentiellement, d'intervenir au niveau de ce que sont les déterminations de ces phénomènes dans ce qu'ils ont de global. (. . .) Et il s'agit surtout d'établir des mécanismes régulateurs qui, dans cette population globale avec son champ aléatoire, vont pouvoir fixer un èquilible, maintenir une moyenne, établir une sorte d'homéostasie, assurer des compensations; bref, d'installer des mécanismes de sécurité autour de cet al éatoire qui est inhérent à une population d'êtres vivants, d'optimaliser, si vous voulez, un état de vie.»
3. The Original French runs as follows: la santé «perd son altérité logique et temporelle avec la maladie pour se redéfinir dans le jeu d'une autre altérité, celle d'un jeu dialectique individu/milieu—ou environnement—dans un holisme bio-psycho-social » et dont la place «semble redéfinir une nouvelle norme, celle d'adaptation».

REFERENCES

Agier, Michel, 'La main gauche de l'Empire: ordre et désordre de l'humanitaire', *Multitudes*, 11, Winter, 2003.

Fassin, Didier and Dominique Memmi (eds.), *Le gouvernement des corps*, Paris: EHESS, 2004.

Fassin, Didier, *L'espace politique de la santé. Essai de généalogie*, Paris: PUF, 1996.

Foucault, Michel, *Il faut défendre la société*, Paris: Gallimard, 1997.

Golse, Anne, 'De la Médecine de la maladie à la médecine de la santé', in P. Artières and E. Da Silva, *Michel Foucault et la médecine. Lectures et usages*, Paris: Kimé, 2001.

Hardt, Michael and Antonio Negri, *Empire*, Paris: Exils, 2000 [English version: Michael Hardt and Antonio Negri, 2000, *Empire*, Harvard: Harvard University Press, 2000.

Lazzarato, Maurizio, 'Pour une redéfinition du concept de 'bio-politique', *Futur antérieur*, issue 39–40, Syllepse, 1997.

Rabinow, Paul, 'Midst Anthropology's Problem', in A. Ong and S.J. Collier (eds.), *Global Assemblages, Technology, Politics and Ethics as Anthropological Problems*, Oxford: Blackwell, 2005.

Sharma, Akhil, 2000, *An Obedient Father*, New York: Farrar, Strauss & Giroux, 2002.

CHAPTER 11

Water and Re-emergence of Epidemics in Chennai (Tamil Nadu): Along the Path of Globalization[1]

SANDRINE BRISSET

Introduction: A Problem of 'Globalized' World Health

'Investing in water means investing in health' (WHO, 2003). More than twenty years after the international statement of 1981, non-drinking water and the lack of sanitation are still among the ten biggest health risk factors worldwide. 'Developing countries almost exclusively bear the brunt of a large number of these risk factors, while others have already had a global impact' (World Health Report, 2002). In fact, mortality and morbidity due to water-borne diseases have not declined commensurate with increase in availability of potable water supply and sanitation. Diarrhoea remains a major health problem with two billion cases a year worldwide and more than 2.2 million deaths (WHO, 2003). The 1990s has at least had the merit of drawing attention to the deplorable sanitation conditions in cities in poor countries and to the concrete reality of the water/health problem rather than to its abstract universal aspect. The distinction is important because, as Aristotle observes, the whole is superior to the sum of the parts (Dauphiné, 1995). In other words, water-related epidemics, taken as a whole, form a system and a series of inter-connected sub-systems. Going beyond the new concept of 'environmental health', the study of the relationship between water and health is particularly relevant both to the 'blurring of traditional scales' and to an account of the globalization process.

None of the world's phenomena—whether they are extreme climatic conditions, global warming, growing poverty levels, the environmental crisis, the inadequacy of health care facilities, new technologies, reforms in water and health provision—considered individually or even in synergy, can explain the renewed outbreak of water-related diseases in certain areas. As G. Salem (2004) points out so well, 'outbreaks of these diseases do not occur just anywhere or at any time'. The 1990s were particularly marked by them because of the concurrent combination of a host of factors, which might account for their intensification, but not their geographical variations. It is, in fact, the combination of various factors that leads to the outbreak of an epidemic in a given place. It is therefore tempting to see a relationship of cause and effect in the economic development of India, one of the major sites of endemo-epidemic diseases and cholera, and to detect here an illustration of the ambivalent relationship between globalization and public health.

Based on the example of Chennai, India's fourth-largest metropolis, we shall insist on the importance of a 'finer analysis of these situations in their totality' (Lévy, 1997: 366). We shall emphasize the relationship between society and environment and try to understand why the health situation deteriorated in the preceding decade, despite capital inflows and all the efforts made. We shall analyse the implications for a given place of what we have called 'The Turning-Point of the 1990s'.

Phase One of the Telugu Ganga or Krishna-Pennar Project is now finally taking shape after 50 years of negotiations. The project aims at using the Krishna River, diverted over more than 500 km, to supply water to the Tamil capital which is particularly affected by water shortages. By 2011 more than 1,000 million additional litres of water should reach the city area daily. No water development project comes without major upheavals and it usually ends up reviving the issue of water-borne diseases. However, neither climatic events (floods, droughts), nor the Telugu Ganga, nor even the water development projects underway can explain the explosion of water-related epidemics in the 1990s. They have certainly punctuated the city's history, but they have become much more complex. The purpose of this article is to describe a 'multifaceted reality', in other words, to analyse a water/health/society interaction, in which the 'local' and the 'global' come together.

Globalized because of its origin (colonial trading post) and its administration (World Bank funding and an appeal to foreign capital investment), and now because of its 'imported' development project (huge water development projects and networking technology), Chennai has nonetheless emerged as one of India's cities least open to globalization and most resistant to the great international private-sector companies. Of course, this may simply be due to the very nature of complex systems, which 'have to remain somewhat closed, in order to continue to exist and to protect their identity'.

THE 1990S—A 'TURNING POINT'

Chennai's nickname, the 'Capital of Extremes' (*The Hindu*, 17 April 1997), has never been as true as it is today. Considerable progress was certainly made at all levels of environmental management during the 1990s. The main city is now equipped with an almost completed water-supply and sewerage system and the municipal water grid covers 98 per cent of the Corporation,[2] as against 86 per cent in Delhi and 66 per cent in Kolkata (Ruet et al., 2002). Above all, piped water supply has more than doubled in some ten years and the management of waste water or drainage, for example, has received special attention.

However, Chennai remains at the top of the list of Indian metropolises facing water and sanitation problems. Its water supply level is much lower than the standard 125 lpcd fixed for urban areas with piped water supply;[3] it has the lowest daily availability of municipal water (4 hours as against 10 in Kolkata); severe water pollution, and despite efforts to 'control' the chronic water shortage, it barely managed to cover 60 per cent of its needs in 2001. While the average daily supply was then 103 litres per inhabitant, as against 68 litres per capita in 1991, very few inhabitants actually receive that quantity of water through their taps. In some areas, the daily water availability is barely 20 lpcd, while it exceeds 150 lpcd in others. The peri-urban areas are not, of course, included in the official general statistics. At best, they receive 40 lpcd and sewerage facility is practically non-existent. As regards the watercourses that cross through the city, they continue to record a Biological Oxygen Demand (BOD) level that is much higher than the standard 30 mg/l and to emit the characteristic nauseating odour of foul water. All in all, Chennai 'resembles most other third world mega-cities' (Tropp, 1998: 64), resulting in a general mortality rate (Chennai City (CC): 9.6 per thousand in 2000) that is much higher than the regional urban average (urban Tamil Nadu: 6.4 per thousand), or even the national urban average (urban India: 6.3 per thousand) and a high prevalence of water-related diseases. Malaria and cholera head the list and present a major health problem especially within the Corporation. Of the total malaria cases reported in state, the share of Chennai has in fact gone up from 42 per cent in 1990 to 75 per cent in 2001. Yet a National Malaria Control Programme (NMCP) was launched in Tamil

Nadu in 1953 as were various centrally sponsored urban malaria control schemes from 1972. The incidence of diarrhoea (acute gastroenteritis + cholera) has risen substantially[4] over a ten-year period (+40 per cent) as compared to the 1980s, during which the city was already badly affected by the disease (Figure 11.1, Table 11.1).

As P. Bourdelais (2003) points out so clearly, 'It is not enough to bring water to the city and increase the number of sewers to resolve the issue of urban epidemics.' In addition, 'environmental health', which can be defined as the link between water management in the wider sense of the term and public health (WHO, 2003), must go beyond the framework of a universalized discourse. It should be an integral part of a real health policy, which admittedly cannot be protected from disruptions in terms of funding, but should incorporate distinctive local identities and true metropolitan management. In the rapidly changing coastal environment, we do not expect immediate control over water-

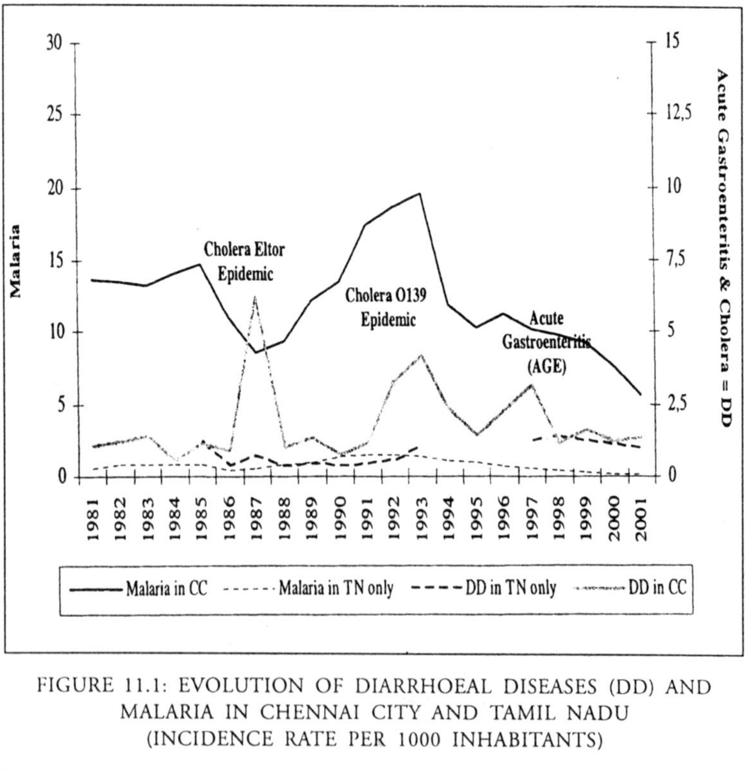

FIGURE 11.1: EVOLUTION OF DIARRHOEAL DISEASES (DD) AND MALARIA IN CHENNAI CITY AND TAMIL NADU (INCIDENCE RATE PER 1000 INHABITANTS)

TABLE 11.1: OUTBREAKS OF ACUTE GASTROENTERITIS AND CHOLERA

(Average Annual Incidence Rate per 1,000 Inhabitants)

	Chennai City				Tamil Nadu only			
	Malaria	Cholera	Age	DD Total	Malaria	Cholera	Age	DD Total
1981–90	12.40	0.58	0.97	1.55	0.79	0.01	0.53	0.54
1991–2000	12.58	0.64	1.54	2.18	0.84	0.004	0.96	0.96

Sources: Compiled from Directorate of Public Health & Preventive Medicine data (number of notified cases).

related diseases, nor, for that matter, do we literally expect a renewed outbreak of ailments arising out of contaminated water that defined the 'pathological style' of the 1990s. The worsening of diarrhoeic epidemics, in fact, as well as the increase in and the specific dating of major health events—the spread of a new cholera strain in 1992–4, subsequently called O139, the explosive diarrhoeic morbidity in 1996–7 (general incidence: 5.44 per thousand) and the atypical flare-up of leptospirosis in 2000 and dengue in 2001—are relevant indicators. We shall see that while these epidemics are no longer simply the outcome of climatic events, they are also not merely the result of a pathogenic impact associated with improvements in domestic water. This is a reality that further underscores the complexity of the pathogenicity/environment/development relationship, while questioning a globalized hygienist vision. Beyond all that, it also accounts for the interdependence of the local and global forces that influence water and health—in a word, for the 'turning point' of the 1990s.

FROM WATER TO HEALTH FOR ALL

'Integrated Water Resources Management models are seen now as an opportunity for encouraging synergies and mainstreaming water-related public health as a cross-cutting issue throughout the decision-making in different sectors and at different levels' (WHO, 2003f). In addition, water (quantity/availability/quality) and health should no longer be managed separately, and the multiplicity of people and institutions involved should not intensify the problems further.

This is a real challenge for Chennai and its region and the Krishna project is no less of a challenge, especially for an urban area defined as being 'intractable to development' (Auclair, 1998: 111), with enormous urban development constraints (sprawling city, high water demand, inadequacy of regional water resources, extreme flatness of the area) and with municipal revenues that are much lower than those of other Indian cities. Now that municipalities have increased responsibilities with the 74th Amendment to the Indian Constitution (1992), the Tamil capital has to find the means to undertake its development and catch up with other cities. Enormously high stakes are involved, since at the same time, the city has to find a sustainable solution to its water shortage, neutralize its ecological problems, eradicate its water-related diseases, restructure its entire water system (supply–disposal–drainage), improve the quality of drinking water and become more autonomous financially.

While it is certainly much easier to act within the framework of a World Bank-assisted federal project, such as the Telugu Ganga Project, which entails a certain number of concomitant modifications and coordinates different levels of action, it chiefly testifies to an increasingly complex water/health reality.

With the transfer of its new water resource, Chennai has, in fact, moved from the intensive exploitation of its hinterland to the management of an inter-state conflict. It is now at the centre of disputes concerning the sharing of the Krishna waters, a dispute dating back to the restructuring of the territory on a linguistic basis in 1953, but regional hydrographical restructuring has recently complicated the dispute.[5] Hydrological borders do not really correspond to state borders and there is no clear definition of the amount of water allocated to each of these basins, which has only enhanced competition concerning this shared resource, not to speak of water competition between the southern states. Although a special tribunal has been formed to resolve conflicts of interest and domestic water has been a priority since 1987 as well as the initiation of the national water policy (1987), we may well ask ourselves whether the 15 thousand million cubic feet (TMC) of Krishna water allotted since 1976 would not inevitably be subject to controversies over time, especially since the various water projects would largely exceed the river's capacity. In fact, the three 'donor' states that the river crosses are claiming a total of 4,269 TMC, i.e. more than double its flow, estimated at 2,051 TMC (with a 75 per cent dependence on the monsoon). In 1999, Karnataka announced that it was reconsidering its supply of 5 TMC to Chennai if Tamil Nadu did not withdraw its objections concerning the sharing of Kaveri waters (*The Hindu*, 19 September 1999).

Despite everything, the Telugu Ganga Project, as well as the different developments taking place at the same time, would gradually allow the Tamil capital to rethink its entire water strategy on different scales and 'make the most of available water' (Brooks, 2002). In other words, it would allow the city to better manage the variation as well as regional specificities regarding water. Today, an attempt is being made to channel and store the maximum amount of rainwater, as the rains are concentrated over a very short period (from October to December), as well as to replenish the over-exploited aquifers by redeveloping the traditional water tanks system. Indeed, this developing city has taken an original path by developing several innovative strategies to save water (rainwater harvesting, water purchase agreements with farmers, desalinization of brackish water, keeping the advancing intrusion of seawater at bay), and by adopting more integrated management practices. It has also modernized its municipal water supply system and delegated some of its services. By restructuring its budget, increasing tariffs and introducing the private sector through subcontracting and for the sale of water, the water company, generally known as Metrowater (or the Metro), has even managed to improve its financial position (Brisset, 2003). Although it had been a loss-making concern, it nonetheless had to pay out more than Rs. 3.50 billion between 1987-2004 (World Bank, 1995, i.e. it had to fund directly 19 per cent of the expenditure necessary for the water and sanitation sector and even begin to repay the loans (estimated at + 65.50 per cent of investments) granted by various local or international bodies.

In about ten years' time, almost all the urban area should be connected to a supply and disposal network managed by Metrowater (as opposed to 29 per cent and 22 per cent in 1991), while earlier the urban suburbs were under the Tamil Nadu Water and Drainage Board's (TWAD) control. While this would be a major breakthrough, the gap between the Corporation and the rapidly growing suburbs would have widened in the meantime. In fact, in the 1990s, the ten-year growth rate was more than six times higher (Urban Area only: 63 per cent, CC: 9.76 per cent) in peri-urban areas. In other words, the modernization of sanitation facilities (drainage, sanitation, domestic water supply, solid waste collection) was taking place too slowly. The Accelerated Urban Water Supply Programme (AUWSP) initiated in 1993–4 for cities with fewer than 20,000 inhabitants in the 1991 Census, as well as the World Bank-assisted Tamil Nadu Urban Development Project, which covers major urban centres in Tamil Nadu (Appasamy, 1993: 90), should gradually relieve the Chennai Urban Area (CUA). Of course, this will only happen if the various metropolitan projects are not carried out separately or—even better—if the main city/suburb schism disappears and proper inter-sector coordination develops between the different bodies involved. The water and sanitation sector must, in fact, be considered in conjunction with environment and health, which is far from the being the case at present, as evidenced by the absence of a joint management structure and the lack of any institutional interface between the water agency and health departments. Of course, this is dependent on the national policy, since the two budgets are now dissociated (GOI, 2002). It was only in 2002 that the national health policy was reshaped and these 'dysfunctions' were officially acknowledged, an attempt finally being made to check global ecological deterioration, rather than look at the problems in isolation.

Likewise, the various outbreaks of water-related diseases in the 1990s underline the inappropriateness of 'control' strategies based solely on the improvement of facilities, as well as the ineffectiveness of the disease surveillance system. And yet, ailments occurring in epidemic form are at the forefront of the national health policy (launched in 1983) and certain pathologies are even the subject of a, sometimes very old, national control programme (filariasis), or even eradication programmes in certain cases (malaria, guinea worm). Nonetheless, water-related diseases remain underestimated for the most part—particularly in suburban areas, or even unrecognized or trivialized by public opinion (as in the case of gastroenteritis). In such conditions it is difficult to provide an appropriate response to early warning signals of outbreaks of communicable diseases. Besides, 'the absence of an efficient disease surveillance network, with real-time information at all levels of the health administration', has been recognized as a major handicap (GOI, 2002). Thus, a National Surveillance Programme of Communicable Diseases (NSPCD), essentially directed towards diseases that can potentially turn epidemic, such as acute diarrhoeal diseases, cholera, viral hepatitis, dengue/DHF, Japanese encephalitis, leptospirosis and plague—was launched in 1997 and a special budget released for beneficiary states.[6] By 2002, about a hundred districts had to be covered, but these did not include the city or the district of Chennai which already had priority under the Telugu Ganga Project.

Thenceforth, water-related diseases were acknowledged as a major health problem and a strategy to control epidemic diseases was gradually implemented. A coordination committee on control of epidemic diseases was also set up (1998) at different levels (state, districts—Chennai city in Tamil Nadu state) and the water/health link was theoretically improved in this manner. However, these health reforms would only have limited impact if peri-urban areas continued to be administered separately. Development also means epidemic control in these peripheral areas with increasingly unsanitary conditions, not just improved water availability. Quality is equally important, especially for a high ground water-consuming urban area. In fact, this was at the heart of the problem of the 1990s, as underlined by the renewed outbreak of water-related epidemics and in particular water-borne epidemics.

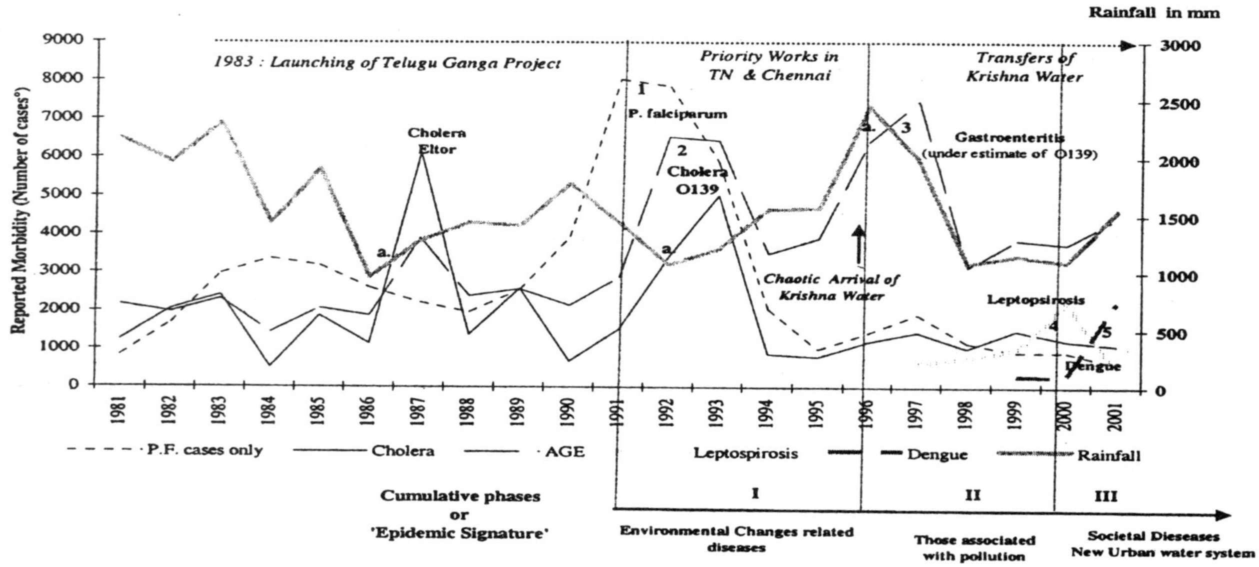

a. Climatic Events (drought - flood)

1 Successive epidemics

° For Cholera & Acute Gastro-Enteritis : hospitalisations

- Rainfall: Nungambakkam Station

Sources : Chennai Corporation - Communicable Diseases Hospital (CDH)

FIGURE 11.2: RE-EMERGENCE OF WATER-RELATED EPIDEMICS IN CHENNAI CITY IN THE 1990S

RE-EMERGENCE OF WATER-RELATED EPIDEMICS

Contrary to expectations, improvements in water availability did not truly stabilize the health situation, nor did they check epidemics, at times triggered by droughts and at others by floods. Conversely, what we witnessed was a resurgence of water-related epidemics, which summarily turned into an 'epidemic of epidemics' (Platt, 1993: 172), an intensification of water-borne diseases and even the emergence of more 'societized' crisis.

No less than five significant episodes were to follow one after another in a period of about ten years (Figure 11.2). From 1991 onwards, the incidence of malaria rose significantly (+ 30 per cent) nearing 20 per thousand in 1993, i.e. a year before the disease once again broke out in the form of an epidemic throughout India (Dhingra et al., 1998). It was more serious this time, since it was due to an eruption of *P. falciparum*, a plasmodial species capable of triggering a cephalic form of malaria that can prove fatal if not treated in time, due to the bursting of red blood cells and intra-cerebral haemorrhage. Generally, such a mani-festation subsides two months after the primary infection (Picq, 1982: 368), but it persisted for more than two years this time (1991–2). Peri-urban areas too recorded a marked increase in malaria over a much longer period (1992–6). Chennai also had to deal with a double diarrhoeic epidemic (acute gastroenteritis-cholera O139), which was asymptomatic given its duration (21 months),[7] its intensity (overall hospitalization rate: 5.5 per thousand as against 2.78 per thousand in 1987) and its form (new type of cholera). This was the first non-O1[8] cholera epidemic, a serovar distinct from the 138 pre-existing forms, which would subsequently be baptized as O139 synonym Bengal, to indicate that it was first isolated from coastal areas of the Bay of Bengal. Until this date, the O1 vibrio (classical biotype, followed by Eltor as of 1964) was recognized as the sole agent responsible for cholera flare-ups and non-O1 was the only offending strain in various sporadic eruptions of gastroenteritis (Kamal, 1971). From October 1992 to June 1994, the new strain even supplanted Eltor and subsequently continued to manifest in spurts without completely disappearing. As for the second half of the 1990s, it was marked by acute gastroenteritis (notably in 1996–7) and a rise in human leptospirosis (2000), an anthropozoonosis transmitted by rodents (especially rats),[9] which cannot be explained solely by excessive rainfall. Without proper management, this pathology can become a major health problem (Albert, 1996: 4), presenting an increasing threat of epidemics. So long as the vector-host-disease cycle continues to be fostered, a disaster like the one in Nicaragua (1998)—when the bacteria (leptospire) affected several thousand people before the disease, initially likened to dengue hemorrhagic fever, was finally recognized—cannot be far behind. In 2001, the incidence of dengue also picked up, with an increase in domestic water storage in open overhead tanks—perfect breeding grounds for vector mosquitoes (Brisset, 2005). These water-related epidemics are therefore very much part and parcel of re-emerging older diseases due to an evolution in the pathogen (cholera O139), a change in parasite formula in favour of *P. falciparum* (Sharma, 1996: 26), an increase in the number of infected human carriers (leptospirosis, dengue) and/or high virulence (acute gastroenteritis).

There is but one step between rising insalubrity and urban epidemics. Considerable progress in terms of hygiene is imperative before we can expect a decline in water-related diseases. In this regard, worsening (in terms of the number of hospitalizations) diarrhoeic outbreaks (Table 11.2) and renewed outbursts of diseases related to contaminated water are particularly significant. Indeed, diarrhoeic morbidity has increased enormously in the last ten years, and this all over the area.[10] On the contrary, the incidence of malaria has only gone up slightly as compared to the 1980s, at least within the Corporation area. These trends have occurred despite a favourable conjunction of circumstances/additional water supply/excessive rainfall/water development projects. On the contrary, the malaria flare-up in 1991–3 occurred during drought years, synonymous with higher levels of storage and the intensive use of wells. However, *Anopheles stephensi*, one of the two vectors prevalent in

TABLE 11.2: INTENSIFICATION OF GASTROENTERITIS & CHOLERA EPIDEMICS IN CHENNAI CITY

	Hospitalizations & Incidence rates per 1,000 Inhabitants					
	1987		1992–3		1996–7	
Acute Gastroenteritis (AGE)	3,898	1.08	12,979	3.33	13,898	3.38
Cholera	6,122	1.70	8,443	2.17	2,630	0.64
Diarrhoeal morbidity	10,020	2.78	21,422	5.50	16,528	4.02

Sources: Corporation of Chennai & Communicable Diseases Hospital (Tondiarpet)

Chennai, breeds in domestic water storage systems such as overhead tanks, sumps, cisterns and wells. As for *A. culicifacies*, it basically grows in ponds and tanks in the periphery. Despite major breakthroughs in the water and sanitation sector, protected water is at best distributed for just a few hours everyday and must consequently be stored. And in areas with no or very little connection to the municipal water system, as well as during the dry season, the use of wells is intense. These hydraulic and ecological changes imply, therefore, 'an enormous potential for *A. stephensi* to multiply and spread malaria and the emergence of two ecotypes: urban malaria transmitted by *A. stephensi* and peri-urban malaria transmitted by *A. stephensi* and *A. culicifacies* (Sharma, 1996: 39). These various transformations undoubtedly influenced the epidemic process of the 1990s—hence the importance of 'thinking in spatial terms' (Giblin, 2000: 31) in order to limit the number of problems.

Beyond the interplay of different environmental, immune or even anthropogenic factors which vary with the pathogenic complex involved, the 'epidemic signature' of the 1990s clearly underlines the paradoxical mechanisms at work between improvements in domestic water supply and accompanying pathogenic crises. Broadly speaking, three major health incidents (*P. falciparum*—cholera O139/acute gastroenteritis/ human leptospirosis—dengue) accompanied the coming into being of the Telugu Ganga Project, from the preparation of the city for the reception of the Krishna waters, through the chaotic arrival of the new water resource in 1996-7 to the emergence of a new urban water system in 2001–2. The time scale allows us to confirm the specific nature of the diseases involved in each of the three stages (Figure 11.2).

Another interesting indicator is that none of these different water-related epidemics are uniquely associated with climate-related events such as drought and flooding. Climatic change is never a factor prior to the outbreak of the epidemic. Climate is, therefore, not the factor that provokes a crisis but a link in the epidemic chain.

All this takes us to a metropolitan scale rarely considered before in discussions of the 'development process within social groups' (Handschumacher et al., 1997). Repercussions on health are indeed increasingly important concerns within the framework of major 'imported' water development projects. However, there is not often much concern about the way the situation has been established within the water-receiving metropolis and the emphasis is placed essentially on vector-borne diseases. In Chennai, the epidemic surveillance system was actually strengthened in 1997, but it was only in 2002 that the national cholera control programme was proclaimed, with a budget of its own and the adoption of multilateral measures combining prevention (anti-cholera inoculations, chlorination of drinking water), ecological hygiene (waste water disposal, solid waste collection) and improvement of facilities. As a major epidemic pole, Chennai has had from the first and retains a major role in the spread of cholera

Apart from deterioration in the health situation, successive epidemic outbursts in the 1990s have demonstrated how impossible it is to act rapidly, even with the support of international organizations in general and, especially, the World Bank. While proving that the water and health dysfunction does indeed exist, these epidemics also show that a 'solution to this problem can create new opportunities for contact between man and water-related pathogens' (WHO, 2003) and they bring the question of development back to the centre of the debate.

THE PRICE OF DEVELOPMENT?

'Increased volumes of water for domestic use do not necessarily translate into increased use or improved health conditions' (White et al., 1972). This explains in a nutshell what happened in Chennai in the 1990s, despite the priority given to domestic water, sanitation and water-related diseases. Behind the drought/treated water shortage syncretism or conversely that of excessive rainfall and contaminated water leading to outbreaks of water-related diseases, lies a much more complex intrinsic reality. Indeed, more favourable climatic conditions did not lead to a more stable situation, nor for that matter did they check the infectiousness of the milieu. Likewise, the arrival of additional quantities of water did not resolve the risk of water shortages in the least and, in fact, increased social inequalities. What actually happened overall to cause such an unstable health scenario and even a pause in the lowering of general mortality?

While urban India has been gradually improving its mortality rate, which has fallen from 7.8 per thousand in the early 1980s to 6.5 per thousand twenty years later, Chennai has recorded an upward trend in the same period (Figure 11.3). This may simply be due to the age structure of the population which causes an uneven distribution of deaths. It is therefore necessary to correct gross mortality rates with rates for different age bands, not forgetting that the male and female mortality rates also show wide differences (Lequin, 1984: 204). Standardized rates allow us to eliminate factors which may cause confusion (age, sex) and to

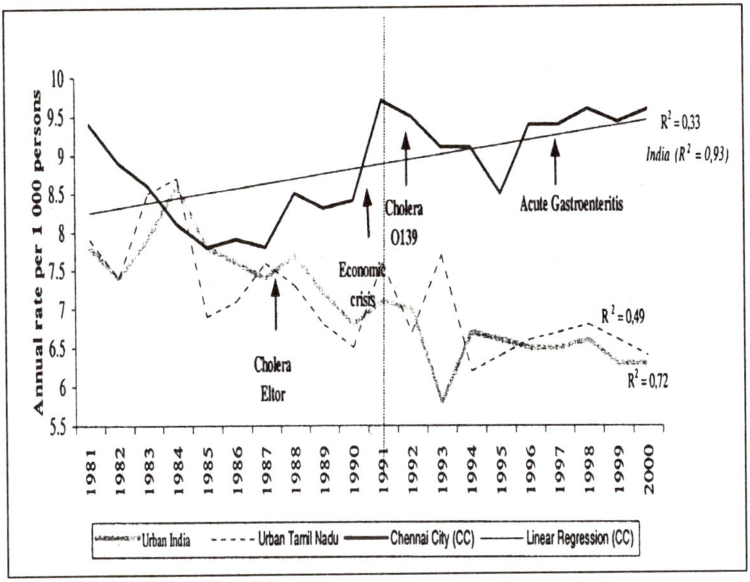

FIGURE 11.3: CRUDE DEATH RATE (CDR) IN CHENNAI CITY, TAMIL NADU AND URBAN INDIA SINCE 1981

concentrate on the local specifics of the phenomena under consideration. In 1995, direct standardization[11] gave a rate of 9.40 per thousand (10.44 per thousand for males) against a specific mortality rate by age band of only 8.68 per thousand. After standardisation, the capital shows an even higher mortality rate, especially for men—all of which confirms that the situation is not improving. The ten-year mortality level was even close to 9.3 per thousand (urban India: 7.62 per thousand) between 1991 and 2000 (Table 11.3), as against 8.4 per thousand (urban India: 6.54 per thousand) in the past and therefore caught up with urban Tamil Nadu's average annual rate for the 1970s. Further, since 1991, the gross mortality rate has not fallen below 8.5 per thousand and the gap with other Indian cities has been widening. By way of information,[12] it was only 7.8 per thousand in Mumbai in 2000 and 6.6 per thousand in Delhi, while it was 9.6 per thousand in Chennai.

All this is certainly neither new nor extraordinary. A temporary rise in the mortality rate (over a period of some forty years) was also apparent in fast-growing cities in the nineteenth century—from 1820 to 1870 in English cities, for example (Bourdelais, 2003: 152). Closer to home, a

TABLE 11.3: NO IMPROVEMENT OF GENERAL MORTALITY IN CHENNAI

Mean Annual CDR/1000	Chennai City	Urban Tamil Nadu	Urban India	All India
1981–90	8.39	7.47	7.62	11.37
1991–2000	9.3	6.77	6.54	9.16

Sources: Corporation of Chennai—The Economic Survey of India (2000–1)–Census of India

number of developing cities saw their mortality rates rise in the 1990s. It is certainly much too soon to attempt to quantify the positive effects of the hydraulic improvements now being undertaken. However, without going further into the debate[13] and, in contrast to the nineteenth-century picture, it is clear that there is no chronological correspondence between the introduction of public health policies and the reduction of infectious diseases, particularly of what can be described as water-borne diseases. According to data collected at Chennai Corporation and then processed, water-borne diseases were still the third leading cause of death between 1990 and 2000 (on average) and diarrhoeal diseases continued to be one of the leading causes of childhood deaths. The revival of water-related diseases and of diarrhoeal diseases is an indicator of the transition-phase problems of a whole hydraulic system as well as of environmental deterioration. But their revival is not simply a question of poor management, even if the choice of providing extra water immediately proved to be prejudicial in 1997, to the extent of renewing the diarrhoeic outbreak already underway. Indeed, if this were the case, the rise in diseases from contaminated water would have been much more explosive between 1997–2001, especially given the excessive rainfall and the unchecked inflow of Krishna waters.

All the public health indicators confirm the total absence of environmental control, or even the inadequacy of measures based solely on standardized health facilities or networking techniques. Indeed, let us not forget that a number of urban interstices remain unconnectable and alternative systems (dry latrines, for example) that are better adapted to local conditions and practices have to be developed. In this regard, the 'main sewerage system, which consists of using water to dilute faecal matter, and then re-concentrates waste water in a processing and purification plant' (Ta Thu Thuy, 1986: 56) does not function well during droughts and is completely overwhelmed in the monsoons, for want of a comprehensive and truly tripartite drainage system.[14] Therein lies the advantage of local projects for setting up simple sanitation systems, especially when there is a lack of requisite funding or to offset environmental constraints.

Clearly, the notion of 'water blindness' used to describe 'the particular engineering culture which has grown out of areas with a comparative abundance of water' (Ohlsson Leif, 1995) is of special significance here. It is not that the Telugu Ganga Project or the network engineering techniques that came down from colonial times are inappropriate, but rather that this huge development project, which is in a transitory phase, has reinforced dysfunctions—maybe even social inequalities—and above all, ground water consumption, as it is more susceptible to contamination. In fact, during the 1990s, the emphasis was primarily on the modern distribution system and the main city area. Now, the Corporation barely provides 45 per cent of the water consumed of which a large proportion is even delivered by tankers to areas that are not connected or are located at the end of the distribution system. All in all, more than 55 per cent of the population still uses wells or hand pumps only, especially in summer (Ramesh, 1999)—paradoxically so, since the arrival of the Krishna waters. Piped water supply has indeed gone up, but only in areas that were already well supplied. At the same time, storage volumes have also increased, as storage is the only way of offsetting irregular supplies. So tanks that are not kept shut and disinfected systematically turn into health hazards for consumers. On the other hand, water supply problems have only worsened for the majority of inhabitants, particularly for the growing number of the poorest of the poor. For want of sufficient pressure or because of excessive pumping upstream, distribution has become even more erratic. Supply problems have therefore become more acute for many inhabitants and this is particularly the case for the poorest of the poor who rely mainly on public water. Indeed, they hardly ever use the private market (on average, five times more expensive than municipal water), except in peri-urban areas, which are not covered by the public distribution system. Various other water strategies have proved to be completely inappropriate, as they were primarily based on the already overexploited groundwater (Brisset, 2003). Despite hopes to the contrary, aquifers have diminished considerably and even deteriorated in many areas. In addition, more than 60 per cent record alarming concentration of TDS, heavy metals (cadmium, lead, chromium) and total coliform count—an indicator of faecal contamination (UNICEF, 1997: 21). In short, the improvements in the hydraulic system had a number of implications on both the societal and epidemiological planes. Water system technology was applied outside any legal, financial and cultural context. As a result, the positive effects of domestic water supply on health have been reduced by the interference of public departments, by inadequate knowledge of local hydraulic strategies and by irregularly distributed sanitation systems.

In fact, the 'Metro miracle', as some have called it (Nair, 2001: 193), not only defined the pathologies of the 1990s but also changed the epidemic risk itself. In that sense, there was a swing from a natural cause to a man-made cause. The price of development was high, since it was, at the least, at the origin of the revival and reinforcement of various diseases. This essentially reminds us that 'water and health are city dependant' and to reply to the question raised by Durand et al. (1993), a 'global problem can never be solved by a global solution'.

Conclusion 1: Local Revitalization of Water and Health

Beyond the totally new problems caused by the water and sanitary policies that were gradually implemented, the water and health crisis of the 1990s underlined the importance of local dynamics. It also showed us how world standards interfere with local situations, through regional conditions.

It is still too early to identify the effects of the reforms that are gradually being implemented or even to speak of issues like 'environmental health'. This occurred only at the end of 1990s with the emergence of a much more comprehensive vision of water and health. Nonetheless, the state influenced local health policies and even allowed the Tamil capital to revitalize the respective sectors. In fact, the Metrowater, a state-run body, which has now become financially more autonomous, is today being congratulated for its efforts in saving water and adopting more integrated management practices. It can manage chronic water shortages better, as evidenced by the example of the 1999–2000 drought. The Metro has now obtained the state's authorization to divert water from Chembarambakkam, a tank included in the second phase of the Telugu Ganga Project and used for agriculture at the time. It has also becaome financially proactive, in particular through a special drought fund. Major progress, therefore, has taken place by focusing attention at the local level and adopting a regional perspective on problems.

However, the 1990s were essentially marked by the gap or even dissociation between water and health considerations, with the interplay between the spectrum of water-related diseases and the weight of internal dysfunctioning at the core. It was believed that the progress made in the water and sanitation sectors would reduce water-borne diseases. On the contrary, they increased substantially all over India, to the point that it became imperative to envisage a national control programme after 2002. Control over water-borne diseases calls for an overall improvement of the environment, as well as a better understanding of their development. As long as peripheral areas are managed separately, the country will always be just a step away from urban epidemics. In other words, while the Metrowater would gradually take over the administration of the entire urban area, the same would also have to be done for the surveillance of epidemic diseases. Only then could these become the 'catalyst of municipal reform and the development of public health' (Arnold, 1986: 118).

Water-related epidemics, then, only represented the tip of the iceberg during the turning point of the 1990s. From then onwards, they stood out from the conventional 'too much or not enough water for health' model (Salem, 1994) and went beyond the framework of new technologies as such, or even new water development projects. These periods of epidemics, which revealed the water-related upheavals taking place in their chronological sequence, correspond, above all, to 'social trajectories'. Therein lies the whole question of pathogenic systems and the problem of their extreme complexity.

FROM ENDEMIC DISEASES TO EPIDEMICS AND VICE-VERSA: A NEW LOOK AT QUANTITATIVE EVIDENCE

In a system that combines improvements in municipal water supply and its pathogenic counterparts, it is necessary to move forward prudently, especially in a context as disrupted as that of the 1990s and where the principle endemic diseases were water borne. The various major health incidents (cholera O139, acute gastroenteritis, human leptospirosis, dengue) sum up what had occurred in the previous decade. Not just because they involved different stages of the domestic water supply chain (supply–disposal–storage), but above all because they marked the high points of a silent evolution.

In fact, an entire process of 'internal globalization' (Beck, 2002: 10) hides behind these specific epidemics, varying according to the transmission cycle of each disease. While many uncertainties remain as regards the origin (place and date of emergence in particular) of cholera O139,[15] the new vibrio found favourable conditions for its very first epidemic manifestation in this fragile coastal ecosystem. In 1997, the decision to increase water supply to the city without any further delay proved to be particularly harmful. The day the Krishna waters reached Red Hills, the terminal tank that supplies the Tamil capital, diarrhoeic morbidity rose at the initial point of supply and the following month, in the areas supplied by the three main distribution stations, which also received water from Red Hills. Simultaneous analyses later confirmed the high presence of pathogenic bacteria—vibrio and Shigella in particular (Kurian, 1998). As for human leptospirosis, it also became a public health problem of, for some observers, en-demic proportions with a mortality rate of 16 per thousand (Sivakami and Asha, 1997). And yet, neither the monsoon, nor the arrival of the new water resource can explain this revival, still less the 2000 peak.

We will emphasize here the most revealing epidemic sequences—those that were not made even more complex by climatic accidents and that showed most clearly the effects of the weakening of society. If we place ourselves at the level of the 'functional scale' of these main water-related epidemics, we can go beyond the stage of C. Nicolle's 'fragile combination of circumstances' (Nicolle, 1993) and demonstrate the ambivalence of societal implications.

Apart from looking at the opportunities the disease had to develop from an endemic stage to epidemic manifestations, ultimately this provides a way of looking at the disease in its environment and examining its pathological progress.

CHOLERA O139: A FIRST SIGNIFICANT EPIDEMIC

The very first cholera O139 epidemic was characterized by a relatively long life-span (2½ years altogether), a high attack rate,[16] an extremely low mortality rate (about twenty cases) and a strong 'geographic revitalization'. Its progress was particularly explosive and rapid, especially in Chennai, which went on to record more than 65 per cent of the notified cases. In fact, the new cholera vibrio triumphed over its host's vulnerability, as well as that of the environment (Figure 11.4).

Cholera is a highly contagious bacterial disease, transmitted by water and contaminated foodstuff. A receptive and non-immune population as well as a primary source of infection are needed for an epidemic to flourish (Rémy, 1988). The absence of cross-immunization among Chennai's inhabitants confirmed that this was a new vibrio and the first condition was met. In fact, in hyper-endemicity areas, children are much more susceptible since adults have already acquired a certain amount of immunity during an earlier exposure. Conversely, cholera O139 affects all age groups, with a specific prevalence among adults (average age: 35 years), a fact that also underlines the extent of inter-human contagion, as soon as the vibrio is present. In a coastal ecosystem, water-based transmission is predominant (Pascual et al., 2002), especially during the monsoons, when water quality becomes increasingly complex, as was the case here.

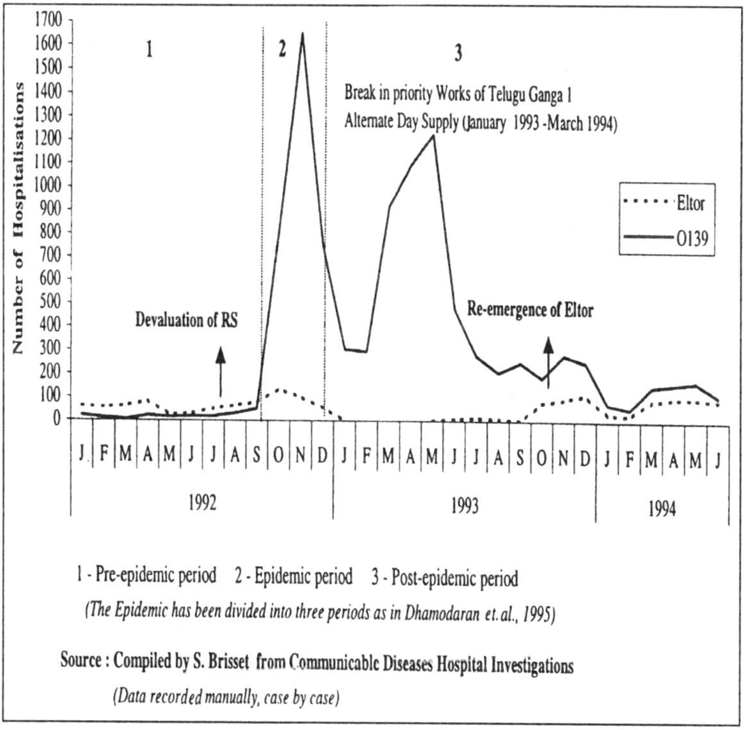

FIGURE 11.4: A RETROSPECTIVE ANALYSIS OF THE FIRST EPIDEMIC OF VIBRIO CHOLERAE O139 IN CHENNAI METROPOLITAN AREA (1992–4)

Water is today known to be the main reservoir for the vibrio (Colwell, 1992). This discovery is of capital importance as man is no longer perceived as a permanent carrier, but as more of an optional host, if not a relay in the cholera cycle. Henceforth, water or the zooplankton with which these bacteria are associated (Colwell, 1996), becomes a continuous medium of dissemination and the water development works underway constitute a real springboard for the disease. In fact, all the *sine qua non* conditions for the emergence and development of this cholera variant—ecological upheavals, higher temperatures, the presence of immigrant workers, water system upgrading, rise in contamination risks—came together. This is particularly true since cholera O139 is capable of surviving much longer in surface waters (Shears, 1994). Significantly, the municipal water distributed since 1991 is taken essentially from the river Korttalaiyar (over 70 per cent) with a view to allowing the northern well fields to refill (Vaidyanathan, 2001: 7). The decision to develop surface resources could well have been a decisive factor in the establishment of this biotope and, indeed, of its revival.

The new infectious agent was more virulent and ecologically more robust than the biovar Eltor of the seventh pandemic. It multiplied much faster and propagated by creating a biofilm on the water surface (Watnick et al., 2001). Temperature (>15 °C), salinity (5.3 per cent), the pH (>8), the method of propagation, are all factors which influence the survival and the proliferation of *V. cholerae* and which explain its dominance at certain periods. The city's three feed tanks (Poondi, Cholavaram and Red Hills), shallow and rich in organic matter, thus offered it a breeding ground of choice, particularly in the dry season (CMWSSB, 1993).

A conjunction of favourable factors and specific societal reactions provoked the epidemic. Contrary to crises in the past, weather hazards were not the triggering factor.[17] There was a clear lack of concordance between the different events, which adds credibility to the hypothesis of a missing 'trigger' link upstream of the epidemic phenomenon. It is true that drought conditions set in in December 1991, but piped water supply was only rotated from January 1993 and it was only from March to August that water was supplied by tanker-trains from the centre of Tamil Nadu (Erode in particular). The epidemic, as such, began in October 1992, before the shortage of treated water and a month before the monsoon. This is possibly a case of a 'threshold' situation in which the disease remains dormant until a critical mass of bacteria has been reached.

The new vibrio in fact began to affect the local population during 1991 and early in 1992 (Albert, 1996). The first cases of cholera O139, acknowledged at posteriori, were reported when development work was on in full swing.[18] The new installations were to be used to replenish the Araniyar-Korttalaiyar wellfields, which was used extensively to supply the capital with domestic water, especially in the dry period, as well as the northern industries. In this pre-epidemic period (January to September), O139 would first appear in the northern industrial suburbs (Attipattu, Ambatur, Manali, Avadi), in Red Hills (Chennai's terminal supply reservoir), and then along the paleoriver before reaching the city (Figure 11.5). A small centre of infection[19] appeared in April in the northern industrial area which was itself partly supplied by northern aquifers, as were the areas in the northeast of the city, which were affected at the same time. The concentration of bacteria rose significantly in Tamaraipakkam and Panjetty, the two aquifers that supplement the municipal water supply, because of the development works underway. From July 1992 onwards, a voluntary 20 per cent devaluation of the rupee led to a rise in prices and had serious repercussions on a population that had already been weakened by repeated droughts, as it was unable to feed itself or pay for potable water, the cost of which rose as the commodity became increasingly scarce. From then on, Chennai offered conditions favourable to the development of this epidemic, which was to affect the non-immune population for a long period, despite the suspension of priority works on Telugu Ganga 1 in January 1993 in an effort to check the crisis.

After a dormant period, the new infectious agent totally replaced Eltor, with the first peak striking during the monsoon and a second in the middle of the dry season (March to May). This was attributed to a shortage of clean water and excessive groundwater consumption. Other factors (domestic storage, impact of the economic crisis, growth of the infectious agent) also led to the resurgence of cholera, since the feed tanks were not yet at their minimum level and neither were water supply quantities. The ineffectiveness of the anti-cholera vaccine and the prophylaxes (popular anti-diarrhoea drugs, some antibiotics, such as tetracycline, in particular) as well as the late official acknowledgement of the disease must also be noted. The epidemic spread rapidly, from a number of very densely populated and highly insalubrious centres (Korukkupet, Vyasarpadi, Tondiarpet in particular) and in 1993, few areas were spared the effect of the new vibrio (Figure 11.6). It is interesting to note, however, that a few 'isolates'—all located in industrial,

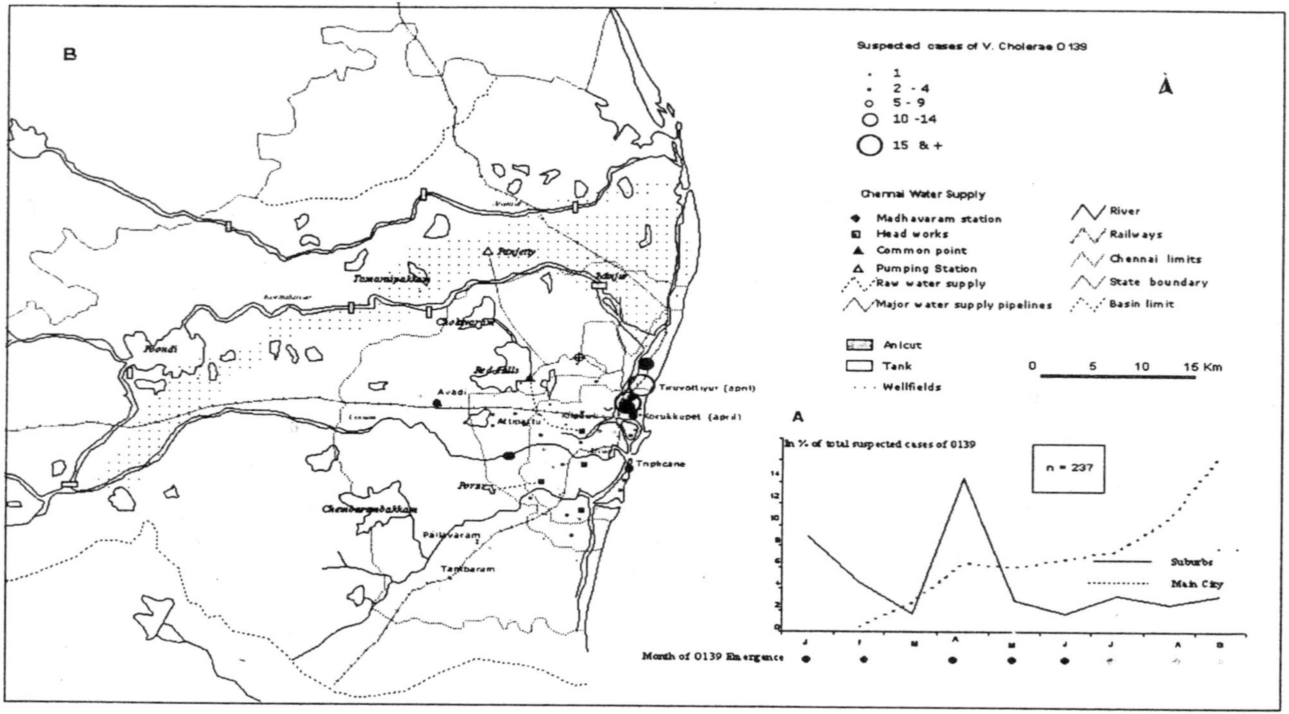

Source: Map realized & data collected (CDH, Tondiarpet) by S. Brisset.

FIGURE 11.5: CHOLERA O139 IN CHENNAI DURING THE PRE-EPIDEMIC PERIOD (JANUARY–SEPTEMBER 1992)—
A: MONTHLY SUSPECTED O139 CASES IN CHENNAI CITY & ITS SUBURBS—
B: SPACES & MONTH OF EMERGENCE

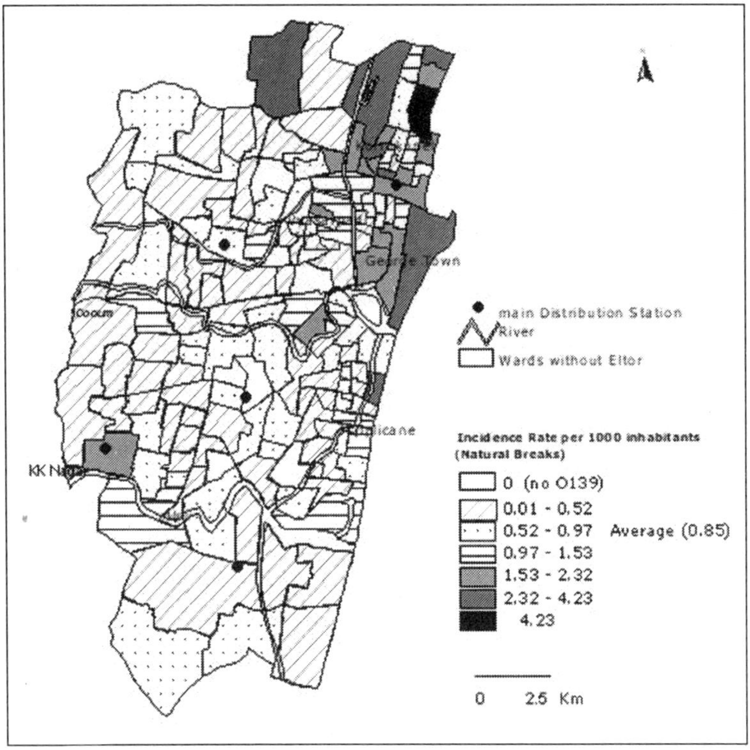

FIGURE 11.6: CHOLERA O139, IN CHENNAI CITY IN 1993

commercial or administrative areas—formed an only slightly pathogenic corridor, along with the Eltor cholera-free wards. Admittedly, these were areas located near major distribution stations and they generally enjoyed sufficient supplies of municipal water, except in 1993, when the water crisis further complicated the transmission chain. Thus, the geographic spread of cholera O139 was as follows: the north-east and a coastal strip that were badly affected, a buffer zone that was totally spared and the West that was much less pathogenic. Only a few secondary pockets (incidence rate of 1–2 per thousand) near watercourses and the south of Adyar—where the picture was in a way reversed from west to east—escaped the general trend. All in all, the high incidence of cholera was essentially due to the conjunction of three elements—ground water consumption, poverty and high population density. The very poor had no choice other than to use local resources, particularly in a period of economic crisis, while those who were better off could opt for more costly solutions.

Admittedly, the first O139 cholera epidemic was the result of the combination of several factors, but, above all, the city found itself facing yet another cholera episode without anyone realizing that this was a turning point in the history of cholera. This also demonstrated the inadequacy of the epidemic surveillance system. The efforts deployed concerned, first and foremost, the recording of cases and not the control of or, indeed, any attempt to understand the cholera vibrio. However, coastal areas, particularly the Tamil capital, played a pivotal role in maintaining cholera's endemicity. As in 1964, Chennai was the initial epicentre if not cholera's 'door' into southern India. Necessarily, other local factors also played a role—if not, cholera would have been endemic in all South Asia's deltaic areas with similar sanitary and demographic conditions.

ACUTE GASTROENTERITIS: CAUSED BY THE ARRIVAL OF THE KRISHNA WATERS BEFORE TIME?

In July–August 1997, the Chennai metropolis recorded an asymptomatic flare-up of acute gastroenteritis and cholera,[20] which was quite significant for this period (the hospitalization of over 3,400 Chennai inhabitants was recorded and there were about 17,000 consultations at the Tondiarpet surveillance centre) and was in no way related to any direct climatic variation.

These diarrhoeic pathologies went up appreciably (+37 per cent) as compared to the same period in the preceding year, which had nonetheless received excessive rains. The reason was immediately ascribed to the lack of hygiene (*The Hindu*, 21 July 1997). Its role was admittedly very crucial, but it did not fully explain the simultaneity of cases in very different areas that were not systematically insalubrious. Broadly, the diarrhoeic sequence was characterized by a gradual intensification, a high concentration of cases (77 per cent) in the city, which was the main beneficiary of the additional water supply, and a specific spatial dissemination. In concrete terms, diarrhoea began to revive with renewed intensity in the wake of the Telugu Ganga Project, before its clear reappearance on the actual arrival of the Krishna waters. Then, a month later, it completely invaded Chennai (Figure 11.7). In short, its evolution took place in three phases, pointing to the Chennai's 'weakening' fabric, if not the reinforced pathogenicity of municipal water.

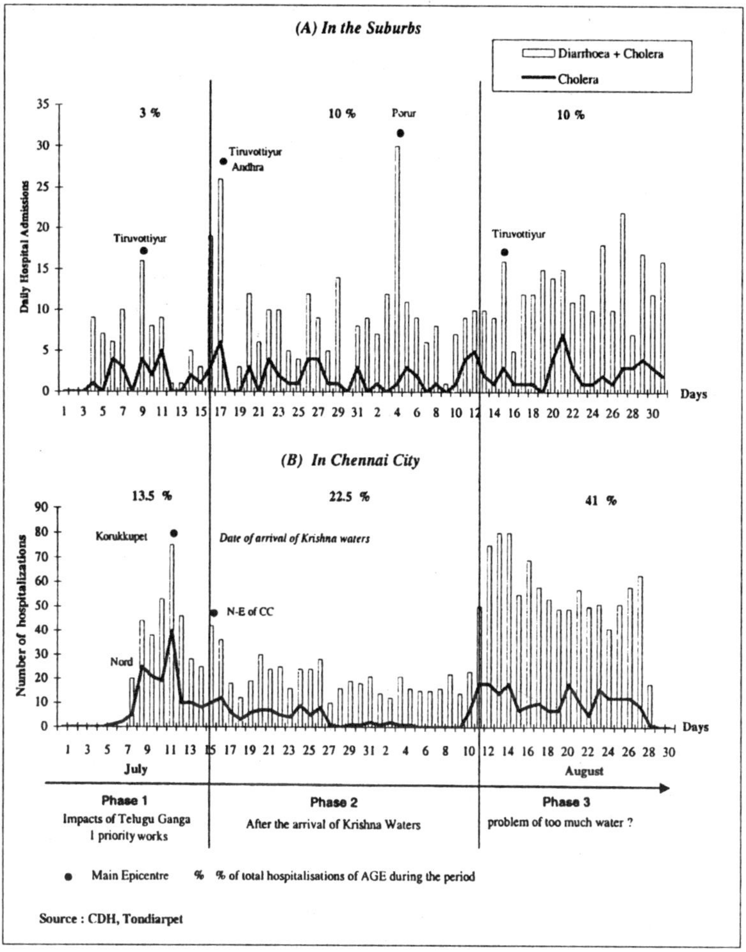

FIGURE 11.7: EVOLUTION OF THE ACUTE GASTROENTERITIS OUTBREAK FROM JULY TO AUGUST 1997

Diarrhoeic morbidity first stepped up (*phase 1*) in areas where improvements in water supply and disposal systems had been carried out first, basically around Red Hills for water supply and Ennore or Perungudi for drainage. The predominance of cholera, a disease associated with contaminated water and lack of hygiene, during a phase when works had been speeded up, was also significant. Admittedly, the first peak spread from not very well integrated localities in Tiruvottiyur and later Korukkupet, often cited with regard to the development of these diseases. According to the Metro team delegated to the site, the municipal supply network in the congested area of Korukkupet was, in fact, under too much pressure and the installation of effluent drainpipes, which were not connected to the houses, enhanced contamination risks (*The Hindu*, 21 July 1997 and private conversations with officials).

This episode of diarrhoea then went on to affect (*phase 2*) the north of the city extensively, according to a specific dissemination pattern, based on the path followed by the new water resource. Small pockets also emerged at the same time in Andhra Pradesh (along the Telugu Ganga canal, not yet consolidated), at the mouth of the Korttalaiyar (Ennore), in Red Hills, in some northern aquifers (especially Panjetty and Minjur), Manali (around the Madhavaram station) and simultaneously in the north-east of Chennai and in the city proper, in particular. In the second phase, the areas that were first served by Krishna waters (mixed water) via Madhavaram station were the most pathogenic. Indeed, this was precisely one of the most vulnerable points in the entire supply system. In fact, it is difficult to understand how Metrowater managed and treated more than 320 mld in July–August 1997. Subsequently, the municipal agency raised the chlorine level and set up 'relay treatment units' in the most vulnerable areas (*The Hindu*, 18 August 1997), in particular Korrukupet, one of the main epicentres of this epidemic. As for the rest of the city, it remained practically untouched by the second peak, except for two secondary pockets in south-west Chennai. The first was around Lake Porur, since the quality of its water had been questioned several times, whenever there was an onset of water-related diseases. The second, in Alandur, had been affected by power problems and a more than erratic supply (*The Hindu*, 3 August 1997), ever since the commissioning of the new supply station in the end of July.

As of 12 August (third phase), Chennai recorded an increase in the number of acute gastroenteritis and cholera cases (1,300 cases in two weeks), directly attributable to an overflow problem. Following heavy monsoon rains, the Krishna waters did rise, successively causing major floods along its course, from the Belgaum district in Maharashtra to Kurnool in Andhra Pradesh. Although a large portion of the surplus water was basically used to irrigate dry lands in Andhra Pradesh and the level of the three tanks supplying Chennai barely rose during this period, the entire regional water system with its multiple interconnections was better supplied and certain particularly vulnerable areas (confluence zones) were completely overwhelmed. Thus, the third diarrhoeic episode essentially affected the areas that were best served by Kilpauk station, which is understandable since water was mainly distributed from this main unit at the time. But these areas were not in the least ready to handle such concentrated water supply. Thus, water overflowed from tanks and main pipes flooded low areas, thereby increasing the number of contamination points. Since the 'overflow' quantities were much lower than estimated, mainly due to ill-timed leaks and overflows, the causes probably lay with drain blockages and deplorable environmental hygiene. An aggravating fact was that these highly pathogenic zones were either extremely vulnerable to floods or were located near waste water treatment plants. Conversely, the areas supplied by the southern headworks station, those at the end of the network (Triplicane–Mylapore) or not very well connected to the municipal water supply, were almost entirely spared (Figure 11.8).

These diarrhoea peaks clearly indicated three types of areas: those revived by the Telugu Ganga, those supplied by Palar or Porur water and the water supply areas incorporated in the private water market. After all, there was but a step between unfinished urban waterworks—or even the availability of water in these areas—and the revival of diarrhoea. For many health professionals, drinking water was the main source of the renewed resurgence of diarrhoea (Sivakami and Asha, 1997: 11). The actual arrival of Krishna waters further reinforced the city's unstable sanitary system. This said, our research, and, by extension, the establishment of a cause–effect relationship, was necessarily done over a limited time period. Since the main supply tanks were already well filled, it would have been wiser to delay the arrival of the Krishna waters, consolidate the system's intermediary stages and change the water management scale. However, given the circumstances, the accounts to be rendered to investors and to society itself, was it not once again more than just a question of choice? In fact, from the very beginning, it had not been possible to respect the Telugu Ganga I schedule and its inauguration had even been delayed by several years. Thus, it was difficult to delay the transfer, especially since the start of the second Chennai water supply and sanitation project depended on it, and so did the release of necessary funding. However, the early arrival of this water was more than detrimental, since it revived the already-destabilized epidemiological situation, with human leptospirosis also finding excellent conditions for development.

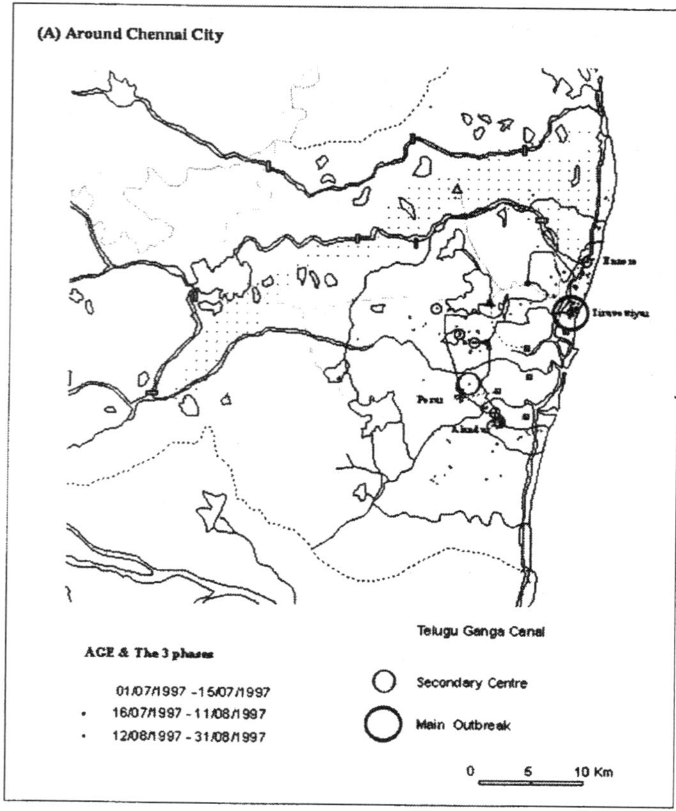

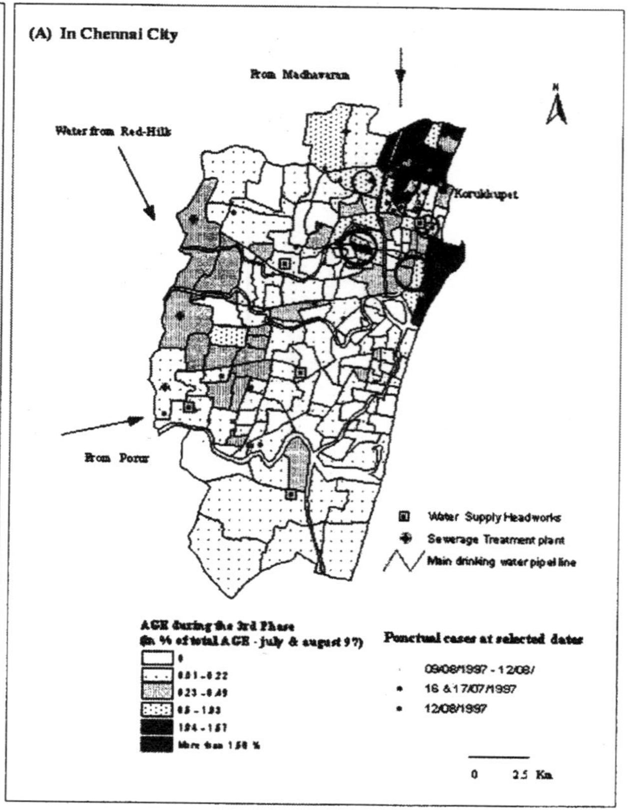

@ S. Brisset, UMR 6063

HUMAN LEPTOSPIROSIS: HEALTH HAZARDS AND DEPRIVED 'FRINGES'

Long considered to be a rare disease and rarely ever diagnosed till the 1990s, leptospirosis was declared endemic in the whole of Tamil Nadu (Muthusethupathi and Sivakumar, 1989). In addition, it was now added to the list of notifiable diseases (*B056*). The Chennai municipality even launched a large-scale programme calling for the eradication of rodents, raising awareness among the people as well as the scientific community, the early detection of the human form and its confirmation by tests, since it is a rather difficult disease to diagnose clinically. Consequently, there is today a tendency to see hidden forms of leptospirosis in the slightest of persistent fevers or other symptoms, leading to a large number of requests for tests. But such a reaction is understandable, considering that a simple antibiotic (penicillin G, amoxicillin) prescribed early enough can prevent death. We shall, therefore, attempt to understand why this anthropozoonosis is affecting more and more people and, through the epidemic of 2000, we shall consider the question of health hazards in deprived areas. The interest of examining this type of pathology lies in the fact that very few studies have been made of it, above all in a precise eco-cultural context and on an intra-urban level.

Caused by a bacteria—most often the spirochete *Leptospira interrogans*[21]—leptospirosis is transmitted to humans (final hosts) from an animal pool, essentially rodents[22] (rats), who discharge leptospires into the environment through their urine. A number of wild or domestic animals can thus become infected, harbouring leptospires in their kidneys for months, if not years, before excreting them in their urine. The survival of the bacteria in nature depends on a number of factors—the pH value (6.2 to 8) in the host's urine, the soil or non-salty water, over which it spreads, as well as the ambient temperature (between 28 °C and 32 °C). Pathogenic leptospires survive particularly well (up to several years) in a shaded and humid area, with a neutral or slightly alkaline pH and when the rainfall is seasonal (Suresh, 1993). This infection, present throughout the world, finds optimal conditions in tropical regions, and particularly in Chennai which is has been destabilized by on-going waterworks.

The presence of leptospirosis in the city and the fact that it periodically affects a number of people is hardly surprising. Indeed, Chennai fulfills all the sine qua non conditions for its development, from the extensive presence of animal pools (rodents, cattle, dogs), to optimal environmental conditions for the survival of leptospires (ideal temperatures, omnipresence of surface waters, existing drains that are never dry, the intensification of problems of water management), to an increased number of man/water interfaces. However, risks of infection go up with the torrential rains at the end of the year. Floods not only cause rodents to migrate, but also promote the dissemination of leptospires and consequently, the contamination of multiple water points and ground water reservoirs the surfaces of which are in direct contact with the ground. In most human outbreaks of leptospirosis, water remains the main source of infection. It is important to note, however, that human infection is not necessary to maintain this zoonotic disease.

It was not easy to determine the growth of human leptospirosis over ten years.[23] In fact, it took until the end of the 1990s to truly identify this pathology. Seeing the large number of patients suffering from this pathocenosis during the manual collection of data at different general hospitals, we listed all the notified cases without realizing that this pathology would recur a few years later. According to all the direct and indirect information collected and processed during our different periods in the field, the number of cases increased visibly from 1995 and particularly with the arrival of the Krishna waters in 1996–7. Nonetheless, it is difficult to link its revival solely to a better screening of leptospirosis, as the disease is no longer limited to certain socio-professional categories (Ratnam, 1994). It is now present throughout the year and has gradually affected all age groups and an increasing number of localities. The epidemic of 2000 (1,012 confirmed cases with more than 70 per cent in the main town, average age of the victims: 23 years) is especially interesting in this light (Figure 11.9). It has, therefore, been the basis of a detailed study based on the confirmed cases of leptospirosis.

Under-fifteens were the worst hit (+ 41 per cent of cases), especially children aged 5–9 (18.42 per cent), that is those most exposed to at-risk environments. The number of deaths (0.40 per cent) decreased compared to previous years which indicates that this zoonosis is now better managed. We have also observed in our studies made over a period of several years that a number of families were able to explain the process of transmission of this disease. In 1997 only the most educated people affected by the illness were capable of giving this information. Neither the rains, nor the arrival of Krishna water, nor the supply of domestic water can explain the monthly omnipresence of cases of leptospirosis, still less their distribution in time and space (Figure 11.10). In fact, it is the social implications of the hydraulic strategies adopted by Metrowater to compensate the lack of rainfall in 1999 that

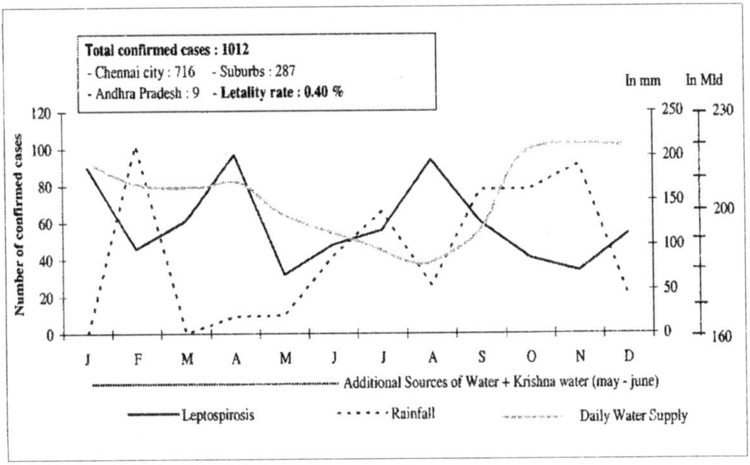

Source: Corporation of Chennai, MGR Medical University.

FIGURE 11.9: RAINFALL, DAILY WATER SUPPLY & HUMAN LEPTOSPIROSIS

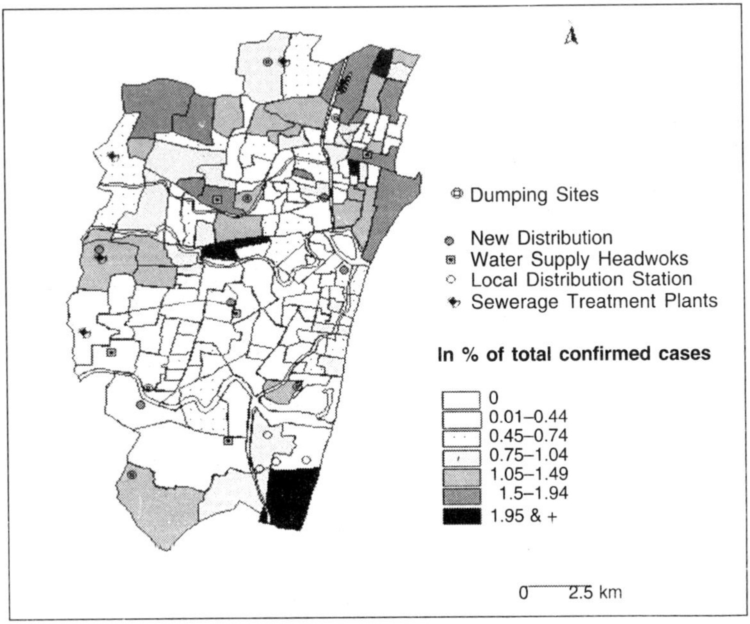

FIGURE 11.10: THE 2000 HUMAN LEPTOSPIROSIS IN CHENNAI CITY

need to be examined. At the time, water from the Chembarambakkam, Rettai Eri and the paleoriver was transferred via the modified and restructured hydraulic system. The Metro managed to preserve its daily water supply all year—as it had not been able to do in previous drought periods—and there was no negative effect on industrial or commercial areas. The spaces that were the most affected in 2000 were all located in the vicinity of waste treatment plants or in highly floodable areas. While the capacity for the evacuation and treatment of used water had practically doubled over ten years, the secondary intermediate network had not been completely restructured. As a result, drinking water was increasingly contaminated with urine from animal vectors (rats in particular), through effluents, water courses or the reflux of waste water, further increased by the works underway. Protected water was the object of a great deal of close attention, however, the Metro did not increase the level of chlorine in the water—a method which destroys leptospires most effectively—until 2001. The real threat of an epidemic came from the deprived areas, especially those slums and suburbs, where growth was at its maximum and environmental problems reached their zenith.

Conclusion 2: 'Old Enemy, New Face'

It is hardly surprising that diseases associated with water management, and intestinal parasitic diseases in particular, have reappeared with renewed vigour in this more than favourable environment and have flared up at a time when society is at its most fragile. Indeed, the ability to manage the health environment is much more crucial than the crisis itself. The cholera O139 epidemic of 1992-3 was certainly made worse by a combination of various elements that appeared at the time, but mostly Chennai Corporation found itself face to face with a new strain of cholera which it had not anticipated and which it could not manage. Yet cholera is one of the diseases which must be reported which, once again, underlines the fact that existing surveillance systems were inadequate. The role of deprived, wet fringes also appears as a background to the epidemic. In fact, it is a whole society's attitude that determines 'the extent of risks incurred and the modes of transmission within an area' (Hanschumacher et al., 1992).

Beyond the overlapping of new waterworks/health projects, the 'epidemic signature' of the 1990s sums up what occurred in Chennai. Briefly, there are three cumulative phases each having its own revealing pathological profile. There is the phase of diseases associated with environmental changes (1991–5), those associated with the infectious nature of the environment (1996–8) and, finally, from 1999, those that we will describe as 'societal' because they were caused by the hydraulic strategies of society as a whole. These three sub-systems, however, make sense only in the context of the global system. The difficulty is that each epidemic is part of the whole. In other words, the silent development in the 1990s is also part of the link between the epidemic and the whole.

Regenerated by the upheavals taking place, cholera O139 and human leptospirosis have gone beyond the stage of 'accidental diseases' (Raoult, 1999) today. They are no longer simply the public health consequences of a changing urban hydraulic network. As G. Rémy pointed out so clearly (1988: 45) in the case of another area altogether, these trace diseases seem to have found 'favourable conditions for epidemization' in Chennai. A certain host/organism balance is necessary, however, if a pathology is to establish itself in the long term. As it advanced step by step, the Telugu Ganga thus became witness to specific pathological processes and to a major 'spatial event' as P. Gentelle puts it (2000: 193). In a way, this epidemiological reality contradicts the theory according to which the rise in the number of cases of water-borne diseases is simply a consequence of major development projects. Their revival can, in fact, be far more clearly attributed to the societal implications of these hydraulic infrastructures.

Cholera O139 was, however, rife at the same time in the entire Indian subcontinent. Similarly, several outbreaks of human leptospirosis were reported from almost everywhere in the world in the 1990s: in Nicaragua, after Hurricane Mitch in 1995, in the continental USA in 1998 or, again in the same year, in Peru and Ecuador following heavy floods. Climatic phenomena unquestionably promoted such eruptions, but do not explain why human leptospirosis, as well as most water-related diseases, re-emerged especially in cities in the developing countries, where sanitation is more than precarious. Along with global changes were a host of local factors, varying according to the pathogenic system in question, which explains why these diseases intensified in one area as compared to another. All in all, every pathogenic system is part and parcel of a much vaster system. And, 'if we enlarge the system, external interactions will, in turn, become internal interactions' (Barbault, 1990).

General Conclusion: The Fourth Epidemic Age?

N. Corner (2002) claimed that, 'plagues are just unfortunate accidents along the path of globalization'. In fact, the re-emergence of water-related epidemics in a given area underlines the ambivalent effect of the globalization process on health as well as the importance of place. We have here a sort of Moebius strip in which global and internal dynamics are equally important and constantly interacting. It is important to remember that 'many global changes depend on micro decisions made at a local level' (Picouet, 2004).

An excellent example of a 'metropolitan health landscape' as defined by S. Curtis, Chennai illustrates the great complexity of under-development and the inappropriate nature of the usual factual approaches to problems. Until the arrival of the Krishna waters in 1997, the Chennai area was well under the threshold of 500 cu.m./inhab./year. It was suffering from 'water stress' (Falkenmark, 1986). In half a century, the population multiplied by 4.5 to 6 in the Chennai Urban Area while municipal water availability only doubled and water drawn from lagoon outwashes was totally unfit for drinking in many areas. It was in this context that the first phase of the Telugu Ganga Project took shape. By 2011, more than 1,000 million litres of additional water is expected to reach the Tamil capital everyday. Nonetheless, it will take the city several more decades to catch up with regard to the availability of drinking water and sanitation facilities and to truly achieve the objective of 'halving the percentage of the population without access to drinking water and the proportion of those without basic sanitation services' (UNESCO, 2003), in other words, for a better situation to emerge. However, the city has chosen an original path by developing several innovative water saving strategies by adopting the system of delegating services to the private sector and by becoming more independent financially. It has, in short, adopted an intermediate model, bringing together decentralization, local initiatives and private operators (often local) reflecting India's position on the management of water, health services or even globalization. The Telugu Ganga has, as it were, brought new life to the water/health sector and encouraged a more global approach to problems.

By insisting on the importance of the transfer and canalization of water, Chennai emphasizes its belief that the quantity of water used is as important as the quality. This concept, suggested by White et al. (1972) questions the purely hygienist approach which concentrates entirely on the purity of the water available and on the management of excreta and it is at the core of strong disagreements between health professionals and their development counterparts. 'Access to sufficient quantities of water could avoid up to 20 per cent of the cases of diarrhoea that we used to believe were due to the poor quality of the drinking water' (Prost, 1996: 238). Yet it is important to make sure that additional water supplies do not worsen an already delicate situation and further encourage social inequality. It is essential to respect the functioning of the societal system.

Far from decreasing, water-related diseases, especially diarrhoeas, have intensified to the point of defining Chennai's 'pathological style'. Of all the public health problems, that of diarrhoea is the most closely linked to water supply and treatment. It can be transmitted both by water and by a lack of water. The most obvious sign of an environmental crisis, these 'diseases of civilisation' (Gudry et al., 1996) underscore the inadequacies of a globalized, hygienist perspective as well as the limitations of models based only on capital and on the solvent sections of the population. It is also clear that the European history of public-health planning is not transferable to Chennai. The work done to improve the drains and the canalization of water in nineteenth-century European cities led to the disappearance of typhoid and cholera and many strains of gastroenteritis. While it is far too early to analyse the positive health effects of the present engineering works, it is clear that water-related epidemics are rife in the great urban areas of the south. Some pathologies like cholera O139 and human leptospirosis in Chennai may well become a permanent presence. Yet the majority of Indian decision-makers subscribe to the views of Illich (Banerjee, 1981) according to which the quality of the general environment is the determinant factor in the health of a whole population. Certainly, it will take time for the cities of the developing countries to be able to manage water-borne diseases as the situation is extremely complex and resources limited.

In the end, the object of this article is to suggest a better way of understanding the notion of 'environmental health' and to question the idea that development necessarily implies the ability to master major epidemics. It attempts to clarify the idea of the 'turning point of the 1990s' and the special role of the big cities, these pathogenic spaces which are open to the world. For 'globalization' to become 'a force for better health' as the *Bruntland Report* (2001) puts it, water-borne epidemics should henceforth be considered differently, both in their globality and as going beyond local specificities. The third epidemic age was that of the 'demystification of the epidemic phenomenon' (Werner, 1999), but the fourth age is that of their redefinition, of their affirmation on a worldwide level, of their endogenous mutations, of, in a sense, their globalization. And, as the Red Queen puts it, the process is never-ending. In Lewis Carroll's Alice in Wonderland, the Queen explains to Alice that it is necessary to run very fast to stay in the same place (Raoult, 1999: 18)—an elegant image to illustrate the paradoxical relationship between evolution and the race to development. As A. Vaguet (2005) so pertinently puts it, our concern should not be tropical diseases but those left behind by development.

NOTES

1. This paper is based on our research work (thesis in progress) which has involved three field trips of 5–6 months each. In brief, the objective is to attempt to understand geographical/water/health changes and to examine the new water/health interface that began to gain ground in Chennai during the 1990s.
2. In 1991 only the city, considered within its old boundaries—but excluding, of course, certain unconnectable areas and slums as well as two of the twelve Panchayats added after 1978—were connected to the municipal supply and drainage system (that is about 87 per cent and 67 per cent of the Corporation). As for other, recent extension areas, they essentially either pumped underground water or were supplied by tankers. Only Villivakkam and Thiruvanmiyur had a main drainage system. See the account of our second field trip (S. Brisset, 'A Geo-Water-Health Crisis in Chennai: A Southern Indian City', 1999, p. 81), especially pages 29 and 44 on this subject.
3. 'The CPHEEO norms are now advised to be 125 lpcd for urban areas where piped water supply and sewerage systems are available, 70 lpcd for urban areas with piped water only and 40 lpcd for towns with standposts', in Richard Franceys, 'Indian Urban Water Supply', Paper no. 35, Birmingham: International Development Department, School of Public Policy, March 1999, p. 14.
4. This is the case in the whole of Tamil Nadu where the incidence of cholera is generally underestimated and many cases taken to be acute gastroenteritis.
5. India was thenceforth divided up into 20 major hydrographical units, further sub-divided into various hydrological basins. Since 1994, Tamil Nadu has had 17 hydrological basins, grouped into 4 regions.
6. An amount of Rs 2.0 crore and Rs 4.85 crore were released to the state authorities in 1997–8 and 1998–9 respectively (TN Heath & Family Welfare, 2001).

7. The period during which vibrio O139 completely supplanted Eltor (from October 1992 to June 1994), and which is termed the 'true' epidemic. However, the pre-epidemic period between January and September should be added. In effect, 're-examination of *V. cholerae* stock stored at the Communicable Diseases Hospital (Chennai) showed that *V. cholerae O139* began to infect the local population as early as January 1992, in M.J. Albert 'Epidemiology and Molecular Biology of Vibrio Cholerae O139, Bengal', *Indian Journal of Medical Research*, 104, July 1996, p.15.
8. To simplify, 'non-agglutinable vibrios' (NAG or Non-O1) do not contain the antigen A (O1) common to O1 vibrios.
9. Leptospirosis are cosmopolitan zoonoses which especially affect rodents (rats, field mice) but also other animals (pigs, cattle, cats and dogs). The contamination of humans may be direct (a bite) or indirect (swimming in or swallowing water contaminated by the urine of vector animals). In its most serious form, the infected subject has high fever, with or without jaundice, digestive system or pulmonary haemorrhage or other bleeding (haemorrhagic meningitis) and low blood pressure.
10. The increase in the number of cases of diarrhoea is less obvious in peri-urban areas because of a clear under-estimation of the number of cases of gastroenteritis and cholera as well as the fast-rising population. These areas will have a major role to play in the epidemics of the 1990s as we shall see in Part 2.
11. The direct standardization method consists in applying specific mortality rates (by age group) to each of the populations analysed compared to a common reference or 'type' population (in this case, that of India), thus eliminating the effect of age weighting on the mortality rate.
12. A lack of appropriate data—and the obvious difficulties in obtaining it—have made it impossible to calculate the respective standardized rates which means, in turn, that it is impossible to compare the different city rates (national or regional rates) with each other.
13. For the three great cities of Paris, Lyon and Marseille, it has been demonstrated that the drop in mortality in the first half of the nineteenth century was contemporary with the work on drainage systems and water suppy (Bourdelais, 2003: 153). For A. Prost (1996) this conclusion of Preston and Van de Walle (1978) are an unconfirmed hypothesis.
14. Domestic, rain and industrial waters have to be treated separately, because they do not require the same level of treatment. Despite these efforts, several bottlenecks persist. Existing drains are never dry, which proves that the separation of drainage systems and wastewater remains largely theoretical.
15. Without entering into a debate, let us simply recall that the new strain seems to have emerged in 1991. Unhappily *V. cholerae* stock cultures have not been preserved, making it impossible to confirm the presence of serovar O139 before January.

16. From January 1992 to June 1994 more than 31,000 citizens of Chennai (CC only: 24,000 or 6.3 per cent) were hospitalized or treated at the Communicable Diseases Hospital of Tondiarpet for acute gastroenteritis and more than 10,000 cases of cholera O139 were confirmed.
17. Unlike the 1987 epidemic, which was a classical model, there was no phenomenon of drought followed by an epidemic of cholera caused by the lack of drinking water.
18. We should specify that the whole period of the epidemic (30 months and some 25,000 cases) has been the object of a detailed space-time analysis based on exact data (sex, age, religion, period and confirmed reason for hospitalization, patient's address) hand-collected at the CDH. This article indicates only the general trends.
19. In fact, cholera appeared simultaneously at two sites in the northern industrial suburb of Tiruvottiyur, one with an Eltor dominant, the other the strain retrospectively identified as O139 which appeared a little further north next to the industrial area itself. 'Infected individuals lived to the north of Madras' (Dhamodaran et al., 1995: 95), but only a micro-analysis allowed us to confirm this hypothesis.
20. To consider cholera alone would have masked a more complicated reality as the type of cholera is no longer specified and the new vibrio is often identified with cases of acute gastroenteritis during this period.
21. Till 1987, the Leptospira genus comprised of only 3 species: *L. interrogans* (with 23 serogroups and 200 serovars), *L. Biflexa* and non-pathogenic *L. parva.* In 1999, there were twelve species.
22. Rodents are, in fact, the main bacterial reservoir, except for some serovars, in particular Ponoma, Tarassovi, grippotyphosa and hardjo, adapted to pet animals—therefore called 'maintenance hosts'.
23. All these findings are the outcome of our spatio-temporal study of human leptospirosis in Chennai during the 1991–2001 period, and especially since 1996.

REFERENCES

Albert, John, 'Epidemiology and Molecular Biology of Vibrio Cholerae O139 Bengal', *Indian Journal of Medical Research*, no. 104, July 1996, pp. 14–27.

Appasamy, Paul P., 'Health and Environment: The Interconnections in Urban Areas: Health and Human Resources Development', *M.I.D.S*, 1993, pp. 281–99.

Arnold, David, 1986, 'Cholera and Colonialism in British India', *Past and Present*, issue 113, November 1986, pp. 118–51.

Auclair, Christine, *Ville à vendre: Voie libérale et privatisation du secteur de l'habitat à Chennai (Inde)*, IFP: Publications du département des Sciences Sociales no. 4, 1998.

Banerjee, D., 'Health for All: Treating the Symptoms', *Economic and Political Weekly*, Bombay, 1 June 1981, pp. 1095–101.

Barbault, R., *Ecologie générale. Structure et fonctionnement de la biosphere*, Paris: Masson Editeur, 1990.

Beck, Ulrich, *Pouvoir et contre pouvoir à l'ère de la mondialisation*, Paris: Editions Flammarion-Département Aubier, 2002.

Bourdelais, Patrice, *Les épidémies terrassées. Une histoire des pays riches*, Dijon-Quetigny: La Martiniere, 2003.

Brisset, Sandrine, 'L'alimentation en eau d'une métropole indienne (Chennai): une lutte coûteuse pour quel développement ?', Publication en ligne (Actes 2003), St-Dié: Festival international de Géographie, 2003.

Brooks, David B., *L'eau : gérer localement*, CRDA, 2002.

Cliff, A.D., *Spatial Diffusion: An Historical Geography of Epidemics in an Island Community*, Cambridge: Cambridge University Press, 1981.

Colwell, Rita R., 'Global Climate and Infectious Disease: The Cholera Paradigm', *Science*, no. 274, 1996, pp. 2025–31.

———, 'The Ecology of Vibrio Cholerae', in D. Barua, and W.B. Greenough (eds.), *Cholera*, New York: Plenum Press, 1992, pp. 107–27.

Corner, N., 'Globalisation: A Biological and Cultural Challenge', 2002 (http://www.Brunonic.org/Nicolaus/globalization.htm)

Dauphiné, A., *Chaos, fractales et dynamiques en géographie*, Montpellier: Reclus Espace mode d'emploi, 1995.

Dhamodaran, S., S. Ananthan and P. Kuganantham, 'A Retrospective Analysis of the Madras Pandemic on Non-O1 *V. Cholera* New Serogroup O139 Bengal', *Indian Journal of Medical Research*, no. 101, March 1995, pp. 94–7.

Durand, M.F. & et al., *Le monde: Espaces et Systèmes*, Paris: Presses de la fondation nationale des Sciences Politiques & Dalloz, 1993.

Falkenmark, M., 'Fresh Water: Time for a Modified Approach', *Ambio*, vol. 15, no. 4, 1986.

Gentelle, P., 'La Chine ou le malaise en périphérie: douze schémas pour une géo-histoire longue', *l'Information Géographique*, no. 3, 2000, pp. 193–218.

Giblin, Béatrice, 'De l'écologie à l'écologie politique: l'enjeu du pouvoir: De la nécessité de savoir penser l'espace', *Hérodote*, 2000, pp. 13–30.

Government of India, *National Water Policy*, Ministry of Water Ressources, 1 April 2002.

Gudry, P., F. Gendreau, and J. Veron (Sous la direction de), *Populations et environnement dans les pays du sud*, Paris: Karthala-CEPED, 1996.

Handschumacher, P., et al., 'Environnement et Santé à Madagascar: une approche globale des déterminants de santé au service des stratégies de développement', in *Table ronde: Maladies transmissibles et environnement*, 1997.

Handschumacher, Pascal and J.P. Hervé and G. Hébrard, 'Des aménagements hydro-agricoles dans la vallée du fleuve sénégal ou le risque de maladies hydriques en milieu sahélien', *Sécheresse*, no. 4, vol. 3, Décembre 1992, pp. 219–26.

Kamal, A.M. 'Cholera in Bengal', *British Medical Journal*, 2 (5763), 19 June 1971.

Kurian, Manju A., 'Bacteriological Analysis of Potable Water from Reservoirs, Treatment Plants and Distribution System of Madras City', University of Madras: Master of Science in Applied Microbiology, 1998.

Lequin, Yves, 'Mouroirs urbains ? Du cycle du choléra à la tuberculose', *Histoire de la France urbaine*, Tome 4, 1984, pp. 287–366.

Lévy, Jacques, *Le tournant géographique: Penser l'espace pour lire le monde*, Mappemonde, Paris: Editions Belin, 1997.

MMWSSB, *Madras Water Supply and Sanitation Project: Master Plan for Drinking Water*, Bombay: Tata Consulting Engineers, 1991.

Muthusethupathi, M.A. et al., 'Leptospirosis in Madras: A Clinical and Serological Study', *Journal of Association of Physicians of India*, vol. 43, no. 7, July 1995, pp. 456–8.

Nair, Shanta Shella, 'The Chennai Experience in Urban Water Harvesting', in A. Agarwal et al. (eds.), *Making Water Everybody's Business: Practice and Policy of Water Harvesting*, Centre for Science and Environment, 2001, pp. 194–8.

Nicolle, Charles, *Destin des maladies infectieuses*, Paris: Lafayette, 1993.

Ohlsson, Leif (ed.), *Hydropolitics: Conflicts over Water as a Development Constraint*, University Press Limited, 1995.

Picq, J.J., 'Epidémiologie du paludisme: Première endémie mondiale (quelques notes)', *Médecine tropicale*, vol. 42, no. 4, juillet-août 1982, pp. 366–81.

Picouet, Michel et al., 'Le renouvellement des théories population-environment', in Picouet et al. (ed.), *Environment et sociétés rurales en mutation: approaches alternatives*, Paris: IRD, 2004, pp. 17–43.

Platt, A.E., 'La lutte contre les maladies infectieuses', in *l'Etat de la Planète*, 1993.

Pascual, Mercedes, M.J. Bouma and, A.P. Dobson, 'Cholera and Climate', *Microbes and Infection*, vol. 4, issue 2, February 2002, pp. 237–45.

Prost, A., 'L'eau et la santé', in F. Gendreau, P. Gudry and J. Veron, *Populations et environnement dans les pays du sud*, Paris: Karthala-CEPED, 1996.

Presto, S.H. and E. Van de walle. 'Urban French mortality in the nineteenth century', *Population Studies*, vol. 32(2), 1978, pp. 275–97.

Ramesh, R., 'Groundwater Quality Management: Pollution Perspectives', *IAHS publication*, no. 259, 1999, pp. 47–55.

Raoult, Didier, *Les nouvelles maladies infectieuses*, Que sais-je ? Paris: Collection PUF, 1999, p. 127.

Ratnam, S., *A Manual on Leptospirosis: A Hazardous Disease of Pet and Dear*, Madras: S.R. Publications, 1994.

Rémy, Gérard, *Paysages et milieux épidémiologiques dans l'espace ivoiro-burkinabé*, Mémoires du Centre d'Etudes de Géographie Tropicale, Paris: Editions du CNRS, 1988.

Ruet, J. V.S. Saravanan and M.H. Zérah, 'The Water and Sanitation Scenario in

Indian Metropolitan Cities: Resources and Management in Delhi, Calcutta, Chennai, Mumbai', Occasional Paper, no. 6, New Delhi: CSH, 2002.

Salem, Gérard, 'Epidémies, pandémies, endémies : quelles géographies?' *Café géographique*, 2004–3.

———, 'L'eau dans les villes du Tiers-Monde: trop ou pas assez pour la santé', *Ville en développement*, no. 23, 1994.

Schubert, A. and I. Lang, 'The Literature Aftermath of the Brundtland Report "Our common future": A Bibliography Based on Citations, in Science and Social Science Journals', in *Environment Development and Sustainability*, vol. 7, no. 1, January 2005, pp. 1–8.

Sharma, V.P., 'Re-emergence of Malaria in India', *Indian Journal of Medical Research*, no. 103, January 1996, pp. 26–45.

Shears, P., 'Cholera', *Ann Trop Med Parasitol*, no. 88 (2), April 1994, pp. 109–22.

Sivakami, Aruna A. and R. Asha, 'The Economic Administration of Biogeo Resources in Urban Cities: A Case Study of Chennai Metropolitan Development Agency (CMDA)', in J. Azariah, H. Azariah and D. Macer (eds.), *Bioethics in India: Proceeding of the International Bioethics Workshop in Madras: Biomanagement of Biogeoresources, 16–19 January 1997*, University of Madras, Eubios Ethics Institute, 1997.

Suresh, B., 'Habitat Study of Leptospires', Ph.D. dissertation, University of Madras, Loyola College, 1993.

Thuy, Ta Thu, 'L'alternatif en assainissement urbain', *Annales de la recherche urbaine,* no. 30, 1986, pp. 53–62.

Tropp, H., *Patronage, Politics and Pollution: Precarious NGO-State Relationships: Urban Environmental Issues in South India*, Sweden: Department of Water and Environmental Studies, 1998.

Vaidyanathan, A. and J. Saravanan, 'Chennai's Water Supply: Problems and Prospects', A Background paper, National Water Harvesters Network–Tamilnadu Unit: Centre for Science and Environment, 2001.

Vaguet, Alain, E. Eliot and S. Brisset (co-eds.), 'L'insoutenable légèreté de la ville durable: la preuve par l'Inde', in M. Jolivet and N. Mathieu N. (eds.), *Qu'est-ce que la ville durable ? Du politique au scientifique,* Collection indiscipline de NSS, 2005, pp. 145–63.

Vaguet, Alain, 'Du système pathogène au système monde', *Cahiers Géographiques de Rouen,* no. 39–40, 1994, pp. 147–54.

Watnick, P. et al., 'The Absence of a Flagellum Leads to Altered Colony Morphology, Biofilm Development and Virulence in Vibrio Cholerae O139', *Molecular Microbiology*, vol. 39, issue 2, January 2001, pp. 223–36.

Werner, A. and H. Goetschel, *Les épidémies, un sursis permanent*, Paris: Atlande, 1999.

White, G.F., D.J. Bradley and A.U. White, 'Drawers of Water: Domestic Water

Use in East Africa', *Bulletin World Health Organization*, 80(1), 1972, pp. 63–73.

World Health Organization, *Emerging Issues in Water and Infectious Diseases*, 2003, p. 22.

———, *Water Sanitation and Health*, Geneva: WHO, 2003f. http://www.who.int/water_sanitation_health/resources/intersectcoll/en/

World Bank, *Second Madras Water Supply Project (India)*, Report no. 14175-IN, May 1995.

PART II

LOW SPEED HEALTH LANDSCAPES

B. Unequal Globalization Landscapes

CHAPTER 12

The Paradox of Proximity: Accessibility to Maternal Care Infrastructure in Rural South India

VIRGINIE CHASLES

Introduction: Reproductive Health Care at the Heart of Gender Issues

One of the most striking indicators of the depreciation of women in India is its population structure, which shows an imbalance in the male-female ratio. With a sex ratio[1] of 933 women for 1,000 men in 2001, India bucked the global trend, since the number of women everywhere else was more or less equal to, if not slightly higher than the number of men. Moreover this feature continues to hold true, for in 1991 it was found that the female population was 32 million less than the male population and in 2001, the figure grew to 36 million (Visaria, 1995). In brief, this is seen as the result of exceedingly high female mortality rates during early childhood. This is principally due to the discriminatory treatment meted out to the girl child, who is not given proper medical care or is given a nutrient deficient diet (Ghosh et al., 2002) due to the preference shown towards the boy child (Burguière, 1986). Secondly, a trend towards selective abortions has been observed over the past several years (Chakrabarty, 2001), and female foeticide (Rao and Jain, 2001) is undoubtedly largely responsible for the continued decline in the female population, as is particularly evidenced in the juvenile sex ratio.[2] Finally, maternity and childbirth constitute just as important a cause for the excess female mortality rate. In fact, despite the real progress made, maternal mortality in India remains among the highest in the world. According to the National Family Health Survey II[3] (NFHS)[4], it was estimated at 437 deaths per

100,000 live births (448 in rural areas and 397 in urban areas) in 1998–9. Thus, whereas the general mortality and infant mortality rates continue to decline, there has been no decline in maternal mortality (Kumar, 2002).

However, due to the measures taken, especially after the Cairo Conference, reproductive health care is now provided to a larger number of women by the authorities, both in rural and urban areas. Thus, despite the still inadequate health care provided during pregnancy, especially in rural areas, there are clear signs of improvement in follow-up since the 1990s. Today, India is a country where highly sophisticated medical technology is available as compared to other developing countries and in no way does it lag behind so-called 'modern' societies. Admittedly, these facilities are by and large concentrated in and around urban areas whereas villages remain largely neglected in terms of skilled health care, but nonetheless, women do have access to a larger and more complete range of medical care. But that does not mean that they make optimal use of it, as we have observed that the presence of a public health centre does not necessarily guarantee its use and does not suffice for the improvement of women's health care. On the other hand, maternal mortality has not declined though we have now known its causes for nearly a century and they generally have not changed (Sundari-Ravindran, 2002) the world over even to this day. The three main causes of maternal mortality are still haemorrhages, anaemia and puerperal infections. Hence, it may seem paradoxical that maternal mortality has not declined.

A gender-based approach would then seem to be justified, since if we look at maternal mortality solely from the reproductive health perspective, which consists of maternal health and gynaecological problems, we are forced to admit that it is reflected both in the differential valence[5] between the sexes prevailing in India as well as in structural dysfunctions. In fact, the devaluation of the female gender can be seen in particular in child marriages and, above all, in their premature entry into reproductive life. This not only enhances maternal mortality risks but also postnatal complications and, from a larger perspective, constitutes a major stumbling block to the optimal progress of reproductive life, all the more so given the young age of the women concerned. Moreover, women have no decision-making powers and together with their low literacy rate, this gives rise to prejudices against seeking medical care, since they are kept away both from health care facilities as well as health-related information. From a more structural point of view, the widespread economic insecurity in India affects women's health at different levels. At the family level, the resources set aside for health care are generally limited and the priority is given to men. Secondly, where the State is concerned, the provision of health care remains a handicap, both in terms of quantity and quality, even though the need for family planning and maternal health services has been clearly established. Despite everything, maternal medical care remains inadequate and inappropriate, more so in rural areas, and is unable to meet the real needs of women, who therefore remain a so-called 'vulnerable' category.

In fact, financial problems seem to be of secondary importance. At least, it seems that way if you compare them to the impact of the subordination of women in the social hierarchy. It is true that India—along with Pakistan or Bangladesh—belongs to the rare category of countries where a woman has been at the helm of affairs.[6] But at the same time, we should not forget that these were exceptional cases, which cannot be taken as the general rule for with regard to the social reality of women. 'Do a woman Prime Minister or a sprinkling of women doctors and lawyers prove that Indian women are liberated? What about the millions of illiterate, ignorant and oppressed Indian women with no recourse due to its feudal customs and traditions?'[7] (Lalitha, 2002: 35). As seen in other societies, India too demonstrates androcentric behaviour, which is found in the highly hierarchical relation between the sexes. In other words, 'The Indian civilisation is seen through the male viewpoint alone in which the woman is forever the lesser mortal' (Biardeau, 1995: 77). To sum up, it can be seen in male supremacy and the notion that the primary role of women is to bear children. This role is the essential element justifying their existence and their identity itself, without ever giving them the necessary individual means to fulfil this function in an exemplary manner.

Therefore, studying the treatments available during pregnancy leads us to consider gender and space, and also to study the issue of gender within the framework of health. The aim is not only to measure the impact of the devaluation of women on women's health, especially those in the reproductive cycle, but also to study the equity in the provision of women's health care. Therefore, it is not enough to talk about women's health alone—we must also take stock of the health infrastructure, in India in general and in Andhra Pradesh[8] in particular, both in terms of quantity and quality.

Finally, based on the twin issues of gender and health care services, we must see whether recourse to health care services can be envisaged. However, while it may be possible to measure the impact of both issues on therapeutic approaches, it is not enough to be able to understand all the social dimensions. In fact, although the conception of men and women enables us to interpret society and divulge its cultural referents, all said and done, it cannot help us to get a proper grip on the kind of recourse to health care that will take place. Therefore, we have to push our study farther afield and analyse the rules that govern Indian social thought and functioning as a whole. For example, we must not only understand the role assigned to each one in the social hierarchy, but also determine the importance given to the individual as compared to the community or, to be more precise, the caste. In fact, there are many things that lead us to believe that all these factors could possibly inspire the decision to avail of health care. At a different level, but still linked to cultural fundamentals, the symbolism surrounding disease could also be one of the factors behind the course of treatment followed. Thus, it would be appropriate to measure the impact of such schema on representations pertaining to maternal pathology and gynaecological dysfunction and, as a result, unearth any future obstacles that they may cause in their health care. In India, as pregnancy and childbirth are steeped in deep-rooted prohibitions and ideologies, it seems that the attachment to these social representations is justifiable if we wish to understand both the material and ideal spatial aspects of maternal health care.[9]

Maternity Medical Care Policy in India—A Recent Priority

Reproductive health has now become an integral part of the national health care system. But the State's involvement in this sector is not a recent phenomenon but was initiated by the colonial authorities. To be more precise, Indians obviously did not wait for the British to grab power before doing something about maternal health, but the latter were the authors of its institutionalization. In fact, remedies—particularly for pregnancy—were thought of and gynaecological practices did prevail in the country since time immemorial. But we should also note that during the entire period, maternal health care was always part of the informal sector and was practiced in an isolated and individual manner. These medical practices were shared and spread through local networks between family members or between villages, and not through global networks that a determined, organized and sustained health care infrastructure can provide. Thus, the space occupied by maternal care belonged to private players exclusively. In other words, it was assigned and entrusted to the family domain. In India, childbirth was considered purely nature's work. The texts dealing with it—basically Ayurvedic texts—are more concerned about the place of childbirth and the necessary preliminary preparations. But in general, Indian medicine and medical practice were a male prerogative, and men were ill informed about female pathology (Krishnaraj and Chanana, 1989: 177). Besides, as childbirth was considered one of the most impure events, the higher castes were never involved in delivering a child. This job belonged above all to folk and magic remedies. It remained the women's domain, although, interestingly enough, women are not present in the Sanskrit Ayurvedic tradition. Therefore, it was only after the British established themselves that maternal care entered the public domain; in other words, this was when maternal health centres were established.

IMPACT OF COLONIAL POLICIES

Rudyard Kipling[10] was one of the first people to cry foul at childbirth conditions and the numerous deaths arising out of them. Judging the prevailing practices as being among the most primitive, the British took over this 'drama' and, playing their role of 'superior beings', took it upon themselves to save the women of this barbaric race. That is how the maternal health care policy saw the light of day in India in the nineteenth century. To be more precise, it was then that maternal health care centres were first established under the aegis of the British and that allopathic medicine entered this sector, while at the same time damning the folk and traditional remedies practiced till then as heretical. The first such British institution was the Zénana Bible, founded in 1852. It later became the Medical Mission of India in 1880. These institutions, which were initially a women's initiative, did not stop at providing care for women but also decided to do away with the practice of traditional midwifery. Calling their methods rudimentary, unhygienic and even dangerous, the British benefactors decided to impart basic techniques to a few 'indigenous' women (Shah et al., 1996)—in other words Western techniques, which alone could be legitimately acceptable and salutary.

Later, the National Association for Supplying Female Medical Aid to the Women of India, better known under as the Lady Dufferin

Fund, was established in 1885 (Krishnaraj et al., 1998). This foundation was first set up in West Bengal, Punjab, Bombay, Madras and Mysore. Under the auspices of women missionaries—and also Queen Victoria (at least this is how the legend goes)—from Great Britain, the United States and Canada, dispensaries, hospitals as well as schools for midwives and nursing were established. In 1888, fifteen women doctor missionaries started working in India, accounting for two-thirds of the women doctors practicing in the subcontinent at the time. Along with this initiative, a Medical Women for India Fund was founded in 1882, this time at the behest of Indian and American businessmen. This foundation invited foreign doctors to practice in India—both men and women. In general, the colonial government at that time promoted the establishment of maternity hospitals by British professionals, who then had the right to practice and head hospitals and dispensaries.

Taken up as a philanthropic activity, the colonization process was made more palatable through such voluntary service. This brand of 'goodness' helped the British authorities to create the image of a caring and charitable government. Moreover, opening these maternity hospitals enabled Western women doctors to work in India, as they could not ply their trade in their own countries due to the gender segregation prevailing at the time and the male monopoly in the health sector. Through this policy, Western women—who were not accepted in medical colleges in their own countries—could gain experience and a degree recognizing their competence in this field. The involvement of the British in the reproductive health sector was, generally speaking, extremely profitable for its practitioners. In fact, in Great Britain, women were excluded from the prestigious field of surgery, which remained exclusively in the hands of men. On the contrary, they were allowed to practice surgery in India. Similarly they were allowed to head hospitals, something unimaginable back in Britain in those days. The problem then was to find 'clients', and it was through small gifts that women were lured to deliver their babies in these centres. Obviously, the various measures taken to help Indians also reflected the sense of superiority that was so natural to the colonizers. The idea was that Indians, truly 'paupers', were obviously unable to save themselves, as they were materially and intellectually destitute. Therefore, only the British could give them salvation.

It was also a mean of introducing allopathic medicine and of having it recognized as a better option than other systems of medicine. But as things often turn out, the British efforts were directed at the affluent sections of society. Despite the desire to focus essentially on the poorest sections, this was not the always the line followed. In fact, in order to make a certain degree of medicalization of pregnancy acceptable—that too through the Western medical system—it was at first necessary to convince the most influential class. Given that this class represents and has always represented the breeding ground for diffusion, convincing them meant winning the others' consent—in other words, convincing the masses. At the same time, it was decided that Indian stakeholders would be included. With this in mind, Indian rajas, businessmen and even the urban elite, though only men, naturally, were appointed to the board of directors of these centres. The irony was that whereas the foreign missionaries had long condemned the discriminatory treatment meted out to women, they themselves were found perpetuating this practice. This was not done out of conviction but out of vested interests. Evangelical persuasion gained upper hand to fulfil the different requirements of the 'benefactors', who found this to be a lucrative activity but, above all, a confirmation of their power. To cite an example, hospitals adopted the *purdah* (veil) system, so as to replicate and maintain the seclusion of women as in the domestic sphere. For the same reasons, Christians and Muslims were not admitted in these hospitals, otherwise it would have distressed Hindu women and more so their husbands. Another example is the separate kitchens that were built in respect of the caste system's commensal rules that were in force and therefore not lose the Brahmin clientele, who were at the top of the caste hierarchy then. Later, it was absence of men in the childbirth sector that was declaimed.

In 1920, the Indian Medical Service's elite held a symposium on this issue in Delhi. The main aim during this event was to demonstrate to what extent Indian men were invisible in this sector, unlike the strong presence of the British. In support, *Mother India*, published in 1927 by the American feminist, Katherine Mayo, gave wide publicity to this state of affairs. She even went to the extent of declaring that the offhand approach of Indian men in this regard was proof enough of their inability to govern themselves! Thenceforth, women's health care served as an argument that was used in debates against Indian nationalism. It was undoubtedly an implicitly racist discourse aimed at showing up Indians as an inferior people (Guha, 1998). Going beyond their systems of medicine, it was the entire social system that was repudiated. Once more, politics were at the very heart of the interest in this field.

After this period and until Independence, the colonial government no longer undertook to better Indian women's lot. Apart from a few specific actions, the maternal care policy made no further progress and stagnated—even regressed. It was only after Independence that, hesitantly at first, it began to be of concern to the authorities—this time Indian authorities.

REPRODUCTIVE HEALTH CARE OF BIRTH CONTROL?

First the Bhore Committee[11] in 1946 and then the National Planning Committee in 1948 raised their voices against the high maternal and child mortality rate in the country. With a view to reducing this problem they insisted upon educating people about health and hygiene. Taking cognisance of the recommendations given in these two reports, the Indian government made maternal and childcare an integral part of its health policy right from the first Five Year Plan (1951–6). Yet, despite this remarkable initiative, sufficient measures were not taken for improving reproductive health. In fact, the measures aimed at reducing maternal mortality announced in the early 1950s were more or less replaced by the fight against communicable diseases and then by birth control and child health care (Bhatia and Cleland, 1996). In fact, maternal health care meant popularizing contraceptive methods and holding inoculation campaigns. Of course, specific programmes to promote antenatal checkups, treat anaemia and train traditional midwives, as well as high-risk pregnancy medicalization were developed, but none of them received the attention due to them, at least not until the World Conference in Cairo.

The World Conference held in Cairo in 1994 set the agenda to be followed by member countries in the reproductive and child health sector. It was then that India added the reproductive and child health programme to the family welfare programme. The programme became operational in October 1997 and encompassed measures aimed at population stabilization, maternal health, child mortality, sexually transmitted diseases as well as reproductive infections. The programme was initially implemented at the grassroots facilities level, i.e. in primary health centres, which are theoretically closer to the people, in order to optimize its effects. The actions taken were real, but were nonetheless inadequate and ran out of steam very soon.

Finally, despite concrete measures, the maternal care programme does not meet the real needs of women in India today. It must be emphasized that planning for this sector is largely in the hands of men and women are generally excluded from discussions aimed at framing the health policy. The policy was too long connected with birth control and neglected both mothers and women, for rarely did it concern gynaecological morbidity and maternal check ups. Thus, maternal care provided will be far from satisfactory as long as women remain largely uninvolved due to an ideology that is above all Malthusian in nature and is not turned towards 'private life'—even that of women.

Moreover, if we take the case of Andhra Pradesh (Figure 12.1) alone, it is evident that the maternal health care policy is not implemented on the basis of women's real needs but rather on the basis of population density. In other words, variables like fertility and the demographic profile of the population are not taken into account. These factors are not spread homogeneously throughout the national territory. Observing the Andhra Pradesh health landscape gives the perfect illustration of this correlation. In fact, it may be noted that the health infrastructure is more or less identical to the state's economic infrastructure. In other words, health care is distributed based on a gradient that is proportional to development levels, and in this case, population density. Andhra Pradesh, the most populous of the India's southern states, is characterized by striking regional contrasts. In a nutshell, we can say that the state comprises of two climatic regions: semi-arid and coastal. The Telangana region spreads over the north-east whereas Rayalaseema consists of four southern districts. Finally coastal Andhra conforms to a delta region made up of the Krishna and Godavari rivers.

Two regions clearly characterized by greater infrastructure density can be found in the state's central portion. The first is spread along the coastal front, characterized in particular by an excessive polarity within the confines of the above-mentioned rivers, and corresponding generally to coastal Andhra and its richest deltas, such as the Godavari delta. Accordingly, special efforts have been made to increase the irrigated land area, so the region was able to achieve relatively prosperous development both in the agricultural and industrial sectors. Therefore, the population density here is higher than elsewhere and, as a result, a growing demand for medical care. It is not our purpose here to see whether these needs have been fully taken care of, but it appears that health care services are most concentrated in this region. It must also be noted that the coastal strip's urban framework consists of numerous small towns. On the other hand, there are only a handful of towns in the state's hinterland, but they are big towns.

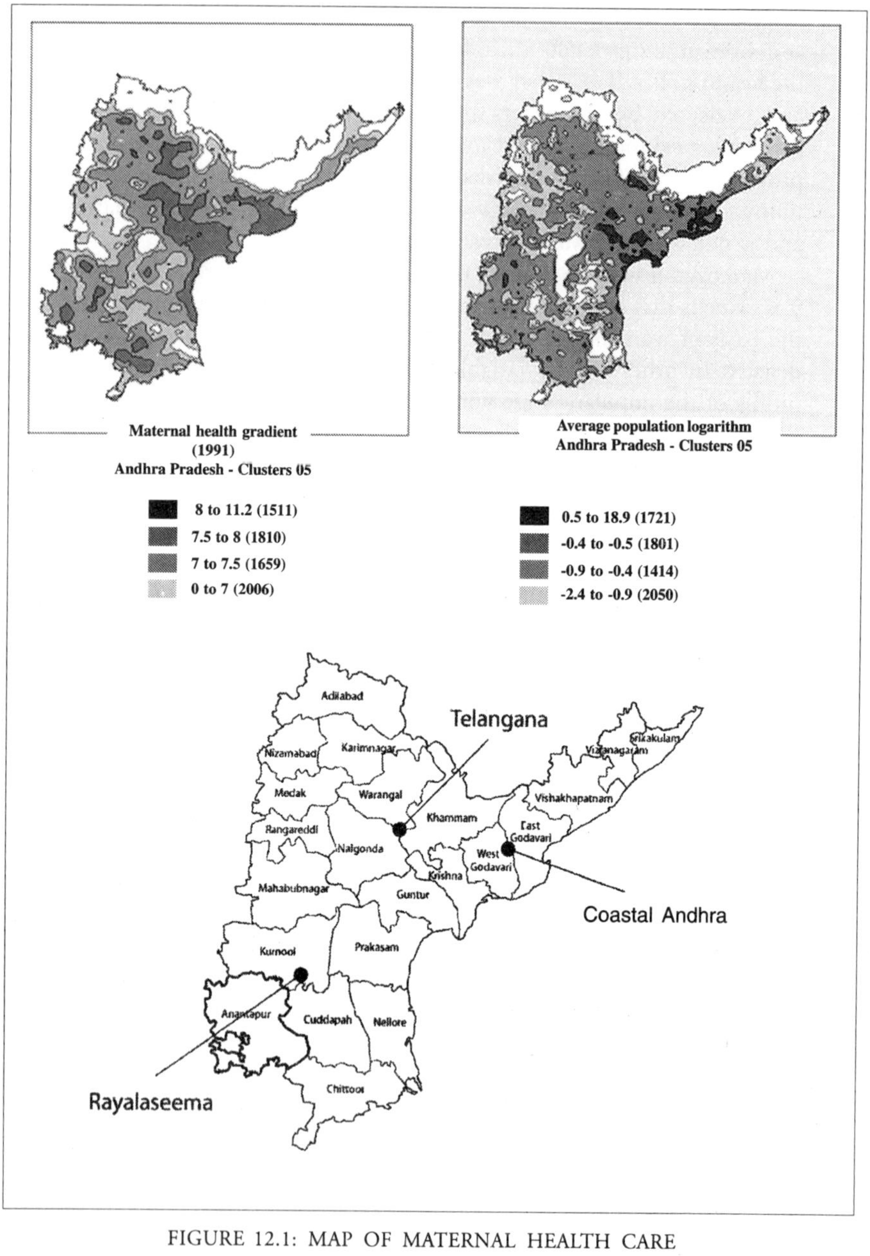

FIGURE 12.1: MAP OF MATERNAL HEALTH CARE IN ANDHRA PRADESH

We can place Telangana in the first sub-group, where Hyderabad, the state capital, is located. Although it has a lower health infrastructure density, Telengana is also privileged and stands out for being so. It can be seen as a kind of coastal extension, above all due to the underlying dynamics of the two rivers that run through it. Telangana is located on the Deccan plateau and is known for its ancient and strong urban, economic tradition. This explains why it is particularly characterized by a relatively better health care infrastructure compared to its neighbouring areas. Nevertheless, glaring administrative contrasts can be seen. Thus, there are two marginalized areas here, marked by their paucity of infrastructure: the Adilabad plateau in the north-west, marked by extreme economic backwardness, and Telangana's south-west, which in its turn suffers from an geographical environment.

In Rayalaseema, the prevailing conditions may be termed enduring or, better still, intermediary. It is characterized by a combination of several major drawbacks. As we have already mentioned, it is known for deficient rainfall—its recorded annual average is 691 mm as against 929 m in Telangana and 1,024 in coastal Andhra. In addition, this region is endowed with very few natural resources and therefore displays slow economic development.

Finally, the most underprivileged regions are actually a few tribal areas in the state's northern and central mountains and forests, which have an extremely low population density and where only minimal infrastructure is available.

To conclude, at present, maternal health services remain concentrated in towns. Rural areas are still largely neglected by the health authorities, since the most effective techniques are found in the urban areas. We shall now examine how both urban and rural women make use of health services.

Women in Rural areas and their Choices of Health Care Facilities

Since 1990s, more than 75 per cent of health care is dependant on the private sector in India (Misra et al., 2003). Though it had a very limited presence until 1970, the private health sector subsequently witnessed a meteoric growth. There were two major reasons for this: firstly, people were looking for quality of care—at least according to their perceptions, and secondly, due to social imitation. More explicitly, private clinics, which were initially accessible to the elite alone, soon began to be identified with quality care. Therefore, while they had been the prerogative of the upper and middle classes thus far, they now began cater to a larger section of the population, comprising the under-privileged classes too (George, 2002). There are several reasons justifying this health care preference, such as the effectiveness of treatment provided by private practitioners.

Thus, both in towns and villages, the private sector is now incorporated in a large number of the therapeutic choices made by patients, as more than 80 per cent of patients consult private practitioners at the national level. And according to a study undertaken in 2002 (George, 2002), it is in Andhra Pradesh that recourse to private hospital and clinics is the highest, much above the national average. In general, it may be said that people use the public sector for minor ailments, but they go to the private sector for serious illnesses. If we direct our attention to rural areas alone, the recourse to the private sector is based on certain novel criteria. But here, it is the location that is important rather than the treatment itself, as people believe that both the quality and diversity of treatment depend upon the location. This being so, distance is no longer a major factor while selecting treatment, but to the contrary, it is not only accepted but also desired as symbolically, it is considered an integral part of quality care. To ensure that they regain their health in the shortest time possible, patients do not mind travelling several kilometres. The nearest health centres in villages mostly belong to the public sector and are therefore not much frequented. It must be said that their rural location does in no way determine their quality. Secondly, public health care is suspect because it is free (Bhatia, 1975). Finally, their proximity itself goes against the perception of quality. Thus, contrary to our hypotheses, proximity does not constitute an attraction. We are thus faced with a real paradox. In fact, we could honestly say that treatments depend on the availability of health care as well the costs to be borne—in other words, the cost of treatment and distance to be travelled. But these 'price' and 'distance' variables seem to be working in the opposite direction: free treatment is suspect and distant locations are preferred for treatment. Finally, the time and effort spent in reaching a far-off health centre are less important than the facility's reputation for quality and fast-acting treatments (Gatrell, 2002). But some distinctions must be drawn in this matter, for though the logic of seeking treatment elsewhere holds good primarily for men and secondarily for children, it is not applied to women (Figure 12.2).

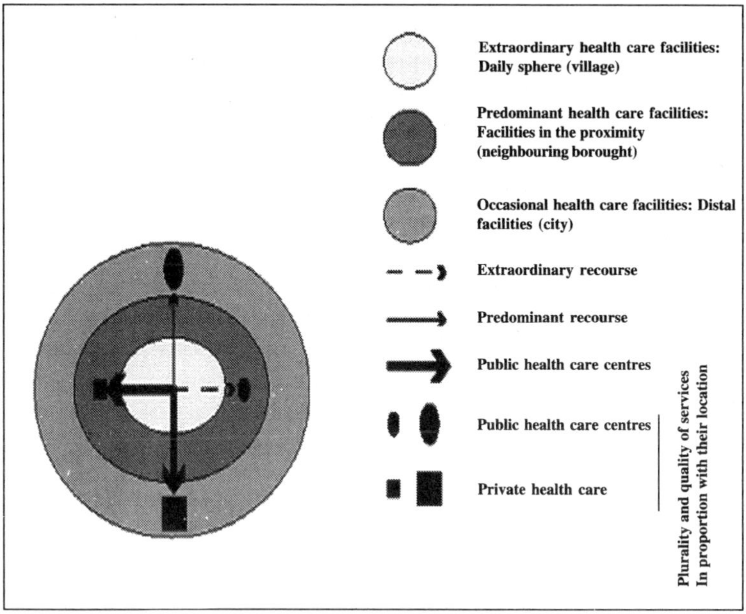

FIGURE 12.2: CHOICES OF HEALTH CARE DESTINATIONS FOR MEN, CHILDREN AND WOMEN IN THEIR FIRST PREGNANCY

RESTRICTED MOBILITY FOR TREATMENT

Women generally seek medical help less often than men and they are also the primary users of poor quality health facilities (Mathur and Sharma, 1995: 176). Further, this is particularly the case for younger women (Madhiwallan 2003). Where reproductive health care is concerned, women generally prefer to consult a doctor located away from their daily space, due to the shyness and discretion that is the custom of villagers, and in order to maintain secrecy. It must be noted that women are afraid of being wrongly accused, especially of sexual deviation, whenever they complain about gynaecological problems. They therefore avoid taking their family into confidence and, if possible, find the farthest possible place for treatment (Barua and Kurz, 2001).

Thus, in this context, the nearest health care facilities are not only under-utilized because they do not fully meet patients' requirements, but also because they can damage a woman's reputation and hence the community's as well. It is anonymity that is more important than the distance factor. To be more precise, women choose the health care institution that enables them to escape the community's gaze and that offers them anonymity. Therefore, it is the 'symbolic' distance from their social sphere that takes precedence over the physical distance. While distance is commonly considered as proof of quality, for women it has the added advantage of anonymity. So it is privacy they seek above all. In the West, a similar attitude can be found in the work done on mental health facilities. In fact, it has been seen that in this case, patients generally shun the nearest institution. It is not only the quality of care, but also confidentiality that weighs on patients' minds in their choice of institution.[12] But in a larger perspective, the fact that women are self-conscious and ashamed of their bodies and sexuality often stops them from getting medical help when they are suffering from gynaecological problems. It should also be mentioned that they give more importance to other family members' health. Thus, they would never hesitate to take their children to a medical centre if it proves necessary, but would rarely do the same for their own ailments (Mukhopadhyay and Savithri, 1998).

Also, their choice of health centre, when they do decide to go to one, is based on novel criteria. In fact, like men, women too have begun to have greater faith in allopathic medicine. While they nonetheless remain the highest consumers of folk remedies and homoeopathy, they rarely consult traditional practitioners. Similarly, although they may invoke God's help to cure illnesses, they do not place all their faith in the Gods and undergo more 'scientific' treatment, along with their prayers. On the other hand, even if their conditions compel them to consult public sector doctors more often, in no way does this diminish their faith in the private sector (Basu, 1992), with the youngest women showing the most marked preference for this sector (Sumaraj, 1991).

From another perspective, the choices of therapeutic treatments available to women are extremely limited. In fact, they consist of very few stages and very few are diversified. To be more precise, whenever women fall ill, they merely take as much rest as possible and practice self-medication. The latter practice is very limited in nature and mainly consists of herbal extract-based beverages and dietary restrictions. Sometimes, albeit very rarely, they take an aspirin their husband may have bought in the neighbouring borough or borrow one from a female neighbour. If the physical discomfort persists, they visit the nearest primary health centre or else await for the certified midwife to make her rounds in the village. It is only when they are unable to perform their daily chores that they may visit a quality health care centre, i.e. a private sector centre, preferably in an urban location. But, the latter situation rarely arises and is by and large more an exception than the rule. In other words, it is only when they feel that their illness is rather serious that they consult a private practitioner, and most often visit the nearest even if they would preferred to go in an urban location. To conclude, their choice of treatment is very limited. It is above all confined to the village and, if necessary, seldom goes beyond the immediate neighbourhood (Figure 12.2).

To sum up, it is evident that medical treatment reflects social norms and value placed on each individual (Conradson, 2003). Thus, we can understand the symbolic place given to women by observing their treatment choices and it becomes all the more evident when we study the medicalization of pregnancy.

EXTRAORDINARY THERAPEUTIC MOBILITY DURING PREGNANCY

As mentioned before women seek medical care away from the community's gaze and in relative anonymity, a decisive element in their decision as to where to go for health care, although this is done only in extraordinary situations as it concerns women's gynaecological health. On the contrary, pregnancy triggers a different logic concerning the recourse to medical care, if not ideologically, at least materially, simply because pregnancy is above all a community issue. In fact, women are anxious about the result of the pregnancy for it is not enough to become pregnant—the community's perpetuation must be ensured. In this situation, the family agrees to provide good health care, both in terms of quantity and quality.

Antenatal Checkups on the Increase

In India, the Reproductive and Child Health Programme lays down at least three prenatal checkups for pregnant women, with the first before the end of second trimester. On the whole, the National Family Health Survey II showed that only 65 per cent of pregnant women underwent this prenatal examination, of which 49 per cent were carried out by a doctor and 16 per cent by a nurse or midwife. Depending on the source of the data, a few variations can be observed in the figures, but they are nonetheless very similar. Thus, according to the Multiple

Indicator Survey (a survey conducted at the national level) for the year 2000,[13] nearly 62 per cent of mothers between the ages of 15 and 49 did undergo at least one prenatal checkup during pregnancy.[14] It is in Andhra Pradesh, Kerala, Tamil Nadu and Maharashtra that these figures are the highest. Generally, such checkups are set up proportionately to the woman's age, but above all based on a parity system. As a result, 78 per cent of women undergo prenatal checkups during the first pregnancy, then the figure drops down to 37 per cent when their parity is more than or equal to six children. On the other hand, it increases with their educational level and standard of living. Also they prefer to do their prenatal checkups with a doctor (preferably a lady doctor), doctors being identified with quality care as compared to checkups done by a nurse, for example.

Finally, an ever-growing number of women are going in for prenatal checkups. This observation is also corroborated by the destination sought for maternal care. In fact, 80 per cent of the women we spoke to had their prenatal checkups done in quality institutions, or at least reputedly so. Such visits, now undertaken by a growing number of women, demonstrate a real willingness on their family's part to give them access to the best possible care, although in practical terms, the progress made in this sector does not fully meet the real maternal care needs. Whatever be the case, the reality is that the destinations sought for prenatal care are the same as those sought for male health care. In fact, for ailments common to both sexes, women always consult doctors in the nearest health centre of dubious quality, whereas for antenatal care, it is not so. In fact, the family affords them destinations at a greater distance and of a better quality for maternal care. The care they enjoy at that time is often identified with the health care enjoyed by men. However, we must point out that antenatal checkups of this kind are mostly restricted to the first pregnancy. To be more precise, if the first child is born in good health, and more so if it is a boy, subsequent pregnancies do not entail the same attention. The primary interest is in the start of the woman's fertility cycle (Navaneetham and Dharmalingam, 2002).

Resistance to Birthing at Home

In India, childbirth is considered a natural process, which partly explains why it takes place so often at home. In fact according to data provided by the National Family Health Survey II, only 34 per cent[15] childbirths take place in maternal care centres, half of them in the private sector.

As regards other women, 50 per cent give birth in their marital homes and a little below 10 per cent in their own parents' homes. The Multiple Indicator Survey gives a higher figure because in 1999 it registered 35 per cent childbirth in maternal care centres, divided into 26 per cent for rural areas and 65 per cent for urban areas.

As for delivery in hospitals, it is Kerala that leads the way once again, registering an average of 96 per cent babies born in hospitals and out of this proportion 76 per cent are in rural areas. In Andhra Pradesh, it is 50 per cent of which 35 per cent is in the private sector, 13 per cent in the public sector and 2 per cent in NGOs. So this clearly shows that the medicalization of delivery most often leads to recourse to quality facilities for the woman giving birth. It must also be added that the private sector is considered more efficient due to its working hours. 'I went to a private hospital for my delivery because it was a Sunday and there are no doctors in the primary health centre on Sundays'![16]

From another perspective, again in Andhra Pradesh, there are twice as many hospital deliveries in towns (79 per cent) as in rural areas (40 per cent). Similarly, this proportion is higher among women below 35 years of age (32–5 per cent) than for women in the 35–49 years age group (20 per cent).

The parity variable must also be noted among the factors of differentiation: 51 per cent hospitalizations for the first child but only 12 per cent from the sixth child onwards. In Andhra Pradesh, this proportion is 60 per cent for the first-born and only 34 per cent for the fourth and fifth children, cutting across caste and educational levels. In the same vein, a study undertaken in Tamil Nadu (Das Gupta et al., 1995) showed that 44 per cent of the first pregnancies in this south Indian state were admitted in the hospital and the proportion declined proportionally to women's parity, despite the increased obstetric morbidity risks and maternal and child morbidity risks, in general, linked with numerous pregnancies. In addition, hospital deliveries are two or four times more frequent among women who have undergone at least four prenatal examinations (70 per cent) as compared to those who underwent just 1–3 checkups (between 18 and 38 per cent). This figure is only 7 per cent for women who never had any prenatal check up. Several factors contribute to the positive correlation between prenatal checkups and delivery in hospitals. In fact, women who go for prenatal checkups are more inclined to have their babies in a hospital because their doctors advise them to do so. In addition, a woman who reserves a hospital room for delivery can be called in for prenatal examinations by the hospital. Another important factor is that of possible complications, for a woman who has complications is more likely to ask for prenatal examinations and subsequently deliver her child in a hospital. Finally, a growing awareness of the advantages of medical care for pregnancies and childbirth can be observed, especially among young, urban and educated women. However, deliveries at home remain customary and are sometimes encouraged for financial reasons, as shown by the following testimony: 'It is very expensive to go to a hospital for delivery. At home, it would cost just between Rs. 250 and 300 whereas in the district general hospital we would have to pay Rs. 6,000.'[17]

Apart from the place of delivery, medical assistance during childbirth is also of importance. The data available with the National Family Health Survey II shows that 42 per cent of childbirths were assisted by health care professionals,[18] 31 per cent by doctors and 11 per cent by midwife-nurses. Traditional midwives, popularly called *dais*, conducted more than 35 per cent of deliveries and friends or family members assisted in 23 per cent of deliveries (Ashtekar, 1996). Amongst women who gave birth in a health centre, 71 per cent were assisted by a doctor in the public sector as against 87 per cent in the private sector. The number of childbirths assisted by a doctor is very low in the case of women in the age group of 35–49 years as compared to younger women. Besides, here too there is a decline in proportion depending on the parity. In fact, in first pregnancies, 46 per cent were physician-aided childbirth cases as against 11 per cent for the sixth child onwards. Similarly, this figure changes according to the place of residence: 23 per cent in villages as against 56 per cent in towns. Physician-aided childbirths depend particularly upon the number of prenatal checkups: among women who never underwent any examination, only 8 per cent had a doctor in attendance, while the figure rose to 33 per cent for women with three prenatal checkups and 62 per cent for those who were examined at least four times. Among those who did not undergo prenatal examinations, 51 per cent were attended by a traditional midwife and 35 per cent by friends or family members.

Whatever be the case, more than 60 per cent of women still give birth at home at the national level. It is interesting to note in this regard that women who underwent several prenatal checkups and who were advised to have their baby in a hospital by medical personnel, nonetheless gave birth at home. But it must be clarified here that women have no say in this matter, more so if they are young, as the family and relatives have the last word. On the whole, home birthing still remains the rule, mainly for two main reasons.

First of all, in society's eyes, a woman's body cannot be seen by outsiders, i.e. the medical staff. Secondly, though pregnancy itself is not considered a polluting process, the same does not apply to childbirth. In fact, it is considered to be of the utmost impurity, highly dreaded by the family circle. Hence, the process has to take place in a confined area, which normally results in the parturient's quarantine. In this situation, it is a question of preserving both the family's honour and holiness. But today, childbirth medicalization is on an upward curve. Nevertheless, as we have seen, along with prenatal care, it too is done only during the first pregnancy, and there is a clear downswing with parity. On the whole, even in this case, childbirth takes place according to the community's customs. It is more of a social happening than an individual's reproductive act and thus the woman is totally overshadowed—not by the mother, but by the society as a whole.

Postpartum Monitoring Spurned

When dealing with maternal care we often forget the postpartum phase. According to estimates, a mere 35 per cent of mothers receive postpartum care, all over the world, whereas 70 per cent receive prenatal care and almost 60 per cent have a qualified person in attendance during childbirth. However, it is possible to prevent both the mother's and baby's incapacitation or death by intervening rapidly during this phase, which begins around one hour after the expulsion of the placenta and includes the six following weeks. Hence, the mother's and newborn's health does not depend merely upon care during pregnancy and delivery, but also upon the care they receive during the first few weeks following delivery.

It is for this reason that the Reproductive and Child Health Programme recommends three postnatal visits. According to data available with the National Family Health Survey II, only 17 per cent of non-institutional births benefit from postpartum examinations in the two months following childbirth. Among those who undergo such a check-up, 14 per cent have it two days after delivery and 31 per cent in the week following delivery. More urban women receive such care than their rural sisters. Also the check up frequency varies according to the mother's educational level and standard of living. The mother's age as well as parity should be appended to these two factors. Also, this figure varies according to the number of prenatal examinations the mother underwent: 7 per cent for those who never underwent one as against 32 per cent for those who underwent at least three. Similarly, mothers who had a health professional assisting them are more inclined to undergo a postpartum examination (29 per cent) as compared to mothers assisted by traditional midwives (15 per cent), friends or family (13 per cent).

More broadly speaking, once again on the basis of the data available with the National Family Health Survey, only one-fourth of women receive postpartum care, most often only women who have delivered through a Caesarean section (Sharrif, 1999). This is the case especially in Dokkalapalle. Figures given by the Multiple Indicator Survey are not very different, as they declare that 24 per cent of mothers received postnatal checkups in 1999, i.e. 20 per cent of those in rural areas in the survey and 41 per cent of those living in urban areas. Obviously those who had delivered in institutions benefit from such care in larger numbers. Thus 52 per cent of women who had delivered in hospitals benefited from a postpartum care, as against a mere 10 per cent whose babies were born at home. Though measures to extend postpartum care were taken up as early as in the 1960s, these aimed more at encouraging the restriction of the number of children a couple had. Therefore, they were a non-starter in terms of reproductive health and maternal mortality. However, it must be said that these were not the objective of these measures (Khan, 2003).

All said and done, maternal care in India is characterized by an infrequent recourse to postpartum care, among other things. At the all-India level, only 16 per cent of women enjoy the privilege of a postnatal examination in the two months following delivery. In addition, there are very few information campaigns on this subject. Moreover, the medical professional itself does not talk about this much. Women follow their mothers' and grandmother's example, who never knew about medical checkups and were no worse off for it. Thus, in general, once the child is born, life goes back to normal, at least for the father and the family, who do not consider the postnatal stage as being crucial, despite the risks the mother is exposed to for several weeks. As regards the new mother, she has to begin various purification processes (isolation, dietary restrictions) before starting her normal community routine without spreading her impurities. As van Gennep explains, the aim of childbirth rituals is to be able to reincorporate the woman into the society she belonged to before, or to give her a new status as a mother in the society, especially when it is the first born and a boy. Even here we can once again see to what extent reproduction is a socially organized process (Mathieu, 2001).

Lastly, sterility[19] problems most often lead to frequent and expensive courses of treatment (UNISA, 1999), but the efforts families are ready to take to treat reproductive dysfunctions are hard to come by. Woman's health *per se* receives very little attention. And by and large, more than financial and accessibility constraints, it is the social constraints that restrict the destinations a woman may seek for treatment (Figure 12.2).

Conclusion: Incomplete Medicalization of Pregnancy

We have been able to see some of Indian society's main fundamentals more clearly by adopting a specifically gender-based approach and by studying the medical care available to women especially during pregnancy. But there again, not only did the androcentric nature of the situation become evident, but also people's representations in the context of medical care as well as the reasons why people travelled longer distances for treatment, both in the case of men and women. The example of the way women use health centres alone throws light on previously not so well-known realities. To be more precise, whereas the general tendency is to give much more importance to variables related to accessibility and service costs, in our study, these proved to be of secondary importance in the choice of destinations sought for different kinds of medical care. In the same vein, the emphasis is on standards of living and education when dealing with developing nations. But in this matter too, we have found additional factors involved. Lastly, the choice of facility for health care still depends upon the position allotted to the person concerned by the social hierarchy. There is a more restricted recourse to health care, and of lower quality, for common ailments in the case of women when compared to men. In the case of reproductive morbidity, female patients often seek distantly located medical facilities, a recourse that is directly related to privacy issues. In this case, therefore, women seek anonymity to escape society's gaze rather than quality health care. On the other hand, the choices made with regard to health care destinations during pregnancy may seem paradoxical, novel or even unsettling. In fact it is the community as a whole and not the pregnant woman herself that is taken into account at such times. In such cases, 'extraordinary' treatment itineraries are chosen, at least when compared to other ailments at other times.

Thus despite the inadequate coverage of pregnancy, more so in villages, there has been a marked improvement in its monitoring. Whereas till recently, the priority remained birth control and the reduction of infantile mortality, health centres today offer quality maternal care. It must also be noted that there has been an increase in recourse to medical care in the case of reproductive morbidity. Despite being a taboo subject, it is more talked about now. Whereas women were fatalistic, they have now become more aware of and informed about this matter. Contrary to what one may believe, State-run health centres cannot take credit for this progress, and this is borne out by the non-performance of primary health centres. In fact, not only do health care workers rarely mention this subject, but what is more surprising, they are not really qualified to treat gynaecological problems. In the same way, the midwife-nurses attached to primary health centres broach this subject rarely during their village rounds. In conclusion, the information channels that contribute to raising women's awareness are primarily the medical awareness campaigns organised by NGOs as well as private clinics. It is not surprising to learn that NGOs undertake this role, but that private clinics also contribute is rather unusual. Yet, a number of private institutions, mostly highly reputed ones, engage in such activities. One cannot have any doubts about their intentions in this case, for beyond health information campaigns lies the vested interest of attracting patients to their fold. In towns on the other hand, it is mostly the media that keeps women abreast on this subject and educates them on how to avoid or get treatment for certain intimate ailments. In rural areas too, the media and especially television have an impact on women's awareness. Besides, village women are in the habit of passing information about their experiences in this matter by word of mouth.

Finally, the differential valence between the sexes and, in particular, the devaluation of women has grave repercussions. It is true that its fundamental realities have changed somewhat nowadays—for instance, more women hold important professional posts or enjoy greater access to health care, but as we have seen, this does not translate into greater social recognition. Also, we should not be misled by the 'Westernized' look of the upwardly mobile classes today. In fact, despite the outward signs of women's liberation, traditional social norms are still respected in reality—for instance, the practice of arranged marriage still prevails among this class.

Thus, we have to admit that androcentric ideologies and, more specifically, androcentric ground rules remain relatively unchanged in

India. It must also be said that women themselves play a role in perpetuating these and, in a way, serve as a link in the discrimination against them. For instance, all you have to do is observe the relationship between mothers-in-law and their daughters-in-law to be convinced. Of course, this is not an Indian invention—on the contrary, we are dealing with a relationship pattern that prevails in most societies the world over. But on the whole, the devaluation of women is very widespread and deep-rooted in India, at least, that is what the sex ratio imbalance as well as the high maternal mortality rate indicate.

NOTES

1. Sex ratio referred to in this paper is actually taken from the female index, in other words number of women per 1,000 men.
2. According to the Indian census, the juvenile sex ratio (0–6 years) was 927 in 2001 as against 945 in 1991 at the national level. But in 2001, this time in Andhra Pradesh, the juvenile sex ratio was 964 girls per 1,000 boys as against 975 in 1991.
3. This data source is presented in the second part of the presentation.
4. The NFHS I (1992–3) estimated the rate at 424 maternal deaths for every 100,000 live births. Notwithstanding statistical errors and a better screening of this mortality rate, the 1991 rate still seems to indicate a marked increase in this kind of mortality.
5. Term borrowed from Françoise Héritier, in *Masculin/Féminin, la pensée de la différence*, Odile Jacob Publications, 1996.
6. Nehru's daughter, Indira Gandhi, was elected prime minister in 1966. She continued in power till 1977, regained power in 1980 and remained prime minister till her assassination in 1984. In Bangladesh, Sheikh Hasina was in power from 1996 to 2001. She lost the 2001 elections to be replaced by another woman, Khaleda Zia. In Pakistan, Benazir Bhutto was elected prime minister in the 1988 elections. Removed from power in 1990, she held office again from 1993 to 1996.
7. K. Lalita, 'Femmes en lutte, analyse historique de l'organisation progressiste des femmes en Andhra Pradesh', in *Enjeux contemporains du féminisme indien* (Contemporary Issues of Indian Feminism), Editions de la Maison des Sciences de l'Homme, 2002, pp. 23–40.
8. A south Indian state, it was possible to assess its health care policy thanks to the 'Espace et Mesure' programme in south India, coordinated by C.Z. Guilmoto.
9. Results of research work done for a doctoral thesis in geography at Rouen University on maternal health care in rural India (Andhra Pradesh), under

the guidance of Alain Vaguet (Rouen University) and supported by the South India Fertility Project, headed by C.Z. Guilmoto (IRD).

10. Rudyard Kipling was born in Bombay in 1865 and died in London in 1936.
11. Committee established by the federal government in 1943 to assess health conditions in the country and give recommendations to improve the situation in future.
12. On this point, refer to: S.M. Taylor & al., 'Attitudes Toward the Mentally ill and Reactions to Mental Health Facilities', in *Social Science and Medicine*, vol. 13, issue 4, 1979, pp. 281–90. A.E. Joseph & J.L. Boeckh, 'Locational Variation in Mental Health Care Utilization Dependent upon Diagnosis: A Canadian Example', in *Social Science and Medicine*, vol. 15, issue 3, 1981, pp. 395-404, C. Philo, 'Across the Water: Reviewing Geographical Studies of Asylums and the Other Mental Health Facilities', in *Health and Place*, vol. 3, issue 2, 1997, pp. 73-89.
13. See Department of Women & Child Development and United Nations Children's Fund, *Multiple Indicator Survey—India 2000*, November 2001, India.
14. To be more accurate, the break-up was 57 per cent in rural areas and 81 per cent in urban areas.
15. This proportion was 20 per cent during the National Family Health Survey I (1992–3).
16. Umadevi, 26 years old, a Hindu patient seeking treatment at the Agai Primary Health Centre, interviewed on 30 August 2000.
17. *Manushi*, no. 105, March–April 1998.
18. This proportion was 33 per cent during National Family Health Survey I.
19. Concerning this point, during our visit to Dokkalapalle, we did not list cases of sterility. However, it must be noted that we only met a few women there. There is much that leads us to believe that among all the women in the village, several could be sterile, but the issue is largely taboo.

REFERENCES

Ashtekar, S., 'Health Care in Bharat, A National Blind Spot', *Manushi*, issue 92–3, January–April 1996.

Barua, Alka and Kathleen Kurz, 'Reproductive Health Seeking by Married Adolescent Girls in Maharashtra, India', in *Reproductive Health Matters*, vol. 9, no. 17, 2001, pp. 53–62.

Barua, A. et al., 'Implementing Reproductive and Child Health Services in Rural Maharashtra, India: A Pragmatic Approach', *Reproductive Health Matters*, vol. 11, issue 21, March 2003, pp. 140–9.

Basu, A. M., *Culture, the Status of Women and Demographic Behaviour Illustrated with the Case of India*, Oxford: Clarendon Press, 1992.

Bhatia, J.C. and J. Cleland, 'Obstetric Morbidity in South India: Results from a Community Survey', *Social Science and Medicine*, vol. 43, issue 10, 1996, pp. 1507–16.

Bhatia, J.C., 'Traditional Healers and Modern Medicine', *Social Science and Medicine*, issue 9, 1975, pp. 15–21.

Biardeau, M., *L'hindouisme, anthropologie d'une civilisation*, Paris: Editions Flammarion, 1995.

Burguière, A., *Histoire de la famille*, Paris: Armand Colin, 1986.

Chakrabarty, L.S., 'Human 'Development in South Asia 2000: The Gender Question', *Economic and Political Weekly*, vol. 36, no. 42, 20 October 2001.

Conradson, D., 'Geographies of Care: Spaces, Practices, Experiences', *Social and Cultural Geography*, vol. 4, issue 4, December 2003, pp. 451–4.

Das Gupta, L.C. Chen and T.N. Krishnan, *Women's Health in India, Risk and Vulnerability*, Bombay: Oxford University Press, 1995.

Gatrell, A.C., *Geographies of Health: An Introduction*, Oxford: Blackwell, 2002.

George, A., 'Quality of Reproductive Care in Private Hospitals in Andhra Pradesh', *Economic and Political Weekly*, 27 April 2002, pp. 1686–92.

Ghosh, S., A. Kilaru and S. Ganapathy, 'Nutrition, Education and Infant Growth in Rural Indian Infants: Narrowing the Gender Gap?', *Journal of the Indian Medical Association*, vol. 100, issue 8, August 2002.

Guha, S., *From 'Dais' to Doctors: The Medicalisation of Childbirth in Colonial India*, Delhi: Kali Editions, 1998.

Gupta, G.R., *The Social and Cultural Context of Medicine in India*, Delhi: Vikas Publishing, 1981.

Joseph, A.E. and Boeckh J.L., 'Locational Variation in Mental Health Care Utilization Dependent upon Diagnosis: A Canadian Example', *Social Science and Medicine*, vol. 15, issue 3, 1981, pp. 395–404.

Khan, M.E., 'Situation Analysis of the Postpartum Programme in India', *The National Medical Journal of India*, vol. 16, supplement 2, 2003, pp. 28–34.

Krishnaraj, M. and K. Chanana, *Gender and the Household Domain, Social and Cultural Dimensions*, New Delhi: Sage, 1989.

Krishnaraj, M., R.M. Sudarshan and A. Shariff, *Gender, Population and Development*, Delhi: Oxford University Press, 1998.

Kumar, R., 'Prevention of Maternal Mortality: Why Success Eludes Us?', *Indian Journal of Public Health*, vol. 46, issue 1, January–March 2002, pp. 3–7.

Lalita, K., 'Femmes en lutte, analyse historique de l'organisation progressiste des femmes en Andhra Pradesh', in D. Haase-Dubosc et al., *Enjeux contemporains du féminisme indien*, Editions de la Maison des Sciences de l'Homme, 2002, pp. 23–40.

Madhiwalla, N., 'Women's Illnesses: Life Cycle Approach', *The National Medical Journal of India*, vol. 16, supplement 2, 2003, pp. 35–8.

Mathieu, N.C., 'Différenciation des sexes', in P. Bonte and M. Iiard (eds.),

Dictionnaire de l'ethnologie et de l'anthropologie, Presses Universitaires de France, 2001, pp. 660–4.

Mathur, I. and S. Sharma, *Health Hazards, Gender and Society*, New Delhi: Rawat Publications, 1995.

Misra, R. et. al., *India Health Report*, New Delhi: Oxford University Press, 2003.

Mukhopadhyay, S. and R. Savithri, *Poverty, Gender and Reproductive Choice: An Analysis of Linkages*, New Delhi: Manohar, 1998.

Navaneetham, K. and A. Dharmalingam, 'Utilization of Maternal Health Care Services in Southern India', *Social Science & Medicine*, 55, pp. 1849–69.

Philo, C., 'Accross the Water: Reviewing Geographical Studies of Asylums and the Other Mental Health Facilities', *Health and Place*, vol. 3, issue 2, 1997, pp. 73–89.

Rao, M. and D. Jain, 'National Population Policy 2001', *Economic and Political Weekly*, vol. 36, no. 16, 21 April 2001.

Shah, A.M., B.S. Baviskar and E.A. Ramaswamy, *Social Structure and Change, Women in Indian Society*, New Delhi: Sage, 1996.

Sharrif, A., *India: Human Development Report, a Profile of Indian States in the 1990s*, New Delhi: Oxford University Press, 1999.

Sumaraj, L., *Women and Medical Care*, New Delhi: Ashish Publishing House, 1991.

Sundari-Ravindran, T.K., 'Maternal Mortality in India: No Room for Complacence', *National Medical Journal of India*, vol. 15, issue 2, 2002, pp. 58–60.

Taylor, S.M. et al., 'Attitudes Toward the Mentally Ill and Reactions to Mental Health Facilities', *Social Science and Medicine*, vol. 13, issue 4, 1979, pp. 281–90.

Unisa, S., 'Childlessness in Andhra Pradesh, India: Treatment-seeking and Consequences', *Reproductive Health Matters*, vol. 7, issue 13, 1999, pp. 54–64.

Visaria, Leela and Pravin Visaria, 'India's Population in Transition', *Population Bulletin*, issue 3, October 1995.

CHAPTER 13

Local Democracy and Access to Health Services in Delhi: Preliminary Remarks[1]

STÉPHANIE TAWA LAMA-REWAL

Local democracy, decentralization and participation have become key-words in the increased emphasis, in the discourse of political actors, on governance in general and 'good governance' in particular. The latter phrase, appearing first in a World Bank report (World Bank, 1989) and widely used by donor agencies, encompasses a set of principles and practices which several Indian chief ministers have been using, for the past years, as an electoral argument.[2] To put it shortly, good governance is generally defined as being characterized by transparency, accountability and participation,[3] and decentralization is supposed to be a major legislative tool in achieving these qualities. But the discourse on decentralization is often ambiguous: the principle of devolving more power to local levels of decision-making can apply to the internal organization of a particular sector, or to public administration, or to political representation.

As far as health care is concerned, discussions about decentralization take into account all three dimensions. In India, decentralization in the health care sector, presented by the World Bank as a most desirable reform, is also advocated by the central government through specific suggestions falling within the new competences attributed to local self-government institutions by the 73rd[4] and 74th Constitutional Amendment Acts (CAAs). Indeed the National Health Policy formulated in 2002[5] repeatedly suggests that local self-government institutions could play a positive role in improving the delivery of public health services: it urges 'all state governments to consider decentralizing the implementation of national diseases control programmes to local self-government institutions by 2005'; it suggests the setting up of a specifically urban, two-tiered health care structure (primary centre and government general hospital), to be jointly funded by local self-government institutions, state and central governments; and it emphasizes the role that local self-government institutions could play, in collaboration with NGOs and other representatives of civil society (such as community leaders) in implementing the IEC component of the policy (GOI, 2002).

I will consider in this paper only the politico-administrative dimension of decentralization, in order to address the question of the impact of local democracy on people's access to health care, with Delhi as a case study. Political life in India's capital city has indeed been characterized since the 1990s by the development of local democracy *lato sensu*, through three main events: (i) the election in 1993 of the first Delhi Legislative Assembly since 1956; (ii) the election in 1997 of 134 councillors to the Municipal Corporation of Delhi, which had been superseded in 1989; and (iii) the implementation by the Sheila Dixit government, since 2000, of the much advertised 'Bhagidari' scheme, which aims at developing people's participation in the management of local affairs.

These three events do not, obviously, have the same historical and political status: the creation in 1991 of the National Capital Territory of Delhi, with its own Assembly and Council of Ministers, is a major step towards the conversion of the former Union Territory into a full-fledged state; municipal elections result from the implementation of a historic policy of decentralization, defined through the 73rd and 74th CAAs passed in 1992; while the Bhagidari scheme, self defined as a 'citizen-government partnership', is only a programme of the current government, giving a new status and role to 'citizen's groups' represented by Resident Welfare Associations (RWAs) and Market Traders Associations. Yet all three combine to provide, within a decade, a remarkable increase in people's representation and participation[6] at the 'local' level.[7]

In a context where access to health services is limited by major constraints on the demand side (such as poverty,[8] lack of education, gender-based discriminations) and on the supply side (by the inadequate provision of medical infrastructures, personnel and products),[9] one of the first consequences of political decentralization seems to be a multiplication of intermediaries, i.e. people who can link a demand to a supply. I shall attempt to characterize the role played by these new intermediaries, namely locally elected representatives and organized civil society, in people's access to health services—the notion of access is here understood as encompassing both the (physical and temporal) availability of health services, and their accessibility in terms of physical, financial, and social barriers.[10]

What can we expect in this regard? I will use the recommendations of the National Health Policy quoted above as a first benchmark. My second benchmark will be the major argument supporting decentralization everywhere, i.e. that local democracy makes policy-makers more responsive to people's demands. Health care, being a very basic service, is assumed to be a good indicator in this regard, particularly in the context of Indian cities: considering the fact that those people who vote en masse in municipal elections, i.e. the slum dwellers, and more generally the urban poor, are also the targeted users of municipal health services, one may expect that elected representatives at the municipal level be subjected to special pressure from their constituents on the topic of health care.

This paper is the first outcome of an empirical survey conducted in Delhi in October–November 2004. Fieldwork was grounded in four municipal wards selected with a view to provide a representative sample of the city in terms of urban landscape, housing pattern and socio-economic profile of the inhabitants: Kalkaji, in the southern residential area of the city; Seemapuri, across the Yamuna river, where many slums have been relocated; Jama Masjid, at the heart of the dense Old City; and Najafgarh, on the western, quasi-rural border of Delhi. This is a qualitative study based on a series of 50 semi-directed interviews with, and direct observation of, the actors concerned with access to health services in India's capital city: elected representatives and officials at the state and at the municipal levels, political party cadres, NGOs' and RWAs' representatives, doctors and public health care users. After a brief presentation of the current scenario concerning decentralization and health care, I will attempt to sketch the configuration resulting from the three events mentioned above by examining successively the respective action, in terms of health care, of the four main actors of local democracy in Delhi: elected representatives (councillors and members of the Legislative Assembly) and organized civil society (RWAs and NGOs).

Decentralization and Health Care in India

Since the economic liberalization of the early 1990s and the concomitant fast development of the private medical sector, one distinguishes between 'for profit' and 'not for profit' health services. More precisely, the

Indian health care system today involves three main types of actors/providers: (i) the public sector (present at all three levels—primary, secondary and tertiary—and highly centralized); (ii) the private sector (mostly under the form of nursing homes providing primary and secondary health care in urban settings, and private hospitals providing tertiary health care); and (iii) NGOs (mostly at the primary level), which constitute a hybrid category in so far as they are akin to 'not for profit', yet private operators. Moreover, while the WHO had been involved in the Indian health care system from the 1970s onwards, since the early 1990s multilateral organizations such as the World Bank, operating through the Union and state governments, seem to have really become a fourth actor.

Private health care is uneven in quality, yet it is preferred by a majority of people, including the poor, because it is perceived as more efficient: thus '80 per cent of health spending is for private health services' (source: World Bank). There is a gross under-utilization of public, primary health care structures (even though the service they offer is free),[11] due to (i) the poor quality of service (absentee staff, shortage of medical and para-medical personnel, unavailability of drugs, obsolete equipment, inconvenient timings), and (ii) to the widely shared perception that such centres actually are devoted to family planning (which was the case, officially, until 1996).

As a sector, the Indian public health care appears to be a case of failed deconcentration: the referral system does not work, therefore primary facilities are underused while hospitals are crowded with cases that could be treated at lower levels. The principle of subsidiarity works neither between different health care levels, nor between the public and private sector (which should cater to the needs of those who can afford it only). Lastly there is a glaring lack of coordination between the three major providers of health care.

The case for decentralization with regard to the delivery of health care must be understood in this context. Often summed up as devolution of functions, functionaries and finances to a more local level of decision-making, decentralization is supposed to make public action more efficient by getting the administration closer to the people.

Ten years prior to the recommendations of the National Health Policy in this regard, local self-governments became statutory authorities with the 73rd and 74th CAAs, which define the new role allocated to local bodies in the rural and urban contexts respectively. As far as cities are concerned, the 12th Schedule of the 74th CAA, which lists the areas of which urban local bodies are in charge, includes 'public health', alongside 'sanitation conservancy and solid waste management'. Considering that most urban local bodies are now well into their second term under the 74th CAA, one may wonder what, then, has been the impact of political decentralization on the delivery of health care in Indian cities?

A review of the literature on decentralization and health care reveals a relative paucity of publications on this theme with reference to India. Moreover most available studies actually focus on rural India (Gupta and Gumber, 1999; Mahal and Srivastava 2000), especially south India (Ramanathan, et al. 2003). There are also a number of studies on the utilization of health care services by the urban poor (Sundar and Sharma, 2002; Yesudian 1999), but these do not include an assessment of the impact of decentralization in this respect. Lastly, the available literature on the topic appears on the whole to be mostly normative and/or prospective in nature: it elaborates on the many advantages that *can* be expected from decentralization concerning health services, but we know very little of what impact the decentralization policy has actually had, so far, on the functioning of the health care system, especially in urban India. It is this research gap that the present article will begin to address.

The Role of Elected Representatives

There is a strong case for considering both the MCD and the government of the National Capital Territory of Delhi when studying decentralization in that city. Given the particular history, geography and political status of India's capital city, both MLAs and councillors qualify as local representatives.

In fact, Delhi, being the seat of the central government, has always had a particular status. Local self-government in that city-state has been characterized, in the five decades following India's Independence, by fluctuations in the democratic nature and in the competences of its two major institutions: the municipal corporation and the 'state'. This particular history makes it necessary to consider both institutions and their interrelationships in order to locate local democracy.

After India's Independence, Delhi was given the status of a 'Part-C State' in 1950, with a Legislative Assembly, a Council of Ministers and a Chief Commissioner appointed by the central government; but in 1956 it was converted into a Union Territory and placed under the direct administration of the president. A year later, Delhi's municipal government went through a major development:

> The Delhi Municipal Committee was awarded the status of a Corporation under the Delhi Municipal Corporation Act passed by the Parliament on 28th December 1957. Nine of the eleven local bodies functioning in Delhi and the Delhi District Board for Rural Areas were amalgamated with the Corporation. The remaining two local bodies, namely, the Delhi Cantonment Board and the New Delhi Municipal Committee continued to function as independent entities. But the MCD was still controlled by the Central Government: the Union Territory administration of Delhi did not have any control over its functioning.
>
> The first general election to the Corporation was held in March 1958. There were 80 councillors in the newly constituted Corporation; . . .
>
> The MCD was constituted on a sound democratic basis: official and nominated members had no place in it. There was a distinct segregation of deliberative and executive functions. The Corporation with its various committees constituted the deliberative wing, which was responsible for policy making, supervision, guidance and control. The work of policy execution was entrusted to professional administrators and technical personnel constituting the executive wing. . . .
>
> [However] the democratic process was repeatedly interrupted due to supersession by the Government. (Ghosh and Tawa Lama-Rewal, 2005)

Meanwhile, at the Union Territory level, demands for a more democratic type of government resulted in the establishment, in 1966, of a Metropolitan Council (composed of fifty-six elected and five nominated members, and presided by the Lieutenant Governor—appointed by the President of India), endowed with the role of providing recommendations to an Executive Council (composed of one Chief Executive Councillor and three executive Councillors). In practice the decision-making power largely remained in the hands of the Lieutenant Governor, and in 1989 the Sarkaria Committee, endowed with the mission of making recommendations for Delhi's administrative set up, recommended that Delhi be provided with a Legislative Assembly and a Council of Ministers responsible to the Assembly, but also that the National Capital continue as a Union Territory, albeit with a special, constitutional status. The National Capital Territory of Delhi (NCTD) was thus created in 1991 through the 69th CAA, but Delhi's major political parties, i.e. the Bharatiya Janata Party and the Congress (I) have been demanding, ever since, full statehood for Delhi—a Bill in this regard is currently pending in Parliament.

When elections were held to the first Legislative Assembly of the NCTD in 1993, the 70 MLAs were thus the most local representatives available to Delhi people—for the MCD, superseded in 1989, had been functioning since then as a purely administrative organization. But subsequent to the adoption of the 74th CAA, the MCD in turn went through a democratizing reform, and elections under the new Act were held for the first time in 1997.

> The Delhi Municipal Corporation Act 1957 was amended in 1993 with fundamental changes in the composition, functions, governance and administration of the MCD, according to the provisions of the 74th CAA. The number of elected councillors was increased to 134. Seats were reserved for the SCs/STs and women as per the provision of the Act. Twelve Wards Committees were formed at the zonal level, and were included in the municipal authority structure. (Ghosh and Tawa Lama-Rewal, 2005)

Just as Delhi's political history, its political geography too is particular: in this mega city (13.8 million inhabitants, 1,483 sq km) municipal wards—the smallest electoral constituency in India's political architecture—are characterized by their huge size: on an average, there are 73,264 people in each ward (Census of India, 2001)—a figure that casts doubts about the meaning of 'local' in 'local politics'. Indeed the municipal and the state levels of government are closer to each other than they are elsewhere in India, geographically and also statutorily. There are only two councilors for one MLA in Delhi (as opposed to six to eight in other mega cities). As a result, a strong sense of competition is perceptible between MLAs and councillors, since every councillor can virtually expect to become an MLA. In terms of competencies also, in Delhi the 'state' has less power and the Municipal Corporation has more power compared to their respective counterparts in other states: the Delhi chief minister does not control land, public order and police, while the MCD's list of departments is one of the largest among municipal corporations.

Concerning the delivery of health services in the city, a division of competencies has been broadly defined between the two levels of government, according to which the MCD is in charge of primary health care and of the preventive dimension of public health, while the Delhi government takes care of secondary and tertiary health care, and more generally of the curative dimension.[12] I will not describe here the administrative organization of the NCTD health secretariat, nor that of the MCD's health department,[13] rather I will focus on the role of elected representatives, as perceived by themselves and by other actors—officials, party workers, RWA and NGO representatives, doctors and users.

MEMBERS OF THE LEGISLATIVE ASSEMBLY

As we saw above, MLAs of the NCTD were the first 'local representatives' elected in the period starting with economic liberalization, which opened a new era in the delivery of health care. Health being on the state list, what has been the role of MLAs as far as health issues are concerned?

MLAs' policy-making work is rooted in a series of thematic 'House Committees'[14] composed of nine MLAs and renewed every year, endowed with the mission to scrutinize and monitor the work of the various departments of the Delhi government. Interviewed MLAs said that health issues take a large place in the debates of the House, and that such issues are usually raised in the framework of the Women and Child Welfare Committee, or the Estimates Committee. The list of Bills discussed in the Delhi Vidhan Sabha between 1994 and 2003, i.e. by the first two Legislative Assemblies, reveals that health care is the third most important issue with twelve Bills discussed in ten years, even though it comes far behind finance (46 Bills) and law, justice and legal affairs (20 Bills).[15] In their collective capacity as policy-makers, then, MLAs display a relative interest for health issues.

Individually, they support the creation of health infrastructure: according to a senior official of the health secretariat, about 60 per cent of infrastructure provision is due to MLAs' initiative. MLAs may also help organize health camps, motivate people to participate in immunization drives, or provide recommendation letters to people seeking admission in one of the hospitals managed by the Delhi government, which helps to reduce the waiting period. But users say that MLAs are much less approachable than councilors for this purpose.

MUNICIPAL COUNCILLORS

Indeed representatives at the municipal level seem to be more interested in health issues than their counterparts at the NCTD level. The MCD is the oldest public provider of primary health care in Delhi; its health department, which has the largest budget, has recently been subdivided into three sub-sections: 'public health', that is preventive health care; 'hospital administration', that is curative health care (encompassing colony hospitals, polyclinics, primary health centres, dispensaries and mobile clinics); and 'veterinary services'.

The MCD's deliberative wing's organization into a series of thematic 'municipal committees', composed of ten to twenty councilors selected for one year by their respective parties, mirrors the executive wing's organization into 'municipal departments'. The MCD's Medical Relief and Public Health Committee, like other municipal committees, gathers about once every month to discuss a number of issues. Its role consists in (i) examining recommendations expressed by the executive wing, and (ii) making new recommendations. A perusal of the minutes of that Committee's meetings reveals that recommendations coming from the administration evoke little debate, and that most recommendations concern specific requests for action in the wards of the Committee's members. The Health Committee therefore appears to be a privileged site for expressing individual demands in terms of health infrastructure, more than a deliberation forum on health issues.

Indeed many of these demands focus on the creation of new infrastructures, such as a new dispensary or a new maternity ward, rather than on the upgradation of existing facilities; actions which require a formal inauguration ceremony seem to be privileged. This tilt towards more visible type of initiatives is considered by many officials as a proof of councillors' obsession with their future re-election, which leads them to favour actions likely to put them in good light, even if those are not the most needed or the most efficient ones, they say. The number of MCD dispensaries being opened every year appears to have substantially increased since 1997, even though official norms governing their distribution over the city's territory (in terms of population density, availability of and distance to other medical facilities) have not changed.

In this regard, the proceedings of the MCD Health Committee meetings between 1997 and 2004 reveal that many councillors demand that Ayurvedic dispensaries[16] be opened, which can be explained by three reasons. One, the Delhi Directorate of Health Services, whose mission is to coordinate the action of health care providers, has recently decided that ayurvedic medicine (as well as Unani medicine) pertains to the MCD's competence because its holistic nature brings it within preventive medicine. Two, the relatively low cost of an Ayurvedic dispensary (which requires no equipments and relies on relatively cheap, herbal type of medication) increases the likeliness of the request to be granted. And three, when allopathic health centres (be they dispensaries or polyclinics) already exist in a given locality, demanding that an Ayurvedic centre be opened allows one to escape the 'overlap' argument.

Councillors act as watchmen, ombudsmen and errand runners: they may make rounds in the various dispensaries and polyclinics of their ward to keep a check on their functioning; they will report people's grievances concerning medical personnel's misbehaviour to the concerned senior officials; lastly, all the councillors I interviewed mentioned the recommendation letters that they provide to people for getting quicker admission into those hospitals managed by the MCD. Indeed one of the defining qualities of councillors seems to be their approachability: users, RWAs and officials insist that councillors are essentially accessible people—more than MLAs, and more than MCD officials. The major change brought in by the 74th CAA might well be that 'there is a big man[17] at hand now', as several interviewees said. While municipal officials are theoretically directly accessible too, they are more distant spatially (being often transferred), but also socially, and above all they are not accountable to the local people. Councillors on the contrary are by definition rooted in the locality; they cultivate a sense of proximity, both spatial and social, with local voters, to whom they are ultimately accountable.

On the whole, however, neither MLAs nor councillors seem to consider health care as a mobilizing theme, worth investing politically. While councillors' capacity as policy makers is limited by structural constraints—the internal equilibrium between the executive and the deliberative wing within the MCD, as well as the MCD's role, largely confined to the maintenance of civic infrastructures—MLAs do not face this type of constraint. Their own relative lack of interest in health issues may be due to the fact that the NCTD government is in charge of secondary and tertiary health care and the presence of national hospitals in the capital city provides it with an exceptional availability of hospital beds (207 for 100,000 inhabitants, as against 95 for India as a whole in 1995).[18] Other sources need to be explored (such as election manifestoes, details of the proceedings of the MCD Health Committee meetings, proceedings of the Vidhan Sabha House meetings) in order to get a finer understanding of this phenomenon. At this stage one can only note that all the interviewed actors—including councillors and MLAs—insist on elected representatives' individual interventions in their own constituency, which suggests that access to health facilities is an object of political patronage, more than an object of policy initiative.

THE ROLE OF CIVIL SOCIETY ORGANIZATIONS

Two types of civil society organizations have been given an official role in the delivery of health care in Delhi: RWAs and NGOs.

RESIDENT WELFARE ASSOCIATIONS

RWAs, as semi-formal groupings of neighbours concerned with the maintenance of local infrastructure, have been in existence since the 1960s in Delhi. But the Bhagidari scheme launched by the Chief Minister Sheila Dixit in 2000 has given a new dimension to these associations, which have multiplied while acquiring a new status, reflected in the frequency of their mention in the media coverage of city news. The Bhagidari scheme relies essentially on RWAs, to involve stakeholders in urban governance: RWAs now enjoy a very official status, provided they follow—at least on paper[19]—a series of rules (like selecting their representatives through a secret ballot election held every three years)—which entitles two of their representatives to become card holding members of 'Team Delhi'. RWAs are also given a very official role, i.e. that of representing the inhabitants of a given area when dealing with the administration, be it the MCD, the police or the Jal Board, on a range of subjects, from monitoring maintenance works to managing community halls.

> [Bhagidari's] operational procedure includes appointment of nodal officers by the participating service agencies in various areas. The Resident Welfare Associations . . . hold regular meetings with the agencies, identify and prioritize local issues and devise follow up programmes. The Chief Minister Office organizes regular review meetings to monitor the progress, remove bottlenecks and ensure support to speed up action. (Maitra, 2003)

As far as health care is concerned, RWAs are a key instrument of communication between local people and the municipal administration, both ways: they inform the administration about local needs, for instance in terms of anti-mosquito measures; and they convey public health recommendations from the administration to the people. Their role is quite formal in this regard: in each of the 12 MCD zones (each zone encompasses a dozen wards), the MCD zonal health officer, and sometimes the deputy commissioner, holds monthly meetings with RWAs in order to exchange information regarding public health issues.

RWAs may also play a central role in local initiatives such as the organization of an informal ambulance service, or the setting up of a health camp in their locality. In this regard, RWAs reveal a capacity to mobilize local resources (money, the use of private cars, private houses or private furniture, the cooperation of local doctors) which is closely related with their ability to ensure the cooperation of elected representatives, and points at several problematic features.

Firstly, RWAs seem to play a prominent role in the localities where they exist, but that is not everywhere. RWAs are a feature of middle class colonies (whether planned or not; indeed the visibility of RWAs in some unauthorized colonies shows that these are not unorganized at all); therefore the Bhagidari scheme, by relying on RWAs, excludes from its scope a substantial part of the population, the slum dwellers (who constitute about 35 per cent of the population).[20]

Secondly, RWAs' role as local relays between the administration and the people puts them in regular interaction with elected representatives, be they councillors or MLAs, depending on the nature of the issue at stake, whenever the support of such elected representative seems likely to facilitate the administrative process. Such regular interaction makes RWA representatives potential support brokers for elected representatives. In the present scenario, RWAs are the only organizations providing a truly local type of representation, characterized by interpersonal interactions. One can therefore suspect that RWAs' ability to mobilize the support of elected representatives is proportional to their ability to mobilize the support of voters in election times.[21] In other words, RWAs appear to be an important element of political patronage.

As far as health care is concerned, this is worrying in so far as RWAs tend to respond to the deficiencies of the public health care system by facilitating the organization of semi-private medical services. I was told, for instance, of a RWA which financed the rehabilitation of a municipal community hall and obtained the services of a private doctor—with the help of the local MLA—to function as a part-time homeopathic dispensary on the condition that access be limited to the colony's senior citizens only.

Lastly, the Bhagidari scheme is often presented as an experiment in participatory democracy, pertaining to the good governance agenda ostentatiously pursued by the Sheila Dixit government. But to construe RWAs as sites of people's participation is certainly misleading: RWAs are not deliberation forums. The only opportunity for a proper debate among the people represented by the RWA comes with elections, which happen once every three years in the best of cases. RWAs' special visibility stems from the fact that they really embody the notion of a local community in a city where the huge size of municipal wards denies them any 'local' quality. The status and role conferred to RWAs through the Bhagidari scheme reflect the recognition of the need for a truly local level of representation, but they may as well manifest the instrumentalization of the currently fashionable notion of participation to promote political patronage under a different name.

NON-GOVERNMENT ORGANIZATIONS

As far as the delivery of public health services is concerned, NGOs may play two different roles: service provider and/or advocacy group.

Most NGOs active in the field of health care are service providers hired by the state or municipal administration to implement a number of schemes pertaining to public health (particularly immunization programmes); as 'not for profit' private operators, their place in the field pertains as much to the privatization process as to the decentralization policy.[22] NGOs' presence is particularly visible in three types of activity, characterized by their stigmatizing nature (for different types of reasons): the management of cremation grounds; the management of public toilets; and the struggle against infectious diseases, particularly AIDS.

NGOs' dependency on the administration to get paid contracts is not conducive, a priori, to their playing an advocacy role. Yet some NGOs act as vigils on health issues, build cases and actually obtain legislative action, as did for instance the Centre for Science and Environment, fighting air pollution in Delhi. The Jan Swasthya Abhiyan (JSA), self-defined as 'a coalition of the networks of voluntary organizations and people's movements involved in health care delivery and health care policy', has been organizing, for the past four years, a national campaign demanding that access to basic health care be given the status of a constitutional right. In this 'Right to Health Care Campaign', the JSA proceeds by organizing public hearings on the denial of the right to health care in different regions, and on different scales (they can involve lay people or community representatives): 'The basic aim of conducting public hearings is to portray the actual state of the public health system and facilitate dialogue between the public and the local government health officials' (JSA-Delhi).

The JSA-Delhi organized one such public hearing in a Delhi slum in December 2004, which consisted of a series of individual cases of denial of health care being exposed by victims (or by their relatives) in front of (i) a panel of 'experts' (legal activists, social workers, academics, doctors working in public hospitals); (ii) a few 'local big men' (the local councillor, local party workers); (iii) local people. The whole event, taking place in the presence of a few journalists, appeared as a dramatization, in the theatrical sense of the term, of people's appeal to the state: the cases being exposed had been selected beforehand for their representativeness, and their protagonists had been prepared to exposing their often intimate, always painful story in front of such a gathering.

This particular *modus operandi* raises a host of questions on the strategies used by advocacy groups to be heard, and on the democratic nature of the whole process. At this stage, however, I will concern myself only with the paradox inherent in the closest thing I could observe to an articulated, collective demand on health care at the local level, namely that this demand relied on global resources. Indeed the demand to recognize access to health care as a basic human right is legally justified, in the JSA's manifesto, in reference to the Alma Ata Declaration, signed by India at the end of the WHO conference held in that town in Kazakhstan in 1978, which took the pledge of achieving 'Health for all by the year 2000'. The JSA is part of a global 'People's Health Movement', born from an Assembly of representatives of 93 countries who met in December 2000 in Dhaka, calling to renew that pledge. In other words, this public hearing illustrates the subtle dialectics between different levels of collective action: the national component of a global movement mobilizing local people to get more leverage in its advocacy.

HEALTH CAMPS

All the actors I interviewed mentioned their participation in health camps—a mode of health care delivery which seems to embody the ambivalent impact of local democracy on the access to health services.

Health camps are an answer to the paucity of public resources *vis-à-vis* the population's needs. In a context characterized by the shortage of medical infrastructure, medical and paramedical personnel and medicine in a city whose population is relentlessly growing, health camps are primarily an economical way to bring health facilities to those people who are most deprived of it: new in-migrants, slum dwellers, more generally the urban poor. They require little logistical means: an open space, a few tents, some basic medical equipment, a few doctors who participate on a more or less voluntary basis. Health camps provide checkups, basic medicine (albeit in very small quantity) and referral to hospitals. They may also be devoted to specific surgery (as in eye care or polio care).

Health camps have the quality of an event: in order to fulfil their mission (usually defined in terms of the number of persons whose health status must be checked) they are preceded by an advertising campaign usually carried out by social workers, be they employed by the NCTD government (*anganwadis*[23]) or by an NGO. This feature makes them a tool of preventive as well as curative health care; indeed camps may include some sensitization to various health issues, for instance through street theatre.

Due to their essential visibility, health camps invite the participation of local notabilities. Elected representatives and RWAs often enough describe health camps as something of a gift that they offer to their constituents; they will visit the camp when it is full-fledged, which suggests that these occasions are used to reinforce political patronage.

Typically, health camps are public initiatives in poor areas, and semi-private initiatives in middle-class areas. They may be the *modus operandi* of a public health scheme—such as the Stree Shakti programme of the NCTD government, aiming at offering health services to those women and children living in areas deprived of basic health infrastructure through monthly health camps held in each of the nine revenue districts of the NCTD. But health camps may also be the result of ad hoc initiatives launched by RWAs or by councilors in middle-class localities, where they are not so much a substitute to basic health care as a sign of the growing concern for one's health; in that case they will usually offer preventive health services (to detect blood sugar or cholesterol, for instance).

Health camps always involve the cooperation of several of the actors observed so far: the state or municipal administration (which may provide the venue, medical personnel, and *anganwadi* workers to mobilize local people); elected representatives (who will rely on party workers to mobilize people); RWAs (who may provide the venue, mobilize local private doctors and local people); and NGOs (who will assist in running the camp).

Finally, health camps are emblematic of the delivery of health services in Delhi today: they reflect the multiplicity of actors involved, the various types of relations binding them, the use of health care as an object of political patronage. Most importantly, they show that beyond the impression of a multiplication of opportunities to get access to health services, there is a tinkering process in which both the permanence of access and the quality of the care provided are quite uncertain.

Conclusion

The above series of observations allows me to sketch a tentative conclusion on the local democracy's contribution to access to health services in Delhi.

Local democracy has multiplied the number of legitimate intermediaries between the people and the administration, both ways: elected representatives, local notabilities and social workers certainly help people get access to curative health care in a context where such access is often denied on account of overload, corruption and neglect; and they are instrumental for the administration to reach out to the people with preventive health care.

At the only truly local level, RWAs appear to play a definite role as an information relay between the municipal administration and the people. Their relationship with the MCD health department, formalized at the zonal level, can be considered as a successful implementation of one of the recommendations of the National Health Policy—with an important caveat however: RWAs are a feature of middle-class colonies; they have a middle-class bias. RWAs also have the capacity to mobilize local resources for the organization of health camps, but in so doing they constitute a coping mechanism with the inadequacy of the public health care supply, which might help perpetuate it.

At the municipal level, councillors certainly contribute to improve people's access to health services: they monitor the functioning of municipal health centres, they support the opening of new facilities, they may contribute to the organization of health camps, and they help people get quicker admission in MCD hospitals by writing recommendation letters. Yet all of these activities are characterized by the individual dimension of the councillors' intervention, which reduces them to political patronage. Indeed those people, such as new in-migrants, who are not registered on electoral rolls, do not have access to the resources of such patronage. Moreover these types of action, just like RWAs', amount to making do with the failures of the health system instead of confronting them. But councillors' role as policy makers is quite limited in any case; the decentralization policy has redistributed status more than power, in Delhi as elsewhere.

This consideration, however, does not apply to MLAs. Yet in the

Vidhan Sabha health care is not being construed as a major political issue, and MLAs too treat access to public health care essentially in the mode of political patronage.

Should we then conclude that local democracy does not necessarily make policy makers more responsive to people's demand? In a city whose walls are increasingly covered with advertisements for private health centres, presenting health care as the ultimate consumer good, the difficulty might lie, paradoxically, in the applicability of the notion of demand to health care. Indeed there are at least two major obstacles to a collective mobilization on health care: the nature of health problems, perceived as being essentially individual; and the structure of the health care market: the availability of private health care allows an exit strategy for unsatisfied users of public health care. As a consequence, 'in the public culture of India, it is epidemics that become occasions for the exercise of citizen's rights in the field of health' (Das, Das and Countinho 2000: 629). Indeed the only case I encountered of an articulated, collective demand for health care relies on the concept of access to health care as a basic right. And this unique example of local people being mobilized on the issue of their access to health care actually proceeds from a global movement.

Finally, the impact of local democracy on people's access to health care is a mixed one. On the one hand, elected representatives (both MLAs and councillors) doubtlessly have a positive impact on the availability of health care through their pressure towards more creation of infrastructure[24] and better performance (in terms of staff presence and behaviour) of existing health centres. On the other hand, the use of recommendation letters certainly improves accessibility for those who get them, but (i) only (some) voters can obtain such letters; (ii) this practice amounts to making do with the chronic inadequacy of health services; and (iii) it helps perpetuate the weight of non-medical considerations in hospital admission.

RWAs' ability to mobilize resources in order to organize health camps (or an informal ambulance service) also amounts to increasing the availability of health services even while confining the accessibility of the same to their own members only.

Lastly, health camps organized by the public administration (whether the NCTD government or the MCD) certainly aim at addressing the problem of accessibility (denied to slum dwellers, particularly when they are new in-migrants, on account of their peripheral situation—in terms of their physical location, their socio-economic and political status). However the very *modus operandi* of health camps implies an essentially precarious availability of the services they deliver.

On the whole, therefore, the development of local democracy seems to have increased the availability of health services (albeit not necessarily their adequacy), even while favouring a conditional type of accessibility.

NOTES

1. This study is part of a larger, pluri-disciplinary project called 'Urban Actors, Policies and Governance. The Decision-making Processes Governing the Supply and Demand of Collective Goods and Services in Four Indian Metropolises'. The project relies on an Indo-European research network associating twelve scholars, who propose to describe and analyse urban governance in the context of an environment transformed by the policies of economic liberalization and political and administrative decentralization. They propose to do this through a study of the decision-making processes pertaining to the supply and demand of a few collective goods and services (health, education, nutrition, water and slum development) in four Indian metropolises: Delhi, Mumbai, Hyderabad and Kolkata. For more information, see the project's website: http://www.csh-delhi.com/UAPG/
2. Indeed the historic re-election of the Sheila Dixit government in December 2003 in Delhi was due, according to many observers, to its performance in terms of governance.
3. More precisely, the UNDP defines good governance through 'nine inter-related characteristics': participation; rule of law; transparency; responsiveness; consensus orientation; equity; effectiveness and efficiency; accountability; and strategic vision (UNDP 1997).
4. The 73rd CAA defines the decentralization policy in the rural context, while the 74th CAA deals with urban India.
5. The previous one dated back to 1983.
6. Even RWAs are to elect their representatives at regular intervals.
7. The inherently relative value of that adjective is obvious here, as it allows us to use it to qualify the Assembly constituency *and* the municipal ward *and* the colony, albeit with different implications in each case.
8. 'The proportion of people unable to afford health care in urban areas has increased from 10 to 21 per cent in the last decade' (*Frontline*, 18 June 2004).
9. See Pierre Chapelet and Bertrand Lefebvre, 'Contextualising the Urban Health Care System', CSH Occasional Paper no. 11, Delhi, p. 135, 2005.
10. For a discussion of the concept of access, see R. Penchansky, and J.W. Thomas, 'The Concept of Access: Definition and Relationship to Consumer Satisfaction', *Medical Care*, 19(2), 1981, pp. 127–40.

11. However at the secondary and tertiary level of health services, user fees are increasingly being introduced as part of the health sector reforms.
12. In this regard, it is interesting to note that the WHO's 'Healthy Cities' project, which claims to 'engage local governments in health development', decided to transfer the second part of its Delhi project (Trans-Yamuna Area, 1998–9) to the Bhagidari scheme, managed by the Delhi government (NIUA, 2004: 104).
13. Beyond these two major providers of public health care, Delhi is characterized by the multiplicity of agencies providing health services (such as the central government, the New Delhi Municipal Council, the Delhi Cantonment Board, the Railways Ministry), alongside voluntary organizations and the private sector.
14. There are three financial committees, fourteen regular committees, and an indefinite number of ad hoc committees.
15. Source: Secretariat of the Delhi Vidhan Sabha.
16. Along with allopathic medicine, alternative systems of medicine, such as Ayurveda, Unani, Homeopathy and Siddha (in south India) have been integrated into the governmental health system since the late 1970s.
17. Or a 'big woman', since both the 73rd and the 74th CAAs provide that one-third of seats be reserved for women. On the implementation of these women's reservations in Indian cities, see Ghosh and Tawa Lama-Rewal.
18. *Source*: Shipra Maitra, *Delhi: The City and the Capital. A Status Report*, New Delhi: Institute for Human Development, 2003.
19. Interviews with RWA representatives reveal that many different realities co-exist behind this common appellation. RWAs are sometimes formed through co-option rather than election, and they raise resources in a variety of ways, which are more or less transparent.
20. *Source*: Directorate of Health Services, Delhi.
21. In the Jama Masjid area, some Market Traders Associations, which are considered as 'citizen's groups' in the framework of the Bhagidari scheme, do participate, as such, in electoral campaigns.
22. The relation between the MCD and NGOs is emblematized in the Basti Vikas Kendra: these small plots, reserved for one NGO to do community development in every slum managed by the MCD, are a major physical and institutional site of collaboration between the local administration and NGOs, and they are the object of intense competition between NGOs.
23. *Anganwadis* are female social workers employed in the framework of the Integrated Child Development Services programme.
24. The involvement of elected representatives in construction work, however, might be related to corruption. It is much more costly (and therefore, more profitable both for contractors and for the people they bribe in order to get contracts) to build a new structure than to repair an old one. In the MCD, officials and councillors regularly accuse each other of taking kickbacks in connection with construction work.

REFERENCES

Das, Veena, R.K. Das and Lester Countinho, 'Disease Control and Immunisation. A Sociological Enquiry', *Economic and Political Weekly*, vol. 35, Issues 8 and 9, 19–26 February 2000, pp. 625–32.

Ghosh, Archana and Stéphanie Tawa Lama-Rewal, *Democratization in Progress: Women and Local Politics in Urban India*, Delhi: Tulika, 2005.

Government of India (GOI), Ministry of Health and Family Welfare, *National Health Policy 2002.*

Gupta, Devendra B., and Anil Gumber, 'Decentralisation: Some Initiatives in the Health Sector', *Economic and Political Weekly*, vol. 34, Issue 6, 6 February 1999.

Mahal, Ajay, and Vivek Srivastava, *People's Participation, Decentralisation and Delivery of Public Sector Services in India*, Working Paper Series no. 71, New Delhi: National Council of Applied Economic Research, 2000.

Maitra, Shipra, *Delhi: The City and the Capital: A Status Report*, New Delhi: Institute for Human Development, 2003.

National Capital Territory of Delhi (NCTD), *Who's Who of Members of Third Legislative Assembly of the National Capital Territory of Delhi*, 2004.

National Institute of Urban Affairs (NIUA), *Mirzapur Healthy City Project: Report on Action Research*, New Delhi, 2004.

Ramanathan, Mala, Aleyamma Vijayan, D. Varatharajan, R. Sukanya and Priya Nanda, 'Political Decentralization and the Primary Health Care System: Examining the Potential for Improving Women's Reproductive Health Care in Kerala', Centre for Health and Gender Equity, 2003, http://www.genderhealth.org.

Sundar, Ramamani and Abhilasha Sharma, 'Morbidity and Utilisation of Healthcare Services: A Survey of Urban Poor in Delhi and Chennai', *Economic and Political Weekly*, vol. 37, no. 47, 23 November 2002, pp. 4729–40.

United Nations Development Programme (UNDP), *Governance for Sustainable Human Development*, A UNDP Policy Document, 1997, available online at http://magnet.undp.org

World Bank, *Sub-Saharan Africa: From Crisis to Sustainable Growth: A Long-Term Perspective Study*, Washington, 1989.

Yesudian, C.A.K., 'Pattern of Utilisation of Health Services', *Economic and Political Weekly*, vol. 34, no. 5, 30 January 1999, pp. 300–4.

CHAPTER 14

Indian Health Landscapes: Concluding Remarks

SARAH CURTIS

The authors are to be congratulated on this collection of papers on 'Indian Health Landscapes' which brings together a series of perspectives on health and health care in India that are fascinating for at least two reasons. First, they give us thought-provoking information and ideas about the contemporary situation in India. In some chapters, this is viewed from an 'insider' perspective, while other authors write as researchers who, as 'outsiders', have immersed themselves quite deeply in the Indian settings they have researched, and are able to consider how the Indian situation relates to health geographies in western Europe. Second, the papers provide reflections on the health geography of India from the standpoint of theories about processes of globalization and internationalization. From these discussions we see how health and health care exemplify and help to explain globalization processes. Also illuminated are developing points of view in health geography which engage with wider geographical debates over globalization from cultural and social perspectives, as well as economic viewpoints on production and consumption.

As I am not a specialist on health geography in India, I am not able to contribute to the interesting debates in this book about conditions in that country. However, as a health geographer I find a number of very interesting themes emerging here which certainly contribute to some of the issues in health geography eluded to in the introduction by Alain Vaguet. Reading this book has prompted me to reflect on the following themes in particular, which frame my remarks below:

- We have moved beyond conventional perspectives in medical geography towards geographies of health which are more sensitive to the social and cultural construction of 'health' and 'health care' and how this varies from one setting to another;

- There is great potential in the 'global north' to learn from the experience and knowledge of societies in the 'global south' (as well as vice versa) and it is important to consider how a more balanced exchange of 'flows' in expertise can be achieved;
- In the 'global north' (comprising higher income countries), as well as the 'global south' (lower income countries), 'spaces of risk' to health are now being construed from a global as well as a local perspective, and this raises very challenging questions about our knowledge and capacity to manage health determinants.

Towards Geographies of Health and Well-being

Geographical perspectives have increasingly embraced social as well as spatial theory, and this is also reflected in geographical research on health and health inequality (e.g. Smyth, 2005; Smith and Easterlow, 2005). This development parallels the recognition that research in public health generally needs to be more receptive to social theory as well as clinical disciplines in order to address disease causation and tackle health inequality more effectively (e.g. Potvin et al., 2005).

The papers in this collection accord with these perspectives, which encourage health geographers to consider health and therapy as socially and culturally constructed, rather than determined solely by Western clinical science. Furthermore these social and cultural constructions will vary among places (settings) and some of the papers in this collection have illustrated, for example, how ideas about health are differently constructed in more or less traditional communities, and in various settings in India. These constructions are shown to depend partly on power relations (notably, in some of the research reported here, between men and women). The research reported here also shows how social construction of health rests upon a complex structure of traditional and modern interpretations of health and well-being. Bodily and mental states and health-related behaviours have varying meanings, with social, as well as medical significance, and they vary according to the setting, as well as the people concerned. Thus, as the authors in this collection have shown, it is possible to develop a more holistic and nuanced understanding of health and health-related behaviour when it is interpreted with reference to the 'landscapes' of power, of social relations, of material poverty, and of consumption in India. Attitudes and behaviours that might seem irrational and uninformed from a Western clinical perspective can be better understood as rational and socially acceptable responses, adapted to these landscapes.

It is particularly interesting to see these more recent concepts of 'landscape' applied to the Indian situation, since the subcontinent has in the past been a focus for more classic medical geographical studies of 'tropical diseases', based in landscape epidemiology and disease ecology (e.g. reviewed by Learmonth, 1988). The geographers contributing to this volume are not only refocusing geography on emerging infectious diseases, such as the HIV/AIDS epidemic, but are also varying the lenses used to view these new challenges for health.

As health geography moves away from modernist and western clinical constructions of health care, there also has been a growth of interest in a wider range of therapies (Doel, 2003; Andrews, 2004; Smyth, 2005) which have varying salience and interpretations, depending on the contexts in which they are experienced. Research on these also brings into relief the struggles taking place at the local level between more traditional therapies and modern medicine. These may have a different significance in countries like India than in European countries; therapies which in the 'global north' are viewed as 'complementary' and 'exotic', may be viewed from an Indian perspective as the 'original', 'indigenous' therapies, deeply rooted in traditional culture and national identity. The papers in this volume suggest that the relationships between different therapies have a particular social and political importance in India. There are echoes in these chapters of the arguments put forward, for example, by Del Casino (2004) who discusses the tensions between modern and traditional medicine in Thailand and describes how these are played out at the local level.

Health geography is expanding to include research on health as well as illness, as illustrated in this book by research on practices like yoga which promote good health and well-being. The interpretations here allow us to interpret yoga as an example of knowledge and practice flowing abroad from India, in contrast to clinical medical strategies imported from (or imposed by) the 'global north'. We see here the significance of dissemination and blending of ideas and cultures in global space, and also the powerful effects of processes of consumption operating at the international scale, as yoga becomes increasingly commercialized to appeal to consumers across the globe. We have seen in this book that part of this process involves the reproduction of 'therapeutic landscapes' (Gesler, 1992) that symbolise and reinforce the principles of yoga, both within India and internationally. These may also be interpreted as 'liminal' spaces of consumption, designed to manipulate consumers from the 'global north' by offering an environment free from some of the constraints of normal life. However, the demand for traditional Indian knowledge and practice also reflects the emergence of the 'smart consumer', able to make informed choices about alternatives to biomedical treatments. Therefore, we might view the international uptake of yoga, Ayurvedic medicine and other health-related practices from India as an illustration of the new opportunities for health care opened up to some individuals through global cultures and economies.

Spaces of Flows in Health-Related Knowledge: The Implications for Health and Medicine

This process of exchange of health-related knowledge and practice between countries of the North and south is seen in this book to have mixed impacts on India and it prompts us to reflect on issues of social injustices generated by what Castells (1996) describes as global 'spaces of flows'. In India, as elsewhere, there are undoubtedly benefits from access to biomedical knowledge and medical services. However, research reported here shows that when these 'flows' involve an international 'brain drain' of qualified doctors towards countries of the 'North', this results in depletion of national resources of expertise and exacerbation of the north/south divide in access to medical care. Similarly, the globalizing mode of production and consumption of pharmaceuticals has powerful and often deleterious impacts on countries of the South, such as India, and these can be disastrous for public health (as evidenced by the failure to make available in poorer countries the drugs needed to contend with the HIV/AIDS epidemic). On the other hand, authors such as Cooke (2004), reviewing the global development of pharmaceutical industries also comment on the increasing proliferation of small, specialized sites for development of new drugs, which are rapidly developing in countries like India and China. Cooke comments that this runs contrary to the view that global economies are totally dominated by large multinational companies; from an economic standpoint, it is the giant pharmaceutical firms based in the 'global North' that are in crisis in the face of such competition in the 'global South'. These contradictory and complex global trends are particularly striking in countries like India, as demonstrated in this collection of essays.

Geographies of Health in the 'World Risk Society'

In the introduction to this book, the reader is prompted by Alain Vaguet to consider the writings of Ulrich Beck and I agree that it is interesting to reflect on these in relation to the sorts of research reported here. Beck (1999) argues that we are faced with potentially large and very uncertain risks to health and well-being because of global threats associated with economic growth and increasing wealth, as well as poverty and inequality, the existence of weapons of mass destruction and other large-scale threats to sustainability. He suggests that it is becoming impossible to govern and insure against risk in conventional ways and that this has major social and political consequences for contemporary societies. Beck (1999: 141–4) also recognizes the significance of local context when he cites Robertson (1992) in support of an assertion that,

> The new types of risk are simultaneously local and global. . . . The point of impact is not necessarily the point of origin. . . . Thus the enormous spatial disjuncture between knowledge and impact: perception is always and necessarily contextual and locally constituted. . . . The impact of the industrial way of life, in contrast, is spatially and temporarily open and tends to extend across the globe. . . .

Beck's argument is put forward primarily from the perspective of countries in the 'global North'. Perhaps these 'new' anxieties troubling citizens of the 'world risk society' are not very different from those which have long been familiar to significant numbers of people in India in the face of severe, widespread poverty and living conditions at or below subsistence level. Undoubtedly, there is a lot that we in the 'North' can learn from the wisdom and experience that helps people in countries like India to be resilient in these circumstances. This is one reason why the local examples discussed in this book make a valuable contribution for readers in high income countries. At the same time, unevenness in distributions of wealth and the means to a healthy life are very striking within countries like India, as demonstrated by some of the discussion in this book. If we accept Beck's argument, then these local manifestations of inequality can only be understood by taking the global perspective that has been adopted by the authors contributing to this volume.

REFERENCES

Andrews, G.J., '(Re)thinking the Dynamics between Healthcare and Place: Therapeutic Geographies in Treatment and Care Practices', *Area*, 36, 3, 2004, pp. 307–18.

Beck, U., *World Risk Society*, Cambridge: Polity Press, 1999.

Castells, M., *The Rise of the Network Society*, Oxford: Blackwell, 1996.

Chacko, E., 'Culture and Therapy: Complementary Strategies for the Treatment of Type-2 Diabetes in an Urban Setting in Kerala, India', *Social Science & Medicine*, 56, 5, 2003, pp. 1087–98.

Cooke, P. 'Regional Knowledge Capabilities, Embeddedness of Firms and Industry Organisation: Bioscience Megacentres and Economic Geography', *European Planning Studies*, 12, 5, 2004, pp. 625–41.

Del Casino, V.J., '(Re)placing Health and Health Care: Mapping the Competing Discourses and Practices of "Traditional" and "Modern" Thai Medicine', *Health & Place*, 10, 1, 2004, pp. 59–73.

Doel, M.A. and J. Segrott, 'Beyond Belief? Consumer Culture, Complementary Medicine, and the Dis-ease of Everyday life', *Environment & Planning D: Society & Space*, 21, 6, 2003, pp. 739–59.

Gesler, W., 'Therapeutic Landscapes: Medical Geographic Research in Light of the New Cultural Geography', *Social Science & Medicine*, 34, 7, 1992, pp. 735–46.

Learmonth, A., *Disease Ecology: An Introduction*, London: Blackwell, 1988.

Potvin, L. and S. Gendron, A Bilodeau and P. Chabot, 'Integrating Social Theory into Public Health Practice', *American Journal of Public Health*, 95, 2005, pp. 591–5.

Robertson, R., *Globalization: Social Theory and Global Culture*, London: Sage, 1992.

Smith, S.J. and D. Easterlow, 'The Strange Geography of Health Inequalities', *Transactions of the Institute of British Geographers*, 30, 2, 2005, pp. 173–90.

Smyth, F., 'Medical Geography: Therapeutic Places, Spaces and Networks', *Progress in Human Geography*, 29, 4, 2005, pp. 488–95.

Wiles, J. and M. Rosenburg, 'Gentle Caring Experience': Seeking Alternative Health Care in Canada', *Health & Place*, 7, 3, 2001, pp. 209–24.

Contributors

SURINDER AGGARWAL is a professor of geography at the Delhi School of Economics. Email: surinder_aggarwal@hotmail.com

RAÏS AKHTAR is a professor of geography at the University of Kashmir. Email: rais@kashmiruniversity.net

SANDRINE BRISSET is a Ph.D. research student in geography at the University of Rouen. Email: SandrineBrisset@aol.com

JULIEN CHAISSE is a Ph.D. research student in law at the University of Aix-Marseille III. Email: julien.chaisse@iep-aix.fr

PIERRE CHAPELET is a Ph.D. research student in geography at the University of Rouen. Email: pierre.chapelet@wanadoo.fr

VIRGINIE CHASLES is a doctor of geography at the University of Rouen. Email: chaslesvirginie@yahoo.fr

MATHILDE CLERC is coordinating the health programmes of Lafarge Cement in East Africa. Email: thildma7@yahoo.fr

SARAH CURTIS is a professor of geography at the University of Durham. Email: s.e.curtis@durham.ac.uk

EMMANUEL ELIOT is an associate professor of geography at the University of Le Havre. Email: emmanuel.eliot@univ-lehavre.fr

SAMIRA GUENNIF is an associate professor of economics at the University of Paris XIII. Email: guennif@seg.univ-paris13.fr

ANNE-CÉCILE HOYEZ is a doctor of geography at the University of Rouen. Email: hoyez@yahoo.com

STÉPHANIE TAWA LAMA-REWAL is a senior research fellow at the Centre for Indian and South Asian Studies (CEIAS), Paris. Email: Stephanie. Tawa-Lama-Rewal@ehess.fr

BERTRAND LEFEBVRE is a Ph.D. research student in geography at the University of Rouen. Email: bertrand.lefebvre@csh-delhi.com

FABIENNE MARTIN is an Anthropologist at Laborative d'Ethnologie et de Sociologie Comparative U.M.R. 7186 CNRS, Paris X. Email: fabmartin92@hotmail.com

ALAIN VAGUET is an associate professor of geography at the University of Rouen. Email: alain.vaguet@univ-rouen.fr

Index